AF770178

MOVING HEALTH SOVEREIGNTY IN AFRICA

Global Environmental Governance

Series Editors: John J. Kirton, Munk School of Global Affairs, Trinity College, Canada and Miranda Schreurs, Freie Universität Berlin, Germany

Global Environmental Governance addresses the new generation of twenty-first century environmental problems and the challenges they pose for management and governance at the local, national, and global levels. Centred on the relationships among environmental change, economic forces, and political governance, the series explores the role of international institutions and instruments, national and sub-federal governments, private sector firms, scientists, and civil society, and provides a comprehensive body of progressive analyses on one of the world's most contentious international issues.

Recent titles in the series (full listing continued at the back of the book)

Africa's Health Challenges
Sovereignty, Mobility of People and Healthcare Governance
Edited by Andrew F. Cooper, John J. Kirton, Franklyn Lisk and Hany Besada
ISBN 978-1-4094-2832-9

Corporate Responses to EU Emissions Trading
Resistance, Innovation or Responsibility?
Edited by Jon Birger Skjærseth and Per Ove Eikeland
ISBN 978-1-4094-6078-7

Renewable Energy Policy Convergence in the EU
The Evolution of Feed-in Tariffs in Germany, Spain and France
David Jacobs
ISBN 978-1-4094-3909-7

The EU as International Environmental Negotiator
Tom Delreux
ISBN 978-1-4094-1182-6

Global Energy Governance in a Multipolar World
Dries Lesage, Thijs Van de Graaf and Kirsten Westphal
ISBN 978-0-7546-7723-9

Innovation in Global Health Governance
Critical Cases
Edited by Andrew F. Cooper and John J. Kirton
ISBN 978-0-7546-4872-7

Moving Health Sovereignty in Africa

Disease, Governance, Climate Change

Edited by

JOHN J. KIRTON
University of Toronto, Canada

ANDREW F. COOPER
University of Waterloo, Canada

FRANKLYN LISK
University of Warwick, UK

HANY BESADA
University of Ottawa, Canada

ASHGATE

© John J. Kirton, Andrew F. Cooper, Franklyn Lisk and Hany Besada 2014

All rights reserved. No part of this publication may be reproduced, stored in a retrieval system or transmitted in any form or by any means, electronic, mechanical, photocopying, recording or otherwise without the prior permission of the publisher.

John J. Kirton, Andrew F. Cooper, Franklyn Lisk and Hany Besada have asserted their right under the Copyright, Designs and Patents Act, 1988, to be identified as the editors of this work.

Published by
Ashgate Publishing Limited
Wey Court East
Union Road
Farnham
Surrey, GU9 7PT
England

Ashgate Publishing Company
110 Cherry Street
Suite 3-1
Burlington, VT 05401-3818
USA

www.ashgate.com

British Library Cataloguing in Publication Data
A catalogue record for this book is available from the British Library

The Library of Congress has cataloged the printed edition as follows:
Moving health sovereignty in Africa : disease, governance, climate change / [edited by] John J. Kirton, Andrew F. Cooper, Franklyn Lisk, and Hany Besada.
pages cm. – (Global environmental governance)
Includes bibliographical references and index.
ISBN 978-1-4094-5048-1 (hardback : alk. paper) – ISBN 978-1-4094-5049-8 (ebook) – ISBN 978-1-4724-0070-3 (epub) 1. World health–Africa. 2. Regional medical programs–Africa. 3. Medicine–International cooperation. I. Kirton, John J., editor of compilation. II. Cooper, Andrew Fenton, 1950– editor of compilation. III. Lisk, Franklyn, editor of compilation. IV. Besada, Hany, editor of compilation.
RA441.M68 2014
362.1096–dc23

2014015633

ISBN 9781409450481 (hbk)
ISBN 9781409450498 (ebk – PDF)
ISBN 9781472400703 (ebk – ePUB)

MIX
Paper from responsible sources
FSC® C013985

Printed in the United Kingdom by Henry Ling Limited, at the Dorset Press, Dorchester, DT1 1HD

Contents

List of Figures

List of Tables

Notes on Contributors

Obijiofor Aginam is a senior research fellow at the United Nations University's International Institute for Global Health (UNU-IIGH) in Kuala Lumpur, Malaysia, an adjunct research professor of law at Carleton University, and a visiting professor in the IR3S at the University of Tokyo.

Hany Besada is a theme leader for the Governance of Natural Resources Program at the North-South Institute, an adjunct research professor with the Institute of African Studies at Carleton University, and a senior fellow at the Centre on Governance at the University of Ottawa. He served as a research specialist for the Secretariat of the United Nations High-Level Panel on the Post-2015 Development Agenda.

Andrew F. Cooper is a professor at the Balsillie School of International Affairs and the department of political science at the University of Waterloo. He is also an associate research fellow at the UNU CRIS, the United Nations University's Institute on Comparative Regional Integration, in Bruges, Belgium.

Pieter Fourie is an associate professor in the Department of Political Science at Stellenbosch University.

Jenilee Guebert is the former director of research for the Global Health Diplomacy Program, the G8 Research Group, and the G20 Research Group.

John J. Kirton is the co-director of the Global Health Diplomacy Program, based at the Munk School of Global Affairs at Trinity College in the University of Toronto, and a professor of political science at the University of Toronto. He is also the director of the G8 Research Group and co-director of the G20 Research Group.

Julia Kulik is a senior researcher in the Global Health Diplomacy Program, the G8 Research Group, and the G20 Research Group, based at the Munk School of Global Affairs at Trinity College in the University of Toronto.

Franklyn Lisk is a visiting professorial research fellow at the Centre for the Study of Globalisation and Regionalisation at the University of Warwick and a senior associate at the Center for Research on Political Economy in Dakar, Senegal.

Rangarirai Machemedze is deputy director of the Southern and Eastern African Trade Information and Negotiations Institute in Harare, Zimbabwe.

Oscar F. Picazo is a senior health economist with the World Bank in Pretoria, South Africa.

Annamarie Bindenagel Šehović is a lecturer at the Willy Brandt School of Public Policy in Erfurt, Germany. She is also collaborating researcher at the Centre for the Study of Globalisation and Regionalisation at the University of Warwick.

Nelson Sewankambo is the principal of Makerere University's College of Health Sciences, president of the Uganda National Academy of Sciences, and chair of the Medical Education for Equitable Services for All Ugandans (MESAU) consortium.

James K. Tumwine is a professor of pediatrics and child health at Makerere University College of Health Sciences in Uganda and founding editor-in-chief of *African Health Sciences*.

Dennis G. Willms is founder and executive director of the Salama SHIELD Foundation.

Siphamandla Zondi is the director of the Africa Programme at the Institute for Global Dialogue in Johannesburg and an honorary professor of politics at the University of South Africa.

Preface

This book began as a follow-on to a project, inspired by the 2003 outbreak of severe acute respiratory syndrome (SARS), on innovation in global health governance. That project developed and tested a framework of "challenge-response-innovation" to analyse global health governance, and published the results in two volumes: *Global Health Governance: Challenge, Response, Innovation*, edited by Andrew F. Cooper, John J. Kirton, and Ted Schrecker, and *Innovation in Global Health Governance: Critical Cases*, edited by Andrew F. Cooper and John J. Kirton.

These works sparked a broader reflection on how the core concepts and institutions of the state-centric, slow-moving Westphalian world were adapting to save human lives in the face of fast-moving, free-flowing disease that so easily penetrated national boundaries on a global scale. Nowhere were these dynamics more advanced than in sub-Saharan Africa, where people dealt with the equivalent of a SARS outbreak every day, where transborder population movements were massive, where state capacity was often slight, and where the toll of disease and death was high. Thus this new project on moving health sovereignty in Africa was launched, under the auspices of The Centre for International Governance Innovation (CIGI) in Waterloo, Canada, the University of Toronto's Munk School of Global Affairs, and Warwick University's Centre for the Study of Globalization and Regionalization.

The authors assembled for an international workshop on "Moving Health Sovereignty: Global Challenge: African Perspective" in Stellenbosch, South Africa, on 21–22 November 2008. Such was the popularity of the project and the quality of the contributions that the editors decided to report the results in two separate volumes. This one presents the general problématique, concepts, and applications in ways that flow from the earlier framework on challenge, response, and innovation. The other volume, *Africa's Health Challenges: Sovereignty, Mobility of People, and Healthcare Governance*, focuses on the particular problem of moving people, as distinct from pathogens, both within and outside Africa, applying concepts of sovereignty to the migration of the healthcare workforce in particular.

Acknowledgements

In producing this book we have acquired an enormous debt to many individuals in many ways.

Our first debt is to The Centre for International Governance Innovation, which provided the funding for the authors' workshop and for the editorial work on this book. The second is to our colleagues at our home institutions, who offered valuable encouragement and support as we worked on this book. We are also grateful to our researchers and research assistants who helped transform rough drafts into finished prose. At the University of Toronto and its Global Health Diplomacy Program, co-directed by John J. Kirton and James Orbinski, these are Madeline Koch, Jenilee Guebert, Caroline Bracht, Julia Kulik, Corinne Ton That, Colleen Keilty, Robin Lennox, Zaria Shaw, Rozalind Theriault, and Baillie McGurn.

At the University of Waterloo, these are Asif Farooq and Ryan Hilimoniuk.

At Warwick University these are Sharifah Sekalala and Penelope Muzanenhamo.

At the North-South Institute, these are Rachael Calleja, Kristen Winters, and Maria Habanikova.

At Tyndale University College and Seminary, we are grateful to Leah McMillan.

At Ashgate, Kirstin Howgate, Margaret Younger, Brenda Sharp, and their colleagues were as always a joy to work with, especially as their patience was a particularly valuable asset this time.

Finally, we are most grateful to our students, for the constant inspiration they have offered as this book was being conceived, researched, written, and revised. It is dedicated to them.

Abbreviations and Acronyms

ACP	Africa, Caribbean, and Pacific
AfDB	African Development Bank
AFRO	World Health Organization Regional Office for Africa
AHIF	Avian and Human Influenza Facility
APOC	African Program for Onchocerciasis Control
ART	antiretroviral treatment
AU	African Union
BAT	British American Tobacco
BRICS	Brazil, Russia, India, China, and South Africa
CEDRA	Climate Change and Environmental Degradation Risk and Adaptation Assessment
CIA	US Central Intelligence Agency
COP	Conference of the Parties
DOTS	Directly Observed Treatment – Short Course
EPA	economic partnership agreement
ESAP	economic structural adjustment program
FCTC	Framework Convention on Tobacco Control
G7	Group of Seven (Canada, France, Germany, Italy, Japan, the United Kingdom, the United States, and the European Union)
G8	Group of Eight (G7 plus Russia)
G20	Group of 20 (G8 plus Australia, Argentina, Brazil, China, India, Indonesia, Korea, Mexico, Saudi Arabia, South Africa, and Turkey)
GATS	General Agreement on Trade in Services
GATT	General Agreement on Tariffs and Trade
GCAP	Global Call to Action Against Poverty
GEF	Global Environment Facility
IDA	International Development Association
IHR	International Health Regulations
IMF	International Monetary Fund
IMHE	Institute for Health Metrics and Evaluation
IPCC	Intergovernmental Panel on Climate Change
LDC	least developed country
LSDI	Lubombo Spatial Development Initiative
MDG	Millennium Development Goal
MDR-TB	multidrug-resistant tuberculosis
MEF	Major Economies Forum on Energy Security and Climate Change

MEM	Major Economies Meeting on Energy Security and Climate Change
MOP	Meeting of the Parties
NAPA	national adaptation program of action
NCD	noncommunicable disease
NEPAD	New Partnership for Africa's Development
NGO	nongovernmental organization
ODA	official development assistance
OECD	Organisation for Economic Co-operation and Development
PEPFAR	United States President's Emergency Plan for AIDS Relief
R&D	research and development
SADC	Southern African Development Community
SAP	structural adjustment program
SARS	severe acute respiratory syndrome
TRIPS	Agreement on Trade-Related Aspects of Intellectual Property
UNDP	United Nations Development Programme
UN ESCAP	United Nations Economic and Social Commission for Asia and the Pacific
UNFCCC	United Nations Framework Convention on Climate Change
UNFPA	United Nations Population Fund
UNSC	United Nations Security Council
WHO	World Health Organization
WHO/AFRO	World Health Organization Regional Office for Africa
WTO	World Trade Organization
XDR-TB	extensively drug-resistant tuberculosis

PART I
Introduction

Chapter 1
Moving Health Sovereignty in Africa

John J. Kirton

The Challenge

Globalization has generated a great upsurge in mobility at an intense pace on a global scale. People visit friends and relatives more frequently and further away. Tourists take off for vacations in distant locales, seeking relaxation, rest, and recovery, and sometimes cheaper healthcare services. Business people routinely travel throughout the global marketplace and professionals and students do so as well. Military personnel go abroad and usually come home. Individuals move across borders legally and illegally to conduct honest and illicit activities. Members of diasporas flow to and often move back and forth among homes in different states. Immigrants and refugees, including conflict refugees, climate refugees, and natural disaster refugees, cross porous borders when shocks arise to drive them from their home. And climate change and other environmental stresses cause pests, other living things, and physical processes to migrate, increasingly on a global scale.

As people and other living things move in proliferating fashion, so too do the pathogens they carry or encounter. Unfamiliar diseases flow rapidly from anywhere to everywhere, to cause death and devastation to vulnerable peoples behind the national borders that were designed to, and once adequately did, keep their citizens safe inside the comfortable confines of their own static, sovereign, exclusive, territorial states (Ruggie 1993). Increasingly the tools traditionally employed by the governments of these Westphalian states – and by the formal intergovernmental institutions that they have ceded slivers of their sovereignty to – are too small, slow, and static to cope with this fast, fluid, far-reaching new world full of mobile people, pests and pathogens, and proliferating disease and death (Ikenberry 2001; Kickbusch et al. 2013). There is thus an urgent need for innovation in global governance to close this great and growing gap between the new physical challenge of a world on the move and the old public policy response from states and their governments fixed in traditional time and territorial space. Moving health meets static sovereignty and too many people die unnecessarily as a result.

Nowhere is this challenge more acute than in Africa, especially in its sub-Saharan parts. Here people move relatively freely, in order to escape economic and ecological deprivation and deadly conflict. They often move to neighbouring jurisdictions where governments are ill equipped to stop them from entering or to meet their often formidable health and other needs. Healthcare professionals in Africa, facing the exceptional burden of world-leading rates of infectious and chronic disease, and lacking the facilities to cope, flow from underfunded and underdeveloped public systems to better endowed ones close at hand, or follow their patients and people to distant developed countries where they will be better off (Cooper et al. 2013). While healthcare workers move into Africa from the governments, foundations, and nongovernmental organizations (NGOs) of the developed world, there are rarely enough of them to fill the gaps left by the departures and to meet the needs of the Africans left behind. And few tourists fly from rich countries to Africa for treatment in facilities with price tags that are so much more affordable there. In a world of such severe, fast-moving challenges, and the inadequate response of static governments, there is a compelling need for far-reaching innovation in global health governance, to save the lives of so many in people Africa, and indeed everywhere else in a highly mobile world that is now only a plane ride away from Africa itself.

Purpose

This book takes up this subject. Its first purpose is to chart the challenges brought by the clash between the new world of moving people and pathogens and the old world of static sovereign states, as the clash affects the health needs of Africans and those beyond. Its second purpose is to assess the existing and emerging responses, in ideas, instruments, and institutions, of the public authorities most responsible, affected, and concerned. Its third purpose is to identify the innovations introduced, needed, and available to improve the health of those inside Africa and outside too.

The Contributors

To fulfil these purposes, this book assembles the contributions of leading scholars and practitioners, from an array of disciplines and professions, from Africa itself and the world beyond. The authors come from a range of relevant public policy disciplines: medicine, public health, medical anthropology, political science, law, economics, and philosophy. They bring experience working, at present or in the past, in academia, think tanks, NGOs, and multilateral organizations. A strong majority of the authors are African, allowing the continent's challenges, responses and innovations to be explored at first hand.

The Analytical Framework

To guide this analysis of how best to govern the health challenges in Africa in an era of growing globalization, this book adapts, for application to the African region, the framework of challenge-response-innovation developed to assess global health governance (Cooper et al. 2007; Cooper and Kirton 2009; Kirton 2009). Its first step is to chart the health challenges posed in particular by this new world on the move. Among the many severe health problems faced by Africans, which challenges are the most acute, thus deserving a priority place in the public policy response? How has the new mobility of pathogens, people, and information, goods, and services compounded the challenges in the contemporary world?

The second step is to consider the governance response, starting with the core idea of sovereignty, in its classic, competing, and changing conceptions, in a region and a world where the Westphalian inheritance of exclusive, territorial sovereign states from 1648 may be transforming in a fundamental way (Ruggie 1993; Linklater 2007; Goodhart and Taninchev 2011). Among the many changes over the centuries in the meaning of sovereignty, both in general and in application to health, which are the most promising as an ideational guide to the global health governance responses and innovations needed to save Africans and others' lives? Does the sovereignty-grounded concept of security, residing at the core of the Westphalian "national security" state, give a mobilizing or distorting frame when applied to health? Does the human right to health offer an innovative advance for a post-sovereign world of movement or merely a normative argument with little force in a continent where the great gap arises from the commensurate responsibilities of communities and governments to meet the profound health needs? Does the common instinct of humanity, aroused by harms to individuals made aware to others anywhere when deadly shocks arise, transcend the traditional concepts of sovereignty and citizenship to evoke a collective global response (Linklater 2007)? Above all, which concepts and approaches will work best in the aftermath of the great global financial and economic crises of 2008–13 that have so assaulted the health resources of Africans and others.

The third step is to examine how and how well the existing array of global intergovernmental institutions that are responsible for Africans' health, or consequential in affecting it, have responded to this new world of movement and adopted the innovative ideas, instruments, and practices to improve the health outcomes of Africans. While Africa possesses in abundance a growing array of relevant regional organizations, the global institutions still largely drive the socioeconomic determinants of health and thus the health of Africans themselves. At the centre stand the major multilateral economic organizations of the international order constructed in the 1940s, above all the World Bank and the General Agreement on Trade and Tariffs that has become today's World Trade Organization (WTO). Yet also important, especially in connecting health with the full array of physical and social forces that intersect with it, are the more recently created, informal, plurilateral institutions for general global governance that have focused on Africa, above all the Group of Eight (G8).

The fourth step is to consider how specialized institutions, concerned with the health needs on a single continent, cope with challenges that are comprehensive, interconnected, and characterized by complexity and uncertainty on a global scale.

Here the challenge of climate change takes pride of place. How can Africans best cope with climate change's health impacts, adapt to its many other consequences, and contribute to the global climate change control cause?

The fifth step is to highlight the innovations that have been introduced, are needed, and are available across all these dimensions. What innovations have been introduced and are most needed in the ever more mobile Africa that lies ahead? The answer comes first in the realm of ideas. Here the need is to invent and introduce new concepts of sovereignty to capture this emerging world of single, dual, and mutual citizens moving among homelands and stateless people and recent non-citizens such as refugee claimants, and to determine the rights they have in their polity of arrival or new residence (including the right to publicly funded health care), the responsibilities they have to their polity of departure, and the rights and responsibilities of the national governments of their jurisdictions of arrival and departure and the international institutions that stand above both.

A second need, in the realm of instruments, is to consider innovations in several fields. These include citizenship, migration policy, official development assistance, remittances, and community care.

The third need, in the realm of institutions, is to examine how governance arrangements and architecture can and should innovate in order to reflect these new conceptions of sovereignty and the changing physical world that it should match. This includes national and sub-federal governments, intergovernmental institutions, and the NGOs of transnational civil society.

The Arguments

Part II of this volume focuses on "Africa's Health Challenges and Concepts". In Chapter 2, "Moving Health Sovereignty: An African Perspective", Obijiofor Aginam discusses the challenges posed by the globalization of public health. In an era of globalization, global health in practice, scholarship, and national health policy is shaped by complex, global forces, and emerging trends from outside the health sector. This comprehensive interconnectedness complicates the task of setting a coherent public health strategy from an authentically African perspective. New actors and institutions, particularly in the global economy, business, and trade, often make it difficult to align health ideals – such as universal protection and the promotion of health – within the confines of a state. The emphasis of public health discourse on the vulnerabilities of geopolitical boundaries to diseases (mainly the transnational spread of infectious diseases) has ignored the equally prevalent threat of noncommunicable diseases (such as heart failure) within a country. In an era of globalization, African domestic healthcare concerns are overshadowed on the global health agenda, leaving Africa to be viewed only as a source and spreader of disease, so much so that national health concerns, such as diabetes and obesity, are neglected. The resulting public health paradigm globalizes health in a manner that supports the isolationist public health diplomacy that the Europeans used in the mid-nineteenth century, as they sought to insulate "civilized" Europe from the world outside. This embedded orthodoxy still frames today's global health diplomacy, leaving Africa marginalized in the international system. The mutual vulnerabilities of public health now require globalized policy responses that shift from a governance architecture built on the pillars of Westphalia, to one that includes nation-states, intergovernmental organizations, private and corporate actors, civil society, and healthcare communities. African actors must thus share their distinct perspectives on the global health agenda to achieve more effective and encompassing health security for its population.

In Chapter 3, "South Africa's Sovereignty and HIV/AIDS", Annamarie Bindenagel Šehović addresses the political-economic impacts of HIV/AIDS for citizens and the state in South Africa, and how issues of sovereignty have been factored into the state response to the pandemic. Despite being intensively studied and treated, HIV/AIDS remains a serious threat to southern African societies, economies, and polities. This is due to insufficient political leadership, and a lack of access to preventive information, condoms, and antiretroviral medications. Compounding the threat is state sovereignty – specifically a state's ability to balance individual rights with those of the state as a whole, while working to enhance international health governance. In South Africa, the sovereign state has been bypassed by local and international organizations in dealing with its HIV/AIDS crisis. The government has thus been constrained in protecting its citizens as it sees fit. The international community has put intense pressure on South Africa to defeat poverty, and to treat all HIV/AIDS patients with antiretroviral treatment. Yet little regard has been given for local, long-term solutions, and the overall responsibility and accountability for these patients. The international community has thus compromised the long-term success of individual survival and state sovereignty. Although the Global Fund to Fight AIDS, Tuberculosis, and Malaria remains promising, it addresses short-term objectives, leaving national governments with reduced power to act alone in the long term. The South African government should be able to assume and enact responsibilities locally and globally. This power should be enhanced, not diminished, by the interventions of those outside.

In Chapter 4, "AIDS and Security in the Twenty-First Century", Pieter Fourie explores the historical development of multilateral efforts in global health governance and the specific impact of HIV/AIDS on national and international political agendas. He deals in particular with the effort to achieve the "securitization" of HIV/AIDS – a concept that is at the core of the raison d'être of the sovereign state. With the complexities brought about by globalization, and the emergence of new, more virulent pandemics, health problems have increasingly been labelled as security issues, or as "collective insecurity" for sovereign states and the global community. This frame presents effective health governance as a matter of national and international security, thus demanding more sophisticated, collaborative, and timely local and global health governance. It views public health through the lens of security. However, most evidence has shown no significant co-variation between HIV/AIDS prevalence and military insecurity, social uprising, macroeconomic failure, electoral instability, or democratic consolidation. Furthermore, securitization of the pandemic has wrongly been framed as a war to be won, with HIV/AIDS as the enemy that must be defeated. This framework has emphasized a process to secure states, instead of primarily providing better health systems around the world and dealing with the long-term reality of HIV/AIDS. Intervention to assist with HIV/AIDS epidemics should focus on better health care, not security, with health systems tailored to each state. In such a way, the securitization of HIV/AIDS would be done in a more conscious manner to facilitate public health interventions, mobilize funds, and create institutions with a long-term agenda. Multilateral consensus on the effective securitization of HIV/AIDS would include the systemic and temporal realities of the pandemic, such as long-term changes required in gender relations, sustainable behaviour change, and memetic cultural adaptation. Doing so would better respond to the reality of the epidemic.

In Chapter 5, "Assessing African Health Governance amid Global Biopolitics", Siphamandla Zondi argues that the transformations brought by globalization have increased the global burden of disease, with Africa at the centre of the problem. Although healthcare funding has increased in the twenty-first century, health systems in Africa remain extremely fragile due to the political economy of the region, ineffective disease control systems, poor disease surveillance regimes, and a lack of communication among relevant actors. African states are thus ill prepared for pandemics. Their populations in practice lack the basic right to health. While organizations such as the Global Fund have greatly assisted populations in need, current domestic health governance in Africa is weak. It requires more effective leadership and efficient systems.

In Chapter 6, "Conceptual Events: Bridging the Epistemological Divide among Stakeholders", Dennis Willms discusses the concepts of health sovereignty and health governance. Willms questions how such concepts can be applied to fragile nation-states, where national governments are not able to provide basic healthcare services for their people. The role of NGOs here is crucial, but how can governments and NGOs best work together to provide necessary healthcare? In Africa today, the need for healthcare is only increasing with the detrimental effects of climate change on the health of populations. A participatory method called conceptual events can address these issues. This method is meant to transcend specific problems, such as individual histories and views of the world, and enable actors to build trust to address health-related concerns comprehensively. In regard to the problem of HIV/AIDS, conceptual events facilitate a collective, participatory process to encourage people with different truth paradigms to construct shared and ethically compelling frameworks for understanding the problem of the disease and the behavioural and social solutions. In Zimbabwe, Malawi, and Uganda this method resulted in a shared understanding among actors of the risks of HIV/AIDS. This highlights the ability of conceptual events to derive a critical moral imperative to alleviate suffering through collective action.

Part III deals with "Global Governance Responses", focusing on the major international institutions of the old, multilateral, hard law world, notably the World Bank and WTO, and the newer, plurilateral soft law one, above all the G8 (Kirton et al. 2010; Bayne 2011; Kirton and Trebilcock 2004).

In Chapter 7, "Doing Things Differently: World Bank Health Governance Innovations in Sub-Saharan Africa", Oscar F. Picazo argues that the complex, transnational health development challenge in sub-Saharan Africa requires continued innovative governance structures and instruments in the areas of grant funding, financing, and technical assistance. The World Bank has long been committed to Africa and its social development. Indeed, in 2007, the World Bank lent $687.3 million to sub-Saharan Africa for health and social services. The World Bank has assisted with HIV/AIDS, malaria, tuberculosis, and avian influenza epidemics. It also works to strengthen national health strategies and system operations, and it supports regional multi-country initiatives to deal with the spread of disease. Regionalizing critical healthcare services is particularly important for smaller African countries that lack funding and skills for the development of a national healthcare sector. For the long term, improving African healthcare systems will require better legislation, policies, planning, coordination, organization, and management.

In Chapter 8, "Can the World Trade Organization Be Trusted? The Impact of Trade Law and Politics in Global Health Governance", Rangarirai Machemedze addresses the impact of trade law and politics in global health governance. He argues that the market fundamentalism practised by major international institutions cannot solve the health crises affecting developing countries. Specifically, the neoliberal economic policies promoted by the WTO have neither improved the standard of living nor reduced poverty in southern Africa. The cost of basic services, which largely determine health, has become an issue in international trade, as opposed to being a responsibility of the national government. The WTO has dictated health policy in place of national governments. This market-driven effort has not only usurped power from governments, but has also made populations poorer and more vulnerable to the dictates of the market. This is far from the goal of universal, equitable health services. Both sovereignty, which requires a single centre of authority and responsibilities somewhere, and health suffer as a result.

In Chapter 9, "G8 Health Governance for Africa" John J. Kirton, Jenilee Guebert, and Julia Kulik argue that until 2011 the G8 had done a solid job of governing global health for Africa. Indeed, the G8 had increasingly and effectively done so, particularly from 2001 to 2010, followed by a sharp decline in 2011–13. From its first deliberation on global health for development in 1979, through a more direct focus on Africa in 1985, its first concrete commitment to improve the health of South Africans in 1991, to the soon customary inclusion of African participants starting in 2001, G8 health governance for Africa became an increasingly integral part of the G8's annual summits. Over time, the G8 addressed a growing number and range of health issues including those that accompanied globalization, such as the migration of health workers and the escalating movement of disease and products. The G8 responded to these challenges by encouraging improved cooperation, the exchange of information, and the coordination of regulation among sovereign states and national, regional, and international bodies. It did so especially at summits through the decade starting in 2000, where global health governance in Africa was frequently a critical component of the agenda. Several key cases, including the 2010 Muskoka Initiative on Maternal, Newborn, and Child Health, highlight how Africa has benefited from the G8's health governance. An application to African health of the concert equality model of G8 governance, and its extension to emphasize civil society, well explains both this rising performance and its sharp drop after 2010.

Part IV turns to "Connecting Health and Climate Change in Global Governance", as the centre of the new complex of interconnected global challenges affecting African's health and the global governance capacity to respond. Here the global ecological determinants of health are highlighted, alongside the more familiar socioeconomic ones.

In Chapter 10, "The Impact of Climate Change on Health Governance and Sovereignty in Africa", Nelson Sewankambo, James K. Tumwine, and Hany Besada deal with the interconnectedness of climate change and health. The scientific consensus states that human activity greatly contributes to the build-up of greenhouse gases in the atmosphere, increasing global temperatures, particularly in the most vulnerable ecosystems. Of the world's 50 poorest states, 36 are in Africa. They will be disproportionately affected by the effects of climate change. These countries, however, are the least responsible for causing climate change and the least equipped to mitigate its impact on their people's health. With limited capacity in Africa, industrialized countries must contribute financial support, technical assistance, and local capacity building. This challenge will be a true test of Africa's resilience, competence, and ability to adapt. Since 2003, the continent has had positive economic growth rates. Moreover, the rate of HIV infections has stabilized, if not declined. It is now critically important to address climate change in order to safeguard these accomplishments. More effective governance is essential – governance that is transparent, accountable, responsive, and equitable. It should be consensus-oriented and participatory, involving all relevant parties in the realm of health and climate change mitigation, with the goal of achieving sustainable development. African governments, the international community, and civil society must work together. The process must involve the local communities that will benefit from better health services. Top-down interventions that do not inform and engage the local population are often unsuccessful. Effective governance will help bring about a progressive health sector, a green and well-functioning economy, increased creativity, innovation, knowledge and education, and a vibrant and sustainable Africa.

In Chapter 11, "Innovation for Integrated Climate-Health Governance for Africa", Franklyn Lisk argues that poor climate change governance and inappropriate health governance have a detrimental effect on the ability of developing countries to mitigate the impact of climate change on health systems.

Existing global governance systems have failed to address contemporary health issues, particularly the link between climate change and health, despite the evidence of the impact of climate change on health. In sub-Saharan Africa these impacts have been most evident. They pose a serious threat to human well-being and sustainable development in the region. State failures to deal with transboundary, public health issues have exacerbated the problem. Governments have often been unwilling to cede any power to international bodies to deal with climate change and health. Efforts to integrate health and climate change must be dealt with by governments, national agencies, and the international community, in a way that does not compromise state sovereignty. To this end, an innovative and integrated global health governance structure is needed that recognizes health challenges related to climate change. The G8 and G20 should work together under the United Nations Framework Convention on Climate Change (UNFCCC) to assist countries with the adaptation process. The December 2009 Copenhagen conference's successors, and the Rio Plus 20 review conference in 2012 could have been instrumental in reaching an agreement on the mitigation of climate change-linked health problems – but were not.

In Chapter 12, "Connecting Climate and Health: The Global Governance Gap", John J. Kirton and Jenilee Guebert argue that climate change and health are integrally connected in compounding, ever more complex ways. Each field can have positive and negative consequences for the other. The negative effects are increasingly felt in Africa. Yet while the connection is scientifically clear, the integrated governance response remains weak. Despite growing efforts to recognize the climate-health link, health and climate actors largely continue to operate independently of each other, leaving major gaps in the governance of this interlinked challenge. Health and climate actors have both failed to make a concerted collaborative effort. Without an improved, coordinated approach, citizens around the world, starting in Africa, will continue to suffer even further as a result.

Finally, Part V's Chapter 13, "Conclusion", summarizes the findings of the chapters arranged according to the analytic framework of challenge-response-innovation, as it has been adapted for this examination of the African case. It argues that there is considerable consensus, but important ongoing disagreements among the authors in addressing the three central purposes of the book and the analytic framework used in this regard. Yet together they show the usefulness of this framework of global health governance in its application to Africa, and how it can and should be enriched by changing concepts and characteristics of sovereignty in a globalizing world on the move.

References

Bayne, Nicholas (2011). "Plurilateralism and Multilateralism: Comparing Institutions". In *The New Economic Diplomacy: Decision-Making and*

Negotiation in International Relations, Nicholas Bayne and Stephen Woolcock, eds. Aldershot: Ashgate, pp. 205–29.

Cooper, Andrew F. and John J. Kirton, eds. (2009). *Innovation in Global Health Governance: Critical Cases*. Farnham: Ashgate.

Cooper, Andrew F., John J. Kirton, and Ted Schrecker, eds. (2007). *Governing Global Health: Challenge, Response, Innovation*. Aldershot: Ashgate.

Cooper, Andrew F., John J. Kirton, Franklyn Lisk, et al., eds. (2013). *Africa's Health Challenges: Sovereignty, Mobility of People, and Healthcare Governance*. Farnham: Ashgate.

Goodhart, Michael and Stacy Bondanella Taninchev (2011). "The New Sovereigntist Challenge for Global Governance: Democracy without Sovereignty". *International Studies Quarterly* 55(4): 1047–68. doi: 10.1111/j.1468-2478.2011.00691.x.

Ikenberry, G. John (2001). *After Victory: Institutions, Strategic Restraint, and the Rebuilding of Order after Major Wars*. Princeton: Princeton University Press.

Kickbusch, Ilona, Graham Lister, Michaela Told, et al., eds. (2013). *Global Health Diplomacy: Concepts, Issues, Actors, Instruments, Fora, and Cases*. New York: Springer.

Kirton, John J., ed. (2009). *Global Health*. Farnham: Ashgate.

Kirton, John J. and Michael J. Trebilcock, eds. (2004). *Hard Choices, Soft Law: Voluntary Standards in Global Trade, Environment, and Social Governance*. Aldershot: Ashgate.

Kirton, John J., Marina Larionova, and Paolo Savona, eds. (2010). *Making Global Economic Governance Effective: Hard and Soft Law Institutions in a Crowded World*. Farnham: Ashgate.

Linklater, Andrew (2007). *Critical Theory and World Politics: Citizenship, Sovereignty, and Humanity*. Abdingdon: Routledge.

Ruggie, John G. (1993). "Territoriality and Beyond: Problematizing Modernity in International Relations". *International Organization* 47(1): 139–74.

PART II
Africa's Health Challenges and Concepts

Chapter 2
Moving Health Sovereignty: An African Perspective

Obijiofor Aginam

Africa, Health, and the Evolving Concepts of Sovereignty: An Overview

Sovereignty, in its classic sense, refers to the competence of a state to exercise exclusive authority within a defined geopolitical territory. This classic notion of sovereignty – founded on the pillars of the Treaty of Westphalia – has remained the dominant architecture of the international system since 1648. Sovereignty has evolved over time since the 350 years of the Peace of Westphalia (Krasner 1999, 2001; Zacher 1992). It is now widely accepted in academic and policy discourses that infectious diseases do not carry national passports and pathogenic microbes do not respect the geopolitical boundaries and sovereignties of nation-states. The classic notion of sovereignty is therefore an alien concept in the microbial world.

Recent intellectual accounts of the globalization of public health explore the vulnerability of national boundaries and state sovereignty to the menace of emerging and re-emerging infectious and non-communicable diseases (NCDs). While the emergent discourse of global health governance has enriched the relevant epistemological and policy communities in the globalization debate, an African response to the challenges posed by the globalization of public health remains poorly articulated. The apocalyptic doomsday messages of AIDS orphans and HIV-driven declining life expectancies in African societies feature prominently in global health governance literature. Yet the discourse is characterized by an appalling lacuna – a total lack of reconstructive and holistic African perspective on global health challenges. Outside the confines of infectious and communicable diseases, the scholarship of global health governance has developed exponentially in the past decade, largely due to the emerging trends outside the health sector – international trading and economic relations including cross-border trade in goods and services; the growing influence and complex transcontinental networks of multinational corporations whose products like tobacco may have serious implications for population health in most developing countries; marketing of unsafe food and illicit drugs; globalization of unhealthy lifestyles; migration; global travel; innovations in biotechnology; and climate change and other environmental factors. These trends require new governance and regulatory tools and approaches, and also involve new actors and institutions, especially in the global economic, business, and trade arenas, where interests are often difficult to align with the goal of universal protection and promotion of public health. Global health diplomacy is no longer driven by public health but by emerging factors and trends outside the health sector (Aginam 2010).

The field of global health, as argued by scholars of global health governance, is now populated by multiple actors and influenced by diverse interests (Aginam 2005; Zacher and Keefe 2008; Cooper et al. 2007; Fidler 2001, 2004; Hein et al. 2007; Lee, Buse et al. 2002). The multiplicity of actors and diversity of interests in the global health arena, as well as the web of disparities in the health of populations in the industrialized and developing regions of the world, has exceedingly complicated the task of articulating a coherent and intellectually defensible African perspective on "moving health sovereignty" in an age of globalization of public health.

Notwithstanding this complicated task, it is useful – as a starting point – to explore whether Africa has been at the margins or periphery of global health governance. This chapter seeks to articulate a coherent African perspective on the evolving concepts of health sovereignty in an interdependent and globalized world where national health policies are continually shaped and reshaped by complex global circumstances and events outside the health sector.

Africa in the Global Health Policy Universe

Among the often discordant voices in the globalization debate, there is some consensus that the complexities of the multifaceted transcontinental phenomenon of globalization affect people in different societies and regions of the world differently (Held and McGrew 2002). Analysing the linkages between globalization and public health, scholars of global health focus on the temporal, spatial, and cognitive pillars of the globalization debate (Lee and Dodgson 2000; Fidler 1997). In the context of global health, these three globalization pillars are firmly anchored in the widely accepted paradigm that the geopolitical boundaries of nation-states have, in very complex ways, become vulnerable to microbes, especially infectious disease pathogens. As Gro Harlem Brundtland (2001) put it: "In the modern world, bacteria and viruses travel almost as fast as money. With globalization, a single microbial sea washes all of humankind. There are no health sanctuaries".

In the context of population health in most African societies, this widely accepted paradigm – the vulnerability of geopolitical boundaries to disease – can be characterized by two analytical deficits. First, the discourse focuses largely on the threat of transnational spread of infectious diseases and ignores the looming global crisis of non-communicable health threats such as obesity, diabetes, hypertension, and heart disease – all mostly threats that are exacerbated by the globalization of unsafe food, unhealthy lifestyles, and the tobacco epidemic (Phaswana-Mafuya and Tassiopoulos 2001; World Bank 2011a). These are all health issues and burdens that are quickly shifting to Africa and other developing and underdeveloped regions of the world as a result of the opportunities offered by international trade and foreign investment norms that serve as the engines of economic globalization.[1] As the World Bank (2011a, 1) has observed, "the rise of NCDs in middle- and lower-income countries, including amongst younger, working-age populations, makes NCDs a challenge that warrants global attention".

Second, the discourse lacks a "core African content". One frequently cited example of such a lack in global health is the apathy in investment in research and development (R&D) to target neglected or orphan diseases that afflict heavy mortality and morbidity burdens on African populations – malaria, African sleeping sickness, trachoma, river blindness, guinea worm, and many others. As James Orbinski (2008, 366) has argued, "a fatal imbalance existed between the health needs of poor people in developing countries and the lack of R&D to develop medicines to treat them". By relegating African issues to the periphery, the contemporary discourse of the globalization of public health either reinvents or unconsciously maintains the orthodoxy of isolationist public health diplomacy of the mid-nineteenth century, which sought to insulate civilized Europe from the exotic diseases of non-European societies (Aginam 2005; Fidler 1999; Howard-Jones 1975).

With respect to Africa, both nineteenth-century public health diplomacy (driven by European cholera outbreaks) and present-day global health diplomacy (driven by networks of global interdependence) are isolationist. Their isolationist tendencies reside in the flawed impression that the "Third World" is a reservoir of disease (Aginam 2004). As a result, there has always been a conscious effort predominant in the industrialized world to create a health sanctuary that maximizes the health security of their populations. One major objective of this health sanctuary is to insulate the industrialized world from the exotic deadly diseases of the Third World. In this embedded orthodoxy, Africa remains a conspicuous candidate in this Third World disease construct. Capturing this image, Robert Kaplan (2000, 16–17) wrote that:

> As many internal African borders begin to crumble, a more impenetrable boundary is being erected that threatens to isolate the continent as a whole: the wall of disease … Africa may today be more dangerous in this regard that it was in 1862 … As African birth rates soar and slums proliferate, some experts worry

1 According to the World Health Organization (2011a, 33), "the rapidly growing burden of NCDs in developing countries is not only accelerated by population ageing; it is also driven by the negative effects of globalization, for example, unfair trade and irresponsible marketing, rapid and unplanned urbanization and increasingly sedentary lives. People in developing countries eat foods with higher levels of total energy. Increasing NCD levels are being influenced by many factors including tobacco use and availability, cost and marketing of foods high in salt, fat and sugar … NCDs are exacerbated in urban areas by changes in diet and physical activity, exposure to air pollutants (including tobacco smoke) and harmful use of alcohol".

> that mutations and hybridizations might, just conceivably, result in a form of the AIDS virus that is easier to catch than the present strain.
>
> It is malaria that is most responsible for the disease wall that threatens to separate Africa and other parts of the Third World from the more-developed regions of the planet in the twenty-first century.

The concept of mutual vulnerability has been used to analyse the implications of South–North health disparities for all of humanity in the emergent "global neighbourhood", as has the concept of the vulnerability of multilateralism to explore the gaps in the international/global health governance architecture in addressing Third World ("African") health concerns (Aginam 2004, 2005).[2] To relate mutual vulnerability to malaria – an isolated disease largely prevalent in tropical Africa where it constitutes major mortality and morbidity burdens – it could be argued that malaria could pose a serious threat to public health in the industrialized societies of the global North through "airport" and "imported" malaria (Aginam 2004, 305). From 1969 to 1999, airport malaria was reported and confirmed in France, Belgium, Switzerland, the United Kingdom, Italy, Spain, Israel, Australia, and the United States (World Health Organization [WHO] Regional Office for Europe 1999, 6).

The ramifications of mutual vulnerability in modern-day public health diplomacy are complex. Historically, although mutual vulnerability has been reinforced by the speed with which infectious diseases criss-cross national boundaries, the speed at which these events take place in the twenty-first century is unparalleled in human history. This is complicated by the rise in NCD threats (obesity, diabetes, heart disease, hypertension, and cancer), especially in developing countries (WHO 2011a; World Bank 2011a). In the globalized world of the twenty-first century, the drivers of mutual vulnerability to public health threats include global travel; international trade in goods and services; globalization of food processing and supply; population growth, increased urbanization and crowding; and population movements due to civil wars, conflicts, drought, and other human-made or natural disasters. Other factors include the migration of skilled workforce and health professionals, especially from developing and underdeveloped to industrialized countries; irrigation, deforestation, and reforestation projects that alter the habitats of disease-carrying insects and animals; human behaviour such as intravenous drug use and risky sexual activities; increased use of anti-microbial agents and pesticides, which hasten the development of resistance; and increased

2 Mutual vulnerability is "the accumulation of the vicious threats posed to humans by disease and pathogenic microbes in an interdependent world, the susceptibility of humans to these threats, and the obsolescence of the traditional distinction between national and international health threats" (Aginam 2005, 46). Vulnerabilities of multilateralism encompass all issues that nation-states consider consistent with their strategic interests in the multilateral health arena (60). Vulnerability of multilateralism therefore refers to the realpolitik of global health that neglects health problems prevalent in Africa.

human contacts with tropical rain forests and other wilderness habitats that are reservoirs for insects and animals that harbour unknown infectious agents (Centers for Disease Control and Prevention 1998; Lifson 1996).

The cumulative consequence of these factors is that public health has emerged as a complex global challenge within the globalization debate. Applied to population health in most African societies, each of these factors raises very complex challenges. Because these challenges are beyond the scope of this chapter, only a brief discussion of some will suffice.

Communicable or Infectious Diseases and Population Health in Africa

The mortality and morbidity burdens of communicable and infectious diseases on African societies are well documented. HIV/AIDS and malaria remain the leading causes of death (Epstein 2007; Hunter 2003; Aginam 2005, 2002; Fassin 2007; Falola and Heaton 2007). However, what is now known as "orphan" or "neglected" diseases also impede the right of African populations to the highest attainable standard of health.[3] Sub-Saharan Africa remains the most severely affected region in the world, accounting for 69 per cent of the 34 million people living with HIV worldwide in 2011 (UNAIDS 2012b). The fatality of HIV is reinforced by the lethal partnership between the virus, tuberculosis, and other opportunistic infections. Indeed, tuberculosis is the leading cause of death among people living with HIV, accounting for almost one in four deaths among people with HIV is due to tuberculosis (WHO 2011c). There were an estimated 1.1 million HIV-positive new cases of tuberculosis globally in 2010, and 82 per cent of patients live in sub-Saharan Africa. Because of the poor healthcare infrastructure in many African countries, efforts to scale up collaborative tuberculosis and HIV treatment are inadequate. The prevalence of leading communicable or infectious diseases as well as the orphan or neglected diseases in most of Africa has perpetuated "global health apartheid" – a world in which about 90 per cent of the global R&D budget is devoted to the diseases of the 10 per cent of the world population in industrialized and wealthy countries (Santoro and Gorrie 2005). As Daniel Callahan and Angela Wasunna (2006, 192). observed:

> The much cited "10/90 divide" – with 90 per cent of medical research going toward diseases for just 10 per cent of the world population – shows the gross neglect of research for diseases afflicting the world's majority poor. The research and development (R & D) pipeline for drugs for diseases like tuberculosis and malaria is virtually empty – even as resistance to drugs for these conditions increases. The bottom line is that the developing world does not represent a

3 Neglected diseases are diseases and conditions prevalent in developing countries that are too poor to attract significant R&D funding as incentives for pharmaceutical corporations to research and produce essential drugs to treat those diseases and conditions.

> profitable market for the international pharmaceutical industry. In effect, the industry is saying that, because of an inability to pay for them, or to properly distribute and monitor them, development of drugs for the diseases of poor countries is a financial loser.

This fatal imbalance has to be holistically addressed in global health policy if African states are to make any gains toward achieving the health-related Millennium Development Goals (MDGs).

Beyond Infectious Diseases: The Shifting Burdens of Non-communicable Threats to Africa

Most African societies are gradually suffering from a "double jeopardy" in terms of the morbidity and mortality disease burdens on their populations. In addition to the suffocating burdens of leading communicable or infectious diseases such as HIV/AIDS, tuberculosis, and malaria that have already cut life expectancy in half in many countries, there is now an increase in the prevalence of NCDs such as obesity, diabetes, cancer, and heart conditions. These are occurring as a result of the opportunities offered by international trade and economic relations for the marketing of tobacco, unsafe food, and globalization of unhealthy lifestyles in developing countries (WHO 2011a; World Bank 2011a). According to Brundtland (2001), "it is not only the infectious diseases that spread with globalization. Changes in lifestyle and diet can prompt an increase in heart disease, diabetes and cancer. More than anything, tobacco is sweeping the globe as it is criss-crossed by market forces". The tobacco epidemic is shifting rapidly to developing countries, including the leading markets in Africa. Because of strict regulation and policies in most developed countries, leading tobacco multinationals have targeted growing markets in Latin America in the 1960s and the newly industrialized economies in Asia in the 1980s, and have increasingly targeted women and young people in Africa in the 1990s (Connolly 1992). As David Fidler (1999, 201) has argued, "Western tobacco companies succeeded in riding the waves of international trade law, liberal triumphalism, and globalizing Western culture in penetrating the markets and lungs of millions of people in the developing world".

In Nigeria, one of Africa's largest markets, British American Tobacco (BAT) is among the leading single foreign direct investor outside investments in Nigeria's vast oil and gas sector. As a result of the memorandum of understanding signed between BAT and the government of Nigeria on September 24, 2001, BAT built a $150 million modern facility to manufacture various brands of cigarettes in Nigeria. At the commissioning of the factory on 17 June 2003, Nick Hales, managing director of BAT Nigeria, stated that, "This state-of-the-art-factory for which $150 million has been committed will compare with any other world class factory in the tobacco industry ... The result of research already conducted shows that products manufactured in this factory are of the highest international quality".[4]

In 2001 and 2002, BAT stated that it paid millions of dollars in taxes to various state and federal governments in Nigeria. The company claimed to have more than 1,000 workers in its marketing and factory operations in many Nigerian cities: Enugu, Jos, Abuja, and Zaria. BAT Nigeria declared itself to be committed to the principles of sustainability and world-class standards of environmental, occupational health, and safety as well as helping tobacco farmers through responsible tobacco leaf production.[5] Emerging facts from its recent multimillion dollar investment strongly suggest that BAT has become the dominant player in the production, marketing, and advertising of tobacco products in Nigeria. Its billboards adorn the strategic locations in major Nigerian cities. BAT now controls 78 per cent of the tobacco market in Nigeria, and its brands – Benson and Hedges, Rothmans, St. Moritz, and Consulate – are the most popular among the soaring number of Nigerian smokers, including young people and new smokers. Smoking is glamorized as a way of being westernized. As smoking and tobacco use increase in Nigeria and most of Africa, the tobacco epidemic will likely emerge as one of the leading contributors to mortality and morbidity burdens of disease and ill health.

Added to the tobacco epidemic is the increased prevalence of obesity caused by the globalization of unsafe food and unhealthy lifestyles. The fast food industry has expanded enormously throughout Africa. In the more developed African cities such as Windhoek (Namibia), Abuja (Nigeria), Kampala (Uganda), Accra (Ghana), and Cape Town and Johannesburg (South Africa), as well as the less developed smaller cities such as Maseru (Lesotho), it is a common to see long queues of mostly young people and families lined up in the fast food restaurants. As with smoking, eating three meals a day in a fast food restaurant is a taste of being western and evidence that one belongs to the upper middle class in these countries.

Moving Health Sovereignty: Toward a Holistic African Perspective

In my previous work, while searching for a "prophylaxis" for global health challenges, especially the place of the "Third World" in that discourse, I proposed what I called "communitarian globalism" (Aginam 2005, 109–30). In the face of the increasing threats of communicable and non-communicable diseases in a globalized world, communitarian globalism represents a pool of efforts, resources, and skills by states, intergovernmental organizations, and civil society toward the protection and promotion of public health. Communitarian globalism

4 Speech by Nick Hales, managing director, BAT Nigeria, at the commissioning of the Ibadan factory, 17 June 2003.

5 See BAT Nigeria website at http://www.batnigeria.com, particularly the section on "Sustainability".

is imperative because global health governance recognizes the emergence and relevance of actors other than nation-states in global health. With respect to infectious diseases, microbial forces do not respect the geopolitical boundaries of states. The phenomenon of globalization has eroded the erstwhile traditional distinction between national and international health problems. The distinction between "us" and "them", between "our disease" and "their disease", has become anachronistic in a globalizing world. As Brundtland (2003) put it succinctly:

> Today, in an interconnected world, bacteria and viruses travel almost as fast as e-mail and financial flows. Globalization has connected Bujumbura to Bombay and Bangkok to Boston. There are no health sanctuaries. No impregnable walls exist between a world that is healthy, well-fed, and well-off and another that is sick, malnourished, and impoverished. Globalization has shrunk distances, broken down old barriers, and linked people. Problems halfway around the world become everyone's problem.

Global health challenges require globalized policy responses involving multiple actors – nation-states, intergovernmental organizations, private and corporate actors, and civil society. Some global health governance frameworks that support this form of public-private partnerships, although by no means unassailable success stories, include the GAVI Alliance (formerly the Global Alliance for Vaccines and Immunisation), the Stop TB Initiative, the Roll-Back Malaria (RBM) Partnership, and the Global Polio Eradication Initiative. These forms of governance approaches and partnerships involving states and nonstate actors have, in complex ways, challenged the state-centric model constructed on the pillars of Westphalia more than three centuries ago. Because Africa is marginalized in the international system, the task of articulating a coherent African perspective on "moving health sovereignty" must grapple with embedded state-centric interests and the structures of the Westphalian system. As difficult as this task may be, it must start by first recognizing that global health is not simply about infectious diseases. Second, it must recognize that most activities that affect public health occur outside the health sector, especially within the international economic and trade relations of states that are often driven by profit-oriented corporate interests. To confront the international system, an African perspective on global health challenges must address the health-related impacts of trade liberalization propelled by the World Trade Organization (as exemplified by the Agreement on Trade-Related Aspects of Intellectual Property Rights and access to essential medicines, and the General Agreement on Trade and Services and the privatization of health services). It must also address the globalization of unsafe food and harmful products (fast food, tobacco, illicit drugs), the migration of African health professionals to the West, increased investment in orphan or neglected diseases by global pharmaceutical corporations, the relegation of African traditional medical therapies to the peripheries of global health policy, and the participation by African states as active players in global health diplomacy. In all of these, African states must take the lead by building effective healthcare systems within their respective countries as way to boost health security and protect the right to the "highest attainable standard of health" of their populations. As Brundtland (2001) rightly observed:

> Enlightened self interest compels both industrialized country governments and private corporations to do what it takes to drastically reduce the current burden of disease in the developing world. To do so will be good for economic growth, be good for health and be good for the environment. Not only for the three billion people who have yet to benefit from the technological and economic revolution of the past fifty years – but for us all.

As health sovereignty continues to shift in dynamic and complex ways in the twenty-first century, there is an urgent need to reconstruct the architecture of global health governance in an age of globalization to reduce the burdens of infectious and non-communicable diseases prevalent in most African societies.

References

Aginam, Obijifor (2002). "From the Core to the Peripheries: Multilateral Governance of Malaria in a Multi-Cultural World". *Chicago Journal of International Law* 3(1): 87–103.

Aginam, Obijifor (2004). "Between Isolationism and Mutual Vulnerability: A South–North Perspective on Global Governance of Epidemics in an Age of Globalization". *Temple Law Review* 77: 297–312. http://www.temple.edu/lawschool/iilpp/Docs/Aginam,%20Final%20to%20Publisher,%2011-23-04.pdf (January 2013).

Aginam, Obijifor (2005). *Global Health Governance: International Law and Public Health in a Divided World.* Toronto: University of Toronto Press.

Aginam, Obijifor (2010). "Health or Trade? A Critique of Contemporary Approaches to Global Health Diplomacy". *Asian Journal of WTO and International Health Law and Policy* 5(2): 355–80.

Brundtland, Gro Harlem (2001). "Globalization as a Force for Better Health". Lecture presented in the Global Dimensions program, March 16, London School of Economics and Political Science. http://www.who.int/director-general/speeches/2001/english/20010316_lselecturelondon.en.html (December 2013).

Brundtland, Gro Harlem (2003). "Global Health and International Security". *Global Governance* 9(4): 417–23.

Callahan, Daniel and Angela A. Wasunna (2006). *Medicine and the Market: Equity v. Choice*. Baltimore: Johns Hopkins University Press.

Centers for Disease Control and Prevention (1998, September 11). "Preventing Emerging Infectious Diseases: A Strategy for the 21st Century". *Morbidity and Mortality Weekly Report* 47(RR-15). http://www.cdc.gov/mmwr/PDF/rr/rr4715.pdf (January 2013).

Connolly, Gregory N. (1992). "Worldwide Expansion of Transnational Tobacco Industry". *Journal of the National Cancer Institute* 12: 29–35.
Cooper, Andrew F., John J. Kirton, and Ted Schrecker, eds. (2007). *Governing Global Health: Challenge, Response, Innovation.* Aldershot: Ashgate.
Epstein, Helen (2007). *The Invisible Cure: Africa, The West, and the Fight against AIDS.* New York: Farrar, Straus and Giroux.
Falola, Toyin and Matthew M. Heaton, eds. (2007). *HIV/AIDS, Illness, and African Well-Being.* Rochester NY: University Rochester Press.
Fassin, Didier (2007). *When Bodies Remember: Experiences and Politics of AIDS in South Africa.* Berkeley: University of California Press.
Fidler, David P. (1997). "The Globalization of Public Health: Emerging Infectious Diseases and International Relations". *Indiana Journal of Global Legal Studies* 5(1): 11–51.
Fidler, David P. (1999). *International Law and Infectious Diseases.* Oxford: Oxford University Press.
Fidler, David P. (2001). "The Globalization of Public Health: The First 100 Years of International Health Diplomacy". *Bulletin of the World Health Organization* 79(9): 742–849. http://www.who.int/bulletin/archives/79(9)842.pdf (January 2014).
Hein, Wolfgang, Sonja Bartsch, and Lars Kohlmorgen, eds. (2007). *Global Health Governance and the Fight Against HIV/AIDS.* New York: Palgrave Macmillan.
Held, David and Anthony McGrew (2002). "Introduction". In *Governing Globalization: Power, Authority, and Global Governance*, David Held and Anthony McGrew, eds. Cambridge: Polity Press.
Howard-Jones, Norman (1975). *The Scientific Background of the International Sanitary Conferences, 1851–1938.* Geneva: World Health Organization.
Hunter, Susan (2003). *Black Death: AIDS in Africa.* New York: Palgrave Macmillan.
Kaplan, Robert D. (2000). *The Coming Anarchy: Shattering the Dreams of the Post Cold War.* New York: Random House.
Krasner, Stephen (1999). *Sovereignty: Organized Hypocrisy.* Princeton: Princeton University Press.
Krasner, Stephen (2001). *Problematic Sovereignty: Contested Rules and Political Possibilities.* New York: Columbia University Press.
Lee, Kelley, Kent Buse, and Suzanne Fustukian, eds. (2002). *Health Policy in a Globalising World.* Cambridge: Cambridge University Press.
Lee, Kelley and Richard Dodgson (2000). "Globalization and Cholera: Implications for Global Governance". *Global Governance* 6(2): 213–36.
Lifson, Alan R. (1996). "Mosquitoes, Models, and Dengue". *Lancet* 347(9010): 1201–2. doi: 10.1016/S0140-6736(96)90730-8.
Orbinski, James (2008). *An Imperfect Offering: Humanitarian Action in the Twenty-First Century.* Toronto: Doubleday.
Phaswana-Mafuya, Nancy and Dmitri Tassiopoulos, eds. (2001). *Non-Communicable Diseases (NCDs) in Developing Countries.* Hauppauge NY: Nova Publishers.

Santoro, Michael A. and Thomas M. Gorrie (2005). *Ethics and the Pharmaceutical Industry*. Cambridge: Cambridge University Press.

UNAIDS (2012). "Global Report: UNAIDS Report on the Global AIDS Epidemic 2012". Geneva. http://www.unaids.org/en/media/unaids/contentassets/documents/epidemiology/2012/gr2012/20121120_UNAIDS_Global_Report_2012_en.pdf (June 2013).

World Bank (2011). "The Growing Danger of Non-Communicable Diseases: Acting Now to Reverse Course". Conference edition, September, Washington DC. http://siteresources.worldbank.org/HEALTHNUTRITIONANDPOPULATION/Resources/Peer-Reviewed-Publications/WBDeepeningCrisis.pdf (January 2013).

World Health Organization (2011a). "Global Status Report on Non-communicable Diseases 2010". Geneva. http://www.who.int/nmh/publications/ncd_report2010/en/ (January 2013).

World Health Organization (2011b). "TB/HIV Facts 2011–2012". Geneva. http://www.who.int/tb/publications/TBHIV_Facts_for_2011.pdf (June 2013).

World Health Organization Regional Office for Europe (1999). "Strategy to Roll Back Malaria in the WHO European Region". Copenhagen. http://www.euro.who.int/__data/assets/pdf_file/0006/98790/E67133.pdf (January 2013).

Zacher, Mark (1992). "The Decaying Pillars of the Westphalian Temple: Implications for International Order and Governance". In *Governance Without Government: Order and Change in Word Politics*, James N. Rosenau and Ernst-Otto Czemiel, eds. Cambridge: Cambridge University Press, pp. 58–101.

Zacher, Mark and Tania J. Keefe (2008). *The Politics of Global Health Governance: United by Contagion*. New York: Palgrave Macmillan.

Chapter 3
South Africa's Sovereignty and HIV/AIDS

Annamarie Bindenagel Šehović

There is little question that HIV/AIDS poses a threat to individual lives. However, it also arguably constitutes a severe challenge to the integrity of societies, polities, and the sovereignty of states. This is especially the case in countries where access to continual and reliable information, prevention, and treatment is intermittent, thwarted by ineffective leadership, stymied by a lack of capacity, or circumscribed by competing local and global priorities that hamper their ability to respond to the epidemic.

The trajectory of the epidemic itself, given its long early phase dogged by ignorance and disinformation, is partly to blame. But so, too, is the unique nature of the threat that HIV/AIDS poses not only for individuals alone, but also for them as members of society, and thus for the economy and polity in which they reside. This is most evident where the disease prevalence rises above the one per cent threshold that marks the onset of an epidemic. Here, the survival of individual lives that constitute citizens of a state intersects with the existence of the state itself as a sovereign entity responsible for those lives and answerable for them both domestically and globally.

Despite widespread acceptance of the social and economic impacts of HIV/AIDS, there has been little effort to identify and to understand its particular political or economic ramifications. As a result, responses to the spread of HIV/AIDS often fail to harness this knowledge to adapt prevention, coping, and eradication initiatives. Yet it is precisely such knowledge that this is needed to support a response that depends upon a state meeting its sovereign obligations to protect the health and welfare of its citizens. It offers, in the words of Solomon Benatar (2001), a "window and a mirror" to state ethics.

Thus sovereignty plays a dual role with regard to HIV/AIDS. The first role is the state's responsibility to the individual lives of its constituents and arguably all those within its borders – and by extension the responsibility of those constituents to themselves and their society through the means of knowing their status, and fostering prevention while limiting transmission. Individual health is a critical component of sovereign sustainability. The second role is the sovereignty of the state, and its accountability to itself and the international community of likewise sovereign states, for should it fail to act responsibly, that international community might intervene – to the detriment of state sovereignty and possibly also to the individuals who live in that state.

This chapter addresses these dimensions of HIV/AIDS in South Africa. It first identifies the individual and societal implications of the epidemic. It then affirms the role of sovereignty and the repercussions in the case of circumscribed sovereignty in South Africa's response to the epidemic. Finally, it highlights developments in responding to HIV/AIDS and the role of sovereignty so as to recommend ways to support both, in South Africa and beyond.

South Africa and HIV/AIDS

HIV/AIDS is one of the most poignant problems confronting southern and South Africa today. An eventually debilitating disease, HIV/AIDS has increasingly affected populations throughout southern Africa for nearly 30 years, although the number of new infections has begun to decline in recent years. The spread of the disease can be attributed to the insidiousness of the virus and to the fact that it is transmitted through the intimate and largely individual life-giving act of sex. In infecting and killing mostly young, economically and socially active human beings of reproductive age, HIV/AIDS threatens not only the lives of infected individuals but also the integrity of societies, economies, and polities.[1] While some may argue that with as much as 30 per cent of a population infected, the impact on familial stability, social cohesion, economic growth, sustainability, and political stability remains negligible; such medical reduction distorts the penetrating and profound crisis inextricably linked to HIV/AIDS. As researchers – virologists, immunologists, epidemiologists, sociologists, economists, and political scientists – have studied the HIV/AIDS epidemic, it continues to claim individual casualties and wreak widespread havoc on the humans it affects. Hence, despite being the most studied and well-understood virus in human history, it remains an urgent and increasing threat to human society and therefore also to states.

1 While some would argue that HIV has become a chronic condition and that AIDS can be forestalled, perhaps indefinitely, it would be a mistake to appropriate this point of view for southern and South Africa. Statistics for this region show that the disease continues to cause the deaths of disproportionate numbers of especially young adults, and the trajectory of the epidemic shows little sign of abating. This prevalence has to do both with persistent problems in access to prevention and anti-retroviral medications, and with ongoing denial and disaffection in acknowledging and therefore treating the disease. The difficulties in access will only intensify with regard to second-line drugs, most of which are not yet able to be universally procured and provided, and will not be. In addition, it stands to reason that national government and international aid budgets that support prevention and particularly treatment will continue to suffer given the current global economy, with foreboding consequences for efforts to stem the tide of the HIV/AIDS epidemic. This, therefore, stands to undermine the ability of the state to act upon its sovereign responsibility to protect its people.

This threat has essentially two key elements, in line with its manifestation at the individual and state levels. The first element is best described in Tony Barnett's (2006) detailed analysis of HIV/AIDS as a long-wave illness with effects stretching over generations. The second element links this intergenerational effort at individual survival with governance, both national and global. This link stems from two sources: on the one hand, the dependence of individuals on state and nonstate global actors to provide a continual supply and access to antiretroviral treatment (ART) and, on the other hand, the sufficient independence of these state and nonstate global actors and activists to guarantee that dependence. If the latter scenario fails, little recourse remains for the sovereign state – in this instance South Africa, especially failing to provide for ART for its HIV-infected populace on its own – to meet this guarantee. Instead, it may find its role circumvented by alliances of nonstate and global actors that do. Yet these do so with one big caveat for the state: they do not assume either sovereign responsibility for the individual health and welfare of HIV-infected individuals, nor do they take on accountability for such a response vis-à-vis either the state's responsibility to respond or that of the international community in the event of failure. As such, as HIV/AIDS erodes the ranks of young, potentially economically and socially active reproductive generations, it also fundamentally alters the relationship between the state, with its sovereign responsibility, and its constituents, eroding the state's sovereignty and potentially further undermining the polity itself and the political system intended to provide for and protect the lives of its citizens.

Three generally posited hypotheses attempt to explain the persistence of the epidemic and the ineffectiveness of existing coping and curative strategies. The first is insufficient access to prevention information, condoms, and ART, as maintained by the Centres for Disease Control, UNAIDS, and the World Health Organization (WHO). The second is a lack of clear and consistent political leadership (Fourie 2006; Nattrass 2007). The third is lack of resources (Bell et al. 2003). Each hypothesis, however, neither identifies nor recognizes the problem of and response to HIV/AIDS as a symptom of a deeper malaise: namely the fragmentation of sovereignty nationally and globally, and also of state capacity to meet its sovereign responsibilities both to its individual citizens as well as to the community of sovereign states.

In order to understand South Africa's responses to HIV/AIDS, and its consequences, it is necessary to analyse the conditions wrought of the spread of the epidemic, and the fraught national and global political-economic context characterized by state and nonstate alliances of actors and activists circumventing the state. The insights gleaned proffer a new view of the necessary role of state sovereignty in providing and protecting human life and welfare in global governance. Applied here, these have profound implications for South Africa, its response to HIV/AIDS, and the life expectancy of its constituents and the longevity of its polity.

The starting point must be state sovereignty, for global governance remains today a state-centric system, wherein the state retains the ultimate responsibility for the lives and livelihoods inside its borders. As such, sovereignty, according to the Westphalian definition, although challenged, and possibly expanded to reflect the concerns of human security, includes the responsibilities of the nation-state to impose and implement rule in order to ensure the territorial and physical security of citizens; to protect lives and livelihoods by providing basic economic stability, health, and welfare; and to assume accountability to the state itself and to the international community (Brühl and Rittberger 2001; International Commission on Intervention and State Sovereignty 2001; Hösle 2004; Risse 2007). Indeed, in South Africa's case, according to its 1994 constitution, the government assumes responsibility for providing health care, housing, education, and fundamental freedoms and human rights, including the provision of information, prevention, and treatment against HIV/AIDS. Yet no particular order of response is stipulated, nor are any prescriptions for inevitable trade-offs written.

To respond to all of these myriad rights, South Africa's first democratic government sought to balance long-term political and economic stability and sustainability with immediate, short-term demands, including slowly expanding initiatives to address HIV/AIDS. At the same time, the state attempted to limit its international liabilities, both economic and political, in terms of its external dependence particularly upon foreign financing to meet its sovereign responsibilities.

However, the short-term demands got ahead of the intentions. The survival needs of South Africa's HIV-infected constituents multiplied, and so too did their recourse and resources through external state and nonstate actors to have those demands met. This recourse and associated resources bypassed the state and shifted the response to the epidemic, although it did not shift any concomitant responsibility or accountability for it. The pressure those state and nonstate actors brought to bear upon South Africa's fledgling democracy arguably circumvented and circumscribed its sovereignty.

State sovereignty carries the responsibility and accountability to respond to the HIV/AIDS crisis to ensure the survival of its citizens – infected and not infected. This raises the stakes in balancing the rights of all citizens, and inextricably ties a successful act to the survival of the sovereign state. In South Africa's case, the state largely failed to strike a successful balance, but the process it went through reflects the contemporary struggle over state sovereignty.

Three Signs of an Inverse Relationship

South Africa's response to HIV/AIDS vis-à-vis its assertion of state sovereignty highlights an inverse relationship. This is reflected in three phases and characterized by three indicators. The first phase began in 2003 when South Africa banked on sovereign economic independence, largely at the expense of an immediate response to the epidemic. By 2008, in the second phase, in the aftermath of failed attempts to respond and under the weight of national and global actors and activists, the state accepted a greater degree of external dependence and circumvented sovereignty in its improved response. The third phase was in the aftermath of the 2008 financial crisis, however, when South Africa began to regain the upper hand, although this time its independence was in more in line with the maintenance of its HIV/AIDS response.

The first indicator of the inverse relationship is illuminated by the thinking behind this precarious balancing act. In 2007, Trevor Manuel, then finance minister, said:

> My purpose has always been to try to remain sovereign. We saw 10 years of remarkable change in Zimbabwe on borrowed money. Then came 1991 and the first structural adjustment loans fell due. It coincided with my appointment as head of the [African National Congress's] department of economic policy. It became a challenge to take decisions to stay out of the clutches of other decision-makers; to not land at the door of the [International Monetary Fund] (Haffajee 2007).

Manuel's emphasis on sovereignty, invoked in terms of financial independence but equally relevant to aid dependence such as for HIV/AIDS funding, and thus to the integrity of state sovereignty, is perhaps one of the most important structural, practical, and perceptive factors influencing South Africa's response to its HIV/AIDS crisis. And Manuel's concerns were justified. Given the degree of such dependence and the decrease in funding after the global financial crisis, he had every reason to want to insulate South Africa from making a promise – of perpetual, life-saving treatment for HIV/AIDS – that he might not be able to keep (see McCoy et al. 2009; Nishtar and Pablos-Mendez 2009).

Indeed, the following scenario showcases the delicate situation in which South Africa manoeuvred. While the government struggled to revive what was a fragile economy inherited at the dawn of South African democracy, it counted on stability instead of restructuring. In doing so it ditched its initial Reconstruction and Development Plan and adopted the Growth, Employment, and Redistribution strategy devised with advice from an international team of experts. The strategy proposed a strict application of the Washington consensus: the gradual elimination of exchange controls, lower inflation, a reduction of the budget deficit, and quicker privatization (De Coning and Cloete 2000). The South African government applied these nearly perfectly in the hope that foreign investment would flow in. It did not.

South Africa did try to partially invoke rights accorded it under the World Trade Organization's Agreement on Trade-Related Aspects of Intellectual Property (TRIPS), to break medical patents in the case of a national emergency – in this case, for antiretroviral drugs to fight HIV/AIDS. But it did not declare such an emergency. So South Africa wound up in its own courts, charged in 1998 by 39 pharmaceutical companies with attempting to illegally break patents. It also faced the wrath of the US government, which threatened to place it first on a watch list and then on a black list, both of which would have had dire effects on its trade relationships. The South African government lost the case, and with it a means through which it might have paid for ART to protect the lives of its citizens, years before this became the case.

Into the void caused by this state impotence stepped alliances of external state and nonstate actors eager to offer their services in the fight against HIV/AIDS. They circumvented the national government. The unintended results circumscribed South Africa's sovereignty because, although the state retained its sovereign responsibility for its citizens' health, the tools to guarantee such health, in the case of HIV/AIDS, remained in the hands of others beyond its control.

The second indicator of the inverse relationship was the South African state's negligence compounded by nationalist denialism. This stance made it easy for leaders to shirk the responsibility of responding to HIV/AIDS. In the end, however, it only helped diminish state sovereignty as the other actors rose to the occasion instead, although again without assuming the responsibility or accountability of a guarantee.

Denialism posits three main premises relevant to the relationship between HIV/AIDS and sovereignty in South Africa. First, it refuses to accept that life-giving behaviour (sex) carries with it death. Second, it alleges a fatalistic futility in interventions for African rights and argues that Africans should provide African solutions. Third, it asserts that HIV/AIDS must not exist, or must be caused by external factors alone such as poverty. Although perhaps intended to be noble in sentiment, these three myths are devastating deterrents to combating HIV/AIDS. They have also resulted in additional political and practical detrimental effects on the fight against HIV/AIDS and, in particular, on the perception of African states and their commitment and ability to protect their people.

In the context of this analysis, these myths remove the responsibility from the individual and state for responding to a hypothetical HIV/AIDS, linking it to poverty (alone).[2] In doing so, they reject external interventions, and rule out a transfer of or shared responsibility with state and nonstate actors nationally or globally. This once again undermines state sovereignty, as the state remains ultimately responsible and accountable for the health and livelihoods of its citizens and the long-term development of the most-affected African states, including South Africa, whose population and socioeconomic and political health are on the line, while forfeiting both the state's legitimacy and its capacity to act.

The third indictor of an inverse relationship is the international pressure for a particular, response to HIV/AIDS, premised mostly on ART. This response connotes dependence for most states that require additional funding or medical support in order to gain access and distribute these drugs. So while the international community, in collaboration with local activists such as the

2 While poverty could be argued to negatively affect and exacerbate the progression and thus the consequences of the virus, it alone does not cause HIV/AIDS. This line of argument also cultivates a fatalistic perspective through which interventions for individual African rights to access to health care and ART are inherently futile without the eradication of poverty.

Treatment Action Campaign, has mobilized unprecedented amounts of money to fight HIV/AIDS, it has also created a conundrum, namely increased dependence and circumscribed sovereignty.

In the fight over access to ART, the South African government attempted to balance the budgetary implications of an unending roll-out, with competing priorities, such as basic health care, housing, crime fighting, and measures to combat unemployment. However, in postponing initiatives to fight HIV/AIDS, the government also failed to secure the rights and heed its responsibilities to the portion of its population infected and affected by the epidemic. It also jeopardized the gains of its macroeconomic prudence, relying on a population increasingly eroded by the effects of HIV/AIDS.

In the interim, alliances of external state and nonstate actors exerted immense pressure on the South African government to respond to HIV/AIDS, notably through the introduction of ART. Those actors finally got their wish: first with the introduction in 2003, then with an expanded roll-out in 2007–08. Still, the state has not done enough to ensure the sustainability of this approach, just as the inverse relationship predicted: more dependence in the response to HIV/AIDS equals less independence to guarantee sovereign responsibility and accountability. Indeed, in losing the TRIPS case, the South African government also lost any future ability to invoke these two provisions (responsibility and accountability). In the aftermath, therefore, the South African government's ability to exercise its sovereignty over HIV/AIDS waned.

Two global examples are worth highlighting here.

In 2001, the United Nations launched the Global Fund to Fight AIDS, Tuberculosis, and Malaria. The Global Fund, in offering financing for HIV/AIDS intervention, took away some of the government's immediate responsibility to its HIV/AIDS-affected citizens. However, it afforded no long-term commitments or promises, nor did it assume ultimate accountability. Indeed, following a series of corruption scandals and problems with its funding system in 2010, the Global Fund suspended grant making, leaving many countries that depend upon it, notably Uganda and Zimbabwe, in the lurch.

In 2003, US president George W. Bush announced the creation of the US President's Emergency Plan for AIDS Relief (PEPFAR). PEPFAR had a $15 billion budget to be dispersed to 15 focus countries, including South Africa, as well as roughly 100 countries in the form of bilateral aid. An emergency fund, PEPFAR initially tied aid to the purchase of US-made patented antiretroviral drugs. It excluded reproductive health programs that offered abortions and instituted a 33 per cent funding earmark for abstinence-only initiatives. When PEPFAR was renewed by the US Congress in 2008 to the tune of $48 billion to be dispersed over the following five years, these earmarks were removed. In 2009 newly elected Barack Obama launched the Global Health Initiative, which included PEPFAR as a significant component.

The draw of this money made it hard to resist, even for South Africa. But such funding has two major consequences: it assumes some of the financial burden of the South African government's response to HIV/AIDS, but in so doing it largely bypasses the South African government, taking over its sovereign decision-making control. Funding applications and approvals went through the US embassy and were managed by US representatives, relieving the South African government of such support and taking over some responsibility. But it did so without assuming accountability to the South African government or its citizenry, and thus compromised the long-term success of the individual survival and the sovereignty of the state. This is because although the South African government has a seat at the Global Fund table, the funding and spending prescriptions were effectively pre-set. In addition, by relying on such external funding, the government set itself up for a dependency against which it could not insure itself; the price became evident in the aftermath of the global financial crisis of 2008.

A New Era of HIV/AIDS and Sovereignty in South Africa

The resignation of South African president Thabo Mbeki on September 23, 2008, brought the end of an era. Mbeki as well as his controversial minister of health, Manto Tshabalala-Msimang – the proponents (at worst) and condoners (at best) of HIV/AIDS denialism – ceded their positions to an incoming political cadre. Although their removal from government coincided with South Africa's second antiretroviral roll-out already in place, additional changes in the national approach to HIV/AIDS loomed.

At the HIV Vaccine Research Conference on October 13, 2008, Barbara Hogan, the new minister of health, stated unequivocally that "we know that HIV causes AIDS". After years characterized by confusion, between outright denial that HIV causes AIDS and deliberate obfuscation over the part played by poverty in the spread of the virus, Hogan's statement marked a stark contrast. The minister did not deny the many factors that influence the spread of HIV/AIDS – citing race, class, gender and sexual orientation as relevant, as well as migrant labour and poverty. She acknowledged the particular vulnerability that abetted the virus in South Africa. Hogan (2008) also acknowledged the failure of the South African government to meet its responsibilities: "We also wasted time despite having one of the best plans to cope with the epidemic adopted by Cabinet under Dr. Nkosanzana Dlamini-Zuma. So indeed we saw this fastest rate of spread of HIV during the first decade of our hard-earned freedom and democracy".

Hogan's successor, Dr. Aaron Motsoaledi, came in with the government of Jacob Zuma, inaugurated May 9, 2009. Motsoaledi and Zuma affirmed South Africa's commitment to fighting HIV/AIDS, and also to remaining sovereign.

> The Zuma government and his Minister of Health, Dr. Aaron Motsoaledi, are now developing a national HIV strategy that aims at preventing further cases, treating those who are infected, and weaning the nation of foreign assistance for not only AIDS but all of the country's health needs. In short, South Africa

aims to be the first African nation to build health for all, independent of foreign donors (Garrett 2009).[3]

Especially in the wake of the 2008 global financial crisis, it still remained to be seen whether South Africa could manage this balancing act better than before. It is made more complicated by the increasing need, and corresponding rise in price, of second- and third-line ART. The state remains responsible for protecting and providing for the health and welfare of its HIV-infected, and all other, citizens. Protecting all citizens, and guaranteeing that protection, is the responsibility of the sovereign state (Tutu 2008)

Sovereignty, South Africa, and HIV/AIDS

Due to the ongoing challenges posed by HIV/AIDS in particular, and due also to the inverse relationship more broadly, South Africa's focus on its ability to meet its sovereign responsibilities is understandable. The new South Africa is a state forged from the fires of liberation. It is conscious of its history and defensive of its freedom and sovereignty. The HIV/AIDS epidemic, a threat to these gains, confronts this South Africa with a psychological threat to its independence and presents a complex health, economic, and political challenge.

HIV/AIDS remains wedged between national demands and international pressures to alleviate poverty, malnutrition, food insecurity, economic exclusion, and power imbalances among individuals and the state. The survival of individuals directly and indirectly affected by HIV/AIDS, their political constituency and representation, their economic contributions, knowledge transfer, and children are all crucial to a stable and sustainable South Africa (see Poku and Whiteside 2004). Political and economic governance has increased with HIV/AIDS appearing on international policy agendas with prescriptions on aid, trade, and investment. These indirect consequences of HIV/AIDS, over the short and long term, have direct effects on the progress toward growth, stability, and sustainability in South Africa.

No state today is completely independent or sovereign, but the world still remains in a state-centric governance system that renders the national state the repository of ultimate sovereign responsibility. That means that state sovereignty still plays a vital role in both national and global health. It must be strong enough to ensure that the right to health, among other rights, is indeed a reality.

Given this reality, there needs to be a reordering of sovereign responsibility and accountability that takes into account the division of labour between states and nonstate actors in national and global governance. The multiplicity of actors and activists is not going to go away: there will continue to be dilemmas in decision

---

3 South Africa has been receiving increased aid from PEPFAR since 2010. This puts it in the precarious position of being dependent, with particular risk due to the financial crisis and funding flat-lining.

making and challenges of choosing inevitable trade-offs. The situation calls for nationally, entwined internationally, regulated responsibility and accountability (see Morris 2009).

Conclusion and Recommendations

The protection of citizens within a sovereign state is the responsibility of that state. Where neither effective state sovereignty nor clear lines of designated responsibility and accountability to external state and nonstate actors exist to meet this need, provisions should be made to transfer responsibility and accountability to protect the population's health and welfare. Otherwise, ad hoc unregulated interventions threaten to circumvent sovereign responsibility and accountability with potentially detrimental effects on both the sustainable lives and welfare of individuals as well as of the sovereign state.

This is evident in the case of South Africa and its struggle to respond to the challenge of its HIV/AIDS epidemic.

HIV/AIDS is first and foremost a life-threatening individual disease. However, as HIV-infected and affected individuals constitute families, societies, economic contributors, and polities, the impact of the virus has widespread implications. While some of the direct impact of HIV/AIDS might be contained by national policies, such as the provision of ART, prevention campaigns, and financial and educational support, particularly for individuals at high risk of infection and orphans, those policies require national and international attention that is weighed against social, economic, and political priorities.

At the individual level, although the annual numbers of deaths attribute to HIV/AIDS and new infections have been dropping globally, the incidence and prevalence of the diseases continues to threaten southern Africa. At the state level, South Africa has lost some of its ability to control the means to provide for its citizens first because of its failure to invoke its sovereign power and provide a full-fledged HIV/AIDS response and then, in circumscribed circumstances, by depending on other actors to provide that response – which is not a sustainable solution. Although the government has tried outsource some of its interventions, it could not insulate itself against eventual donor fatigue or disinterest or the consequences of the global financial crisis. Thus, South Africa still finds itself caught between its sovereign responsibilities and its circumscribed sovereign inability to meet them.

There are five possible remedies for this crisis.

First, a culture of responsibility at the individual, national, and international levels needs to be cultivated. Unless people and their governments internalize and actualize their own integrity, survival worth, and the value of their lives and livelihood, the fight against HIV/AIDS will be lost.

Second, the rising incidence and prevalence rates indicate that current best-practice models of prevention are inadequate. These should be updated to include greater emphasis on local languages, coordination with local healers, such as South Africa's *sangomas*, and the provision of ART. Clear and consistent leadership is needed to emphasize the value of life and integrate concern for food security, disease prevention, basic health care – seen in the global drive for universal health care – and ART, at the local, national, and international levels.

Third, greater efforts should be made to speed up and avoid duplication of pharmaceutical approval processes by WHO and the US Food and Drug Administration. Such efforts are being addressed in part by the fast-track initiative for HIV/AIDS medications put in place by George Bush and extended by Barack Obama, to be purchased with US funding and used abroad, as well as in a more targeted fashion in the renewed PEPFAR legislation. Still more should be done to institutionalize the approval processes, which should also make special provisions for and require more generic medications. Provisions should also be made to take into account and utilize the patent pool and to make best use of funding from UNITAID, an international initiative funded mainly by levies on air travel to help tackle inefficiencies in the global pharmaceutical market. Subsidies and preferential regional trade agreements might be instituted to promote locally produced generic drugs such as in Brazil and South Africa, to encourage and accelerate local production in other parts of Africa. Such agreements are especially important as India moves up the innovation chain and adopts all the TRIPS provisions, which might reduce global access to erstwhile Indian-produced generic drugs.

Fourth, global donors, including the Global Fund and PEPFAR, should continue in the current vein of "country ownership" and partnership frameworks, to strengthen national input as well as independent responsibility and accountability. They should also invest in strengthening health systems as another means of guaranteeing the sustainability of interventions (see also Swidler 2006).

Fifth, if a sovereign state is unable to provide security, in this instance including health and welfare, to its citizens, provisions should be made for other actors to fill the vacuum. This might be done through international regulation of responsibility and accountability through an oversight institution such as WHO (Lisk 2010). Or it might involve the ceding of sovereign responsibilities through delegation or a system of shared governance. In any instance, it needs to be clarified, who and what is responsible and accountable, in the short and long term, for the right to human health.

References

Barnett, Tony (2006). "A Long-Wave Event. HIV/AIDS, Politics, Governance, and "Security": Sundering the Intergenerational Bond?" *International Affairs* 82(2): 297–313.

Bell, Clive, Shantayanan Devarajan, and Hans Gersbach (2003). "The Long-Run Economic Costs of AIDS: Theory and an Application to South Africa". World Bank, Washington DC. doi: 10.1596/1813-9450-3152.

Benatar, Solomon (2001). "South Africa's Transition in a Globalizing World: HIV/AIDS as a Window and a Mirror". *International Affairs* 77(2): 347–75.

Brühl, Tanja and Volker Rittberger (2001). "From International to Global Governance: Actors, Collective Decision-Making, and the United Nations in the World of the Twenty-First Century". In *Global Governance and the United Nations System*, Volker Rittberger, ed. Tokyo: United Nations University Press, pp. 1–47.

De Coning, Cedric and Fanie Cloete (2000). "Theories and Models for Analyzing Public Policy". In *Improving Public Policy: From Theory to Practice*, Fanie Cloete and Cedric De Coning, eds. Pretoria: Van Schaik.

Fourie, Pieter (2006). The Political Management of HIV and AIDS in South Africa: One Burden Too Many? London: Palgrave Macmillan.

Garrett, Laurie (2009). "Global Health Update". December 23, Council on Foreign Relations, New York. http://www.cfr.org/content/thinktank/GlobalHealth/GHU_Copenhagen_Dec2309.pdf (July 2013).

Haffajee, Ferial (2007). "Not in My Father's House: Trevor Manuel". *Mail and Guardian*, December 13.

Hogan, Barbara (2008). "Speech by the Minister of Health at the HIV Vaccine Research Conference". Cape Town, October 13. http://www.tac.org.za/community/node/2421 (July 2013).

Hösle, Vittorio (2004). *Morals and Politics*. Translated by Steven Rendall. Notre Dame, IN: University of Notre Dame Press.

International Commission on Intervention and State Sovereignty (2001). "The Responsibility to Protect: Report of the International Commission on Intervention and State Sovereignty". December. http://responsibilitytoprotect.org/ICISS%20Report.pdf (December 2013).

Lisk, Franklyn (2010). Global Institutions and the HIV/AIDS Epidemic: Responding to an International Crisis. London: Routledge.

McCoy, David, Gayatri Kembhavi, Jinesh Patel, et al. (2009). "The Bill and Melinda Gates Foundation's Grant-Making Programme for Global Health". *Lancet* 373(9675): 1645–53.

Morris, Kelly (2009). "USA Failing on HIV/AIDS Accountability and Action". *Lancet Infectious Diseases* 9(1): 14.

Nattrass, Nicoli (2007). *Mortal Combat: AIDS Denialism and the Struggle for Antiretrovirals in South Africa*. Scottsville, South Africa: University of KwaZulu-Natal Press.

Nishtar, Sania and Ariel Pablos-Mendez (2009). "The Global Financial Downturn – Imperatives for the Health Sector". *Lancet* 373(9658): 124.

Poku, Nana K. and Alan Whiteside, eds. (2004). *The Political Economy of AIDS in Africa*. Aldershot: Ashgate.

Risse, Thomas (2007). "Paradoxien der Souveränität". *Internationale Politik* 7/8: 40–47. https://zeitschrift-ip.dgap.org/de/ip-die-zeitschrift/archiv/jahrgang-2007/juli-august/paradoxien-der-souver%C3%A4nit%C3%A4t (July 2013).

Swidler, Ann (2006). "Syncretism and Subversion in AIDS Governance: How Locals Cope with Global Demands". *International Affairs* 82(2): 269–84.
Tutu, Desmond (2008). "Responsibility to Protect". *International Herald Tribune*, February 20, p. 6.

Chapter 4
AIDS and Security in the Twenty-First Century

Pieter Fourie

This chapter explores the historical development of multilateral efforts in global health governance and the specific impact of HIV/AIDS on national and international political agendas. Specifically, it deals with the effort to achieve the "securitization" of HIV/AIDS – a concept that is core to the raison d'être of the sovereign state.

With the complexities brought about by globalization, and the emergence of new, more virulent pandemics, health problems have increasingly been labelled as security issues, or as "collective insecurity" for sovereign states and the global community. This frame presents effective health governance as a matter of national and international security that demands more sophisticated, collaborative, and timely local and global health governance. It views public health through the lens of security.

However, most evidence has shown no significant co-variation between HIV/AIDS prevalence and military insecurity, social uprising, macroeconomic failure, electoral instability, or democratic consolidation. Furthermore, securitization of the pandemic has wrongly been framed as a war to be won, with HIV/AIDS as the enemy that must be defeated. This framework has placed the emphasis on a process to secure states, instead of primarily providing better health systems around the world and dealing with the long-term reality of HIV/AIDS.

Intervention to assist with HIV/AIDS epidemics should focus on better health care, not security; on health systems, tailored to each state. In such a way, the securitization of HIV/AIDS would be done in a more conscious manner to facilitate public health interventions, mobilize funds, and create institutions with a long-term agenda. Multilateral consensus on the effective securitization of HIV/AIDS would include the systemic and temporal realities of the pandemic, such as long-term changes required in gender relations, sustainable behaviour change, and cultural adaptation. Doing so would respond well to the reality of the epidemic.

Security and Health: Past Is Prologue

Until the Industrial Revolution of the nineteenth century, state-centred interventions to limit the spread and impact of disease focused mostly on isolated epidemic outbreaks. This was the case with the quarantining of people and goods suspected of harbouring infectious disease, a practice that originated in the Port of Venice during the plague epidemics of the fourteenth century (King 2002, 764). According to Mark Zacher (2007), global health collaboration has evolved through three historical periods.

First, from the mid nineteenth century to the early twentieth century, a treaty to control the international spread of epidemic disease was negotiated, mostly by European states. This happened in parallel with the Industrial Revolution, as colonial masters interacted more frequently with and were more exposed to the diseases of other parts of the world. The negotiations followed a conference held in Paris in 1851 to address cholera. They culminated in the acceptance of the International Sanitary Regulations of 1903, which were later renamed the International Health Regulations (IHR).

The second major development in the search for an international health regime was the establishment of the World Health Organization (WHO) in 1948 under the aegis of the United Nations. WHO championed and approved revised versions of the IHR in 1951, 1969, 1973, and 1981.

Third, since 1990 there has been a dramatic expansion in multilateral efforts at global health cooperation. After the severe acute respiratory syndrome (SARS) scare of 2003, the IHR were again amended. The revised version was formally adopted in May 2005 and came into force in June 2007. A key thrust of this evolving health regime is health surveillance, along with emergency interventions to control epidemic outbreaks (Davies 2013, 308–13). David Fidler and Laurence Gostin (2006, 86) argue that the new IHR constitute a paradigm shift compared to the old version, to the extent that they will transform and "expand the scope of the IHR's application, incorporate international human rights principles, contain more demanding obligations for states parties to conduct surveillance and response, and establish important new powers for WHO" (Fidler and Gostin 2006, 86).

Fidler (2007) points out that this regime is noted for its embrace of health problems as security issues. He postulates that the world now operates in a "post-securitisation phase", in which "viewing public health through the lens of security has become an integral aspect of public health governance in the 21st century" (41). He further argues that the contemporary securitization of health is the result of post-Cold War fears regarding the proliferation of bioweapons and the global spread of communicable diseases (especially HIV/AIDS, but also the SARS and H5N1 scares of recent years), as well as mounting sensitivities regarding the vulnerability of populations in both rich and poor countries in the context of rapid globalization. Zacher (2007, 21ff) contends that there is no simple explanation for the change in the international health regime, but adds that contributing factors have been the emergence of new and more virulent pandemic diseases, the greater understanding of the costs of disease to economies and societies that are more deeply linked through processes of globalization, the expanding participation of civil society and private actors (many via public-private partnerships) in global health governance, and the improvement of disease detection and surveillance via the internet.

Health has thus come to be viewed as an exemplar of humanity's "new collective insecurity" (Shaw et al. 2006, 5). According to Dennis Pirages (2007, 625), such "growing complexity requires more sophisticated forms of governance", as well as the move from a state-centric to a supranational level of global public health governance to address what are, in essence, health issues that transcend national borders. Emerging from these new realities is the tension between the broader human-centric perspective on health, which views health as a basic individual human right linked to broader rights of citizenship and health's social determinants, and the understanding of health that links health to securitization.

Securitization was introduced into political science discourse in the 1990s, when Ole Wæver, Barry Buzan, and other members of the so-called Copenhagen School of security coined the term to advance discourse regarding security "beyond a focus on the nation-state and on the provision or analysis of military security issues only" (Kelle 2007, 218). Barry Buzan and Ole Wæver (2003, 71) summarize the securitization process as follows (see also Cook 2010):

> A security issue is posited (by a securitising actor) as a threat to the survival of some referent object (nation, state, the liberal international economic order, the rain forests), which is claimed to have a right to survive. Since a question of survival necessarily involves a point of no return at which it will be too late to act, it is not defensible to leave this issue to normal politics. The securitising actor therefore claims a right to use extraordinary means or break normal rules, for reasons of security.

Since the fall of the Berlin Wall on November 9, 1989 – 11/9 – and the terrorist attacks on the United States on September 11, 2001 – 9/11 – UN agencies in particular as well as the members of the G8 are in the throes of what could potentially be an interesting marriage between a traditional, militaristic way of thinking about security, and the more contemporary, human security perspective alluded to above. The war on terror and "the war on HIV/AIDS" are seen as two sides of the same coin. Both have been constructed by the US State Department as risks requiring the rapid mobilization of resources and have become a central subject of foreign policy requiring US leadership and international collaboration.

Three Decades of AIDS

On June 5, 1981 the Centers for Disease Control (CDC) published its *Weekly Morbidity and Mortality Report*, chronicling for the first time the symptoms among a few urban gay men of what was set to become the most deadly plague known to humanity. The HIV/AIDS pandemic has since then killed more than 30 million individuals worldwide. Around 34 million people are currently infected globally;

of these, 23.5 million live in Africa south of the Sahara, representing 69 per cent of the global HIV burden (UNAIDS 2012b). In terms of mortality this translates into more than 5,500 deaths among the citizens of the states in the Southern African Development Community (SADC) every single day of 2011.[1] Although the number of infections has started to decline, these numbers mean that SADC experiences the equivalent of a 9/11 attack every day of the year, all year round.

To make matters worse, epidemiologists say that the AIDS epidemic (since it results from HIV, a *lentivirus*, meaning that it acts slowly) is a "long-wave event". Among other implications, this means that it is an insidious phenomenon that might take up to 50 or even 120 years to play itself out (Barnett 2006, 304). Humanity has never experienced anything comparable in its history. The world does not know what the long-term impact of the pandemic will be.

How does one respond to such a threat in an effective and appropriately scaled way? One key response has been to polemicize the epidemic: a master narrative has been created to "securitize" AIDS. By making appeals to states' security, and by crafting AIDS as an "enemy" that needs to be "battled" and "defeated", a number of effects can be achieved. These include the inculcation of a sense of imminent danger or threat, the creation of an identifiable and common villain, the rapid mobilization of the required state or governmental resources required to respond to that threat, and mythmaking about who the saviours or victors might be. Since AIDS first made newspaper headlines in the early 1980s, this narrative or culture of securitization has come to be associated with the epidemic. In the context of the "war against terror" after September 11, 2001, many people are becoming increasingly familiar with the super-patriotic proclivities and nationalistic pathologies that securitization can enable. Thus a closer look at the powerful constructivist role of specific conceptualizations of the pandemic is in order, and timely. Laurie Garrett (2005, 64) observes that,

> in the aftermath of September 11, 2001, the United States tends to define all national security concerns through the prism of terrorism. That framework is overly limited even for the United States, and an absurdly narrow template to apply to the security of most other countries. The HIV/AIDS pandemic is aggravating a laundry list of underlying tensions in developing, declining, and failed states. As the burden of death due to HIV/AIDS skyrockets around the world over the next five to ten years, the disease may well play a more profound role on the security stage of many nations, and present the wealthy world with a challenge the likes of which it has never experienced. How countries, rich and poor, frame HIV/AIDS within their national security debates today may well determine how well they respond to the massive grief, demographic destruction, and security threats that the pandemic will present tomorrow.

1 See AIDSinfo database published by UNAIDS at http://www.unaids.org/en/datanalysis/datatools/aidsinfo.

Since 1998 there has been significant academic interest in the construction of metaphors and myths (including the securitization) of disease and even of the AIDS epidemic in recent years (Altman and Buse 2012; Elbe 2006, 2009; WHO 2007; Ingram 2007; Poku et al. 2007; High-Level Panel on Threats 2004; Altman 1999, 2003; Sontag 2002; Fourie and Schönteich 2001). This analysis is happening within the context of a mostly discreet yet exceedingly influential battle between individual state sovereignty and its concomitant epidemic response imperatives on the one hand, and, on the other, the multilateralization of the pandemic, via the World Bank's Multisectoral AIDS Program, the US President's Emergency Program for AIDS Relief (PEPFAR), the Global Fund to Fight AIDS, Tuberculosis, and Malaria, and UNAIDS.

The scene is set for great tension between autonomous, state-centred interventions on the one hand and multilateral initiatives on the other. Discursively, one of the ways in which this tension has been playing itself out has been through appeals to either a (hard) securitization agenda that appeals to the dangers that AIDS imply for state survival or an agenda that appeals more directly to a softer, human security approach, which underlines the nefarious implications of the epidemic for individual human rights to health. The latter approach has been most closely associated with a developmental agenda.

Changing Global Conceptions of Security

In terms of power politics – politically as well as economically – words and institutions matter. They have had significant impacts on the manner in which ideologies have shaped elites' mental maps, descriptions, and prescriptions about the allocation of scarce resources in society. The multilateralization of AIDS as a security issue has recently come into its own: "the intervention of the Security Council in 2000 was a critical move in securitizing HIV/AIDS, *constructing* the disease as something extraordinary which demanded international attention and action" [emphasis added] (McInnes 2006, 315).

In these terms, the current global order is the result of three major ideological developments that inform everything from international law to the manner in which multilateral institutions and states conceptualize and respond to new threats such as HIV/AIDS. The first major ideological development was the Treaty of Westphalia of 1648, which ended the 30-year religious war in Europe and established the modern state system. Modern notions of state sovereignty and the search for a global balance of power in the absence of a global government resulted from this development. It continues to permeate the way in which states relate to each other. Normatively, the realist ideology that emanated from the Treaty of Westphalia emphasizes the centrality of state autonomy and security – notions that have become embedded in international law and inform the ways in which governments in particular respond to external and other threats.

This realist notion of traditional security has since been questioned and in some ways challenged by liberal notions regarding global power. The French Revolution in 1789 shifted the state-centric view toward greater empathy for a humanistic and individually based level of analysis. The state was now seen as secondary or complementary to the interests of its citizens, whose rights it was obligated to protect. These notions have also become embedded in international law and other conventions – among them UN conventions on individual human rights (including rights to health and other forms of security).

This human-centred approach was supported by a greater developmental focus emphasized by Marxian thinkers, who base their ideological prescriptions on notions of security and what it is that humans need to be "safe from" in the original writings of Karl Marx and others in the mid to late nineteenth century. Rather than focusing on the individual unit of analysis, as the liberals would, proponents underline the importance of economic class and exploitation resulting from material inequalities and structural deficiencies at the national and global levels.

This ideological history is important, as it has had a direct impact on the evolution of multilateral custodians of peace and security after World War II, as well as the ideological underpinnings informing perspectives of health as a security issue in the twenty-first century. The champions at the end of the war wanted to create an organization that would assist in establishing a global order based on the notion of "collective security" (Nye 2000). States would become each others' keepers, not allowing any individual member of the UN to abuse economic or politically nationalistic notions to drag the world into a third world war.

This new system of collective security was entrenched institutionally through the creation of the UN. It was in turn couched in the context of an evolving global legal system based broadly on guarantees of state sovereignty, collective state security, and individual human rights. The ideal thus became a rather interesting hybrid of realist and liberal discourses applied within the multilateral organization, with members of especially the new Second and Third Worlds emphasizing (discursively at least) notions of greater global class equity and fairness. The post-World War II multilateral context thus created a political arena in which the three main ideologies (realism, liberalism, and Marxism) pertaining to evolving notions of security could be tested and played out.

After 1989 and the end of that ideological conflict, however, conceptions of security were reconsidered. No longer was the world subject to conventional notions of conflict; new or other threats would come to permeate the orthodox description of *realpolitik*. The global context had moved on from narrow notions regarding an ideological battle between the First and the Second Worlds played out through proxy wars in mainly the developing world. After 1989, nationalism was reasserting itself: from intra-state conflicts in the Balkans and in Africa to the appearance of a new kind of terrorism wrought of 2 to crises by mobilizing resources – "there is more than a suspicion that the securitizing move was part of an attempt to gain greater political attention for the HIV/AIDS crisis" (McInnes 2006, 326). Other analysts warned that securitization might actually have a counterproductive effect: by "othering" and "enemizing" selective aspects of the pandemic (such as homosexuality, commercial sex workers, intravenous drug users, insidious "big pharma", and so on), a dangerous space could be created for increased stigmatization of especially persons living with HIV (see Elbe 2006; Sontag 2002).

In the short term the securitization of AIDS achieved exactly what many said it needed to: after a visit by Richard Holbrooke, the US ambassador to the UN, to Africa in December 1999 to witness the impact of the growing AIDS epidemic, on January 10, 2000, the UN Security Council (UNSC) for the first time in its history debated what was ostensibly a health issue in terms of security (Behrman 2004, 158–65). This meeting was followed in July 2000 by UN Resolution 1308, which formalized the securitization of HIV/AIDS. It is important that these developments took place within the UNSC: in the days of the Cold War, this was the UN body where global powers could do their posturing; the UNSC is a state-centric vehicle *par excellence*. However, in terms of how Resolution 1308 formally securitized the pandemic, the language of human security was to a large extent evoked. One year after Resolution 1308, in mid 2001, the UN General Assembly held a special session on HIV/AIDS, which went even further to putting the pandemic on the multilateral agenda. During the special session, Colin Powell, US secretary of state and a former chair of the Joint Chiefs of Staff in the Department of Defence, declared that "there is no enemy in war more insidious than AIDS" (Behrman 2004, 266).

The Ideological Utility of Securitizing AIDS

AIDS only became a biomedical issue in the 1980s, and then only appeared on the public agenda in the 1990s. As a result, this context of normative contestation regarding the securitization of AIDS is a recent phenomenon. The consequence has been that various AIDS watchers have been making claims and counter-claims regarding the link between the pandemic and its impacts. This discourse is constantly revised – a process that takes place in an increasingly political global and particularly multilateral environment; this is understandable given the high stakes: billions of dollars have been made available to counter AIDS and other chronic diseases. This has given rise to a nascent AIDS industry (in both financial and ideological terms) as the battle for the control over who can and should shape global efforts to combat AIDS has taken hold (Garrett 2007). In the high political discursive environment regarding the purported link between AIDS and state security there have been significant developments.

As mentioned above, in 1990 the CIA added HIV to its "state failure watch list" as a variable that contributes to state collapse. In 2002 the US National Security Strategy identified failing states as the US's main threat, arguing that failed or failing states provide a fertile breeding ground for terrorism, and also leading to regional spillover effects (United States 2002). This approach dragged more than only the failing states into a condition of anarchy – this conclusion was reiterated by the 2006 US National Security Strategy document (Patrick and Brown 2006, 2; Carment 2003, 407). But in 2005 the US National Intelligence Council (2005, 2) stated that "it is not clear if AIDS can be directly tied to state collapse in the way that was feared and anticipated a few years ago".

Even in the US homeland security environment there thus appears to be no consensus regarding the link between AIDS and state fragility. This in itself is not problematic, given that Kuhnian scientific revolutions are based on the testing and revision of theses. However, it is problematic that the discourse is shaped by a surprising lack of attention to conceptual clarity and, importantly, empirical enquiry. The result has been that the debates about the purported link between AIDS and state fragility have been informed by (mostly unsubstantiated) normative and ideological agendas.

The central polemic can be summarized as follows. First, loose and unsubstantiated statements are made about the co-variance of mature AIDS epidemics on the one hand, and state fragility on the other. In other words, there is an assumption that state fragility itself creates an enabling environment for the vectoring of HIV. Rising prevalence levels in turn are seen to be contributing to state fragility and ultimate state collapse. This first polemic is for the most part untested.

Integrated with this first polemic is an implied polemic that provides the ideological environment for a broader problématique: state fragility in itself is seen as contributing to global insecurity (particularly as it is seen to act as a vector for terrorism) (Krasner and Pascual 2005). In turn it is argued that this global insecurity provides an enabling environment for further instances of state fragility and eventual collapse.

Given the obfuscation and contestation associated with these arguments and the general AIDS-state failure discourse thus far, it is worth exploring what states are, in fact, supposed to do, as well as what is meant by state fragility. Once this has been more firmly established one should be able to speak more confidently to the possible causal links between AIDS and state stability.

States and Fragility

Essentially the core functions of the state are, first, to provide physical security to everyone living in its area of jurisdiction; second, to build and maintain legitimate political institutions to implement government programs and sustain the whole; third, to provide sound and consistent economic management; and, fourth, to provide mechanisms of social welfare to those who need them (Patrick 2006; Eizenstat et al. 2005, 136).

Analysts of state fragility stress a number of qualifications to be borne in mind. For instance, it should not be assumed that the weakest states are necessarily the poorest; weak states tend to have bouts of political instability in common; state weakness spillovers are not linear, but vary by threat (Patrick 2006, 31–2). In other words, any analysis of state fragility as an independent variable is contingent; except for the manifestation of political instability, state fragility manifests itself in exceedingly granular ways. It is thus easier initially to describe fragile states in terms of what they are not. Stable or resilient states have effective institutions, the political will, and capacity to fulfil the core statal functions referred to above; they achieve and maintain a greater degree of social cohesion, social equality, and the ability to withstand exogenous and endogenous shocks. Fragile states, however, are broadly associated with social dissent, lack of border control, predation by the state on their own constituents, flawed institutions, deteriorating infrastructure, endemic corruption, a declining gross domestic product, food shortages, loss of legitimacy, a high rate of infant mortality, a closed economic system, and a general informalization of the economy toward localized subsistence rather than commercial surplus production (Patrick 2006, 45–9; Vallings and Moreno-Torres 2005, 4).

According to this logic, those who argue that AIDS is a security threat by weakening the state should be able demonstrate that the pandemic is directly eroding and reversing the very existence and effectiveness of the state functions described above. However, among those states about which there is general consensus regarding their fragility or their danger of failing, AIDS does not appear as a common feature.[2] In fact, AIDS is not an issue in most of these states at all. Recent studies have shown that there are no empirically demonstrable data that prove any significant co-variation between AIDS prevalence and military insecurity, social uprising, macroeconomic failure, electoral instability, or democratic consolidation (de Waal 2006; Fourie 2007; O'Keefe 2012). This is the case even in national contexts of high-prevalence, mature epidemics.

Given this reality, it is prudent to ask whether the link between AIDS and state fragility in general is not more a matter of ideology than description:

> At bottom, the entire literature on fragile or failed states assumes a particular normative model of the state—a liberal democratic state that is market-friendly, transparent, and accountable, with very specific institutional requirements—without analyzing that model at all. It is a given in identifying failure (Woodward 2004, 6).

---

2 Although there is no universally agreed definition of weak and failing states, there seems to be consensus that the following states are fragile or in danger of failing: Afghanistan, Angola, Bangladesh, Burkina Faso, Burundi, Cambodia, Cameroon, Central African Republic, Chad, Comoros, Congo Kinshasa, Congo Brazzaville, Côte d'Ivoire, Djibouti, Eritrea, Ethiopia, Guinea, Guinea-Bissau, Haiti, Iraq, Kenya, Lao PDR, Lesotho, Liberia, Madagascar, Malawi, Mali, Mauritania, Moldova, Mozambique, Myanmar, Nepal, Niger, Nigeria, North Korea, Pakistan, Papua New Guinea, Rwanda, Senegal, Sierra Leone, Solomon Islands, Somalia, Sudan, Tajikistan, Timor-Leste, Togo, Uganda, Uzbekistan, Yemen, Zambia, and Zimbabwe.

Significantly, the meta-theoretical or ideological prescriptions resulting from this normative model also form the basis of an evolving multilateral or "Geneva consensus" not only for good governance, but also for good AIDS governance. This has exceedingly political implications for the purported links between HIV and democracy, democratic remedies and vaccines against HIV, the inferred links between HIV and fragile states, and (as mentioned above) the evolution of the discourse of securitization regarding both state failure and HIV after 9/11.

Quo Vadis the New AIDS and Security Agenda?

This chapter as a whole teaches the research and policy community two critical lessons, complemented by a number of implications for a required future research agenda. The first lesson is that words matter. How HIV/AIDS – the "problem" – is defined, and by whom, makes a fundamental difference in terms of how responses to the pandemic are conceptualized and implemented (Ostergard and Barcelo 2005). This is the case on a national as well as on a global level. The AIDS policy environment in South Africa was in disarray for years because of contending and contested definitions of the problem (Fourie and Meyer 2010). As demonstrated above states as well as multilateral institutions are working toward coming to grips with the rapidly shifting ontological demands that the pandemic implies. On a continental level, Africa needs to find its own voice regarding perceptions and conceptualizations of the purported links between AIDS and security (de Waal 2003).

The second lesson is that reliable numbers matter. Inductive research can all too quickly lead intellectual elites into a trap of "wag-the-dog" result seeking. Malleable conceptual clarity requires action based on reliable empirical evidence – and the AIDS research community has seen precious little of that. The result has been that scholars have been at war with each other over semantics and dollars rather than with the virus itself. Researchers everywhere need greater accountability to the clients implied by contemporary conceptions of the marriage between heterodox conceptions of security. Such accountability should galvanize the move toward evidence-based policy making, rather than policy-based evidence making.

With these two insights at the macro level in mind, several specific research areas requiring urgent enquiry vis-à-vis the link between AIDS and security present themselves.[3]

This first is the search for better data. Given the dearth of AIDS-related data relating to issues of security, there is a need to establish an integrated surveillance system for recording rates of HIV and AIDS in uniformed services globally within obvious constraints of confidentiality and security. To complement such a system,

3 This list was compiled with reference to the insights gleaned from Tony Barnett and Gwyn Prins (2006), Solomon Benatar (2005), the Netherlands Ministry of Foreign Affairs (2005), and Laetitia van den Assum (2005).

it is necessary to establish a data base of the demographic structure of armies and other uniformed services, their experiences with antiretroviral medicines, terms of access for serving members and their households, and service policies in relation to HIV/AIDS issues in general, to include testing, treatment, and care while in and after leaving the service. Also, empirically based analysis is needed of the role of HIV/AIDS in relation to the issue of force/mission ratios that cannot be met.

The second area is the relationship between AIDS and evolving conceptions of security. Scholars need much more careful testing of the hypothesis that in situations of civil disorder the isolation of civil populations may reduce rates of transmission. AIDS analysts need to move beyond orthodox qualitative and empirical data-gathering methodologies and include the innovative use of scenarios and other futures methodologies to explore the possible impact and expand thinking about this and other long-wave events.

The third area is the relationship between AIDS and governance. Scholars need to recognize the new type of emergency that AIDS causes in high-prevalence countries, and develop policies and programs designed to counter this trend as well as to mitigate the impact on communities, service providers, and vital public sector functions. Comparative studies are needed of HIV/AIDS in irregular forces and in situations of civil peace, with particular emphasis on potential development of appropriate prevention measures and programs. This implies a more careful testing of the hypothesis that AIDS in high-prevalence countries threatens the stability of the state, thus increasing state fragility. It also requires a review of the hypothesis that rising populations of orphans and vulnerable children may lead to more instances of civil disobedience and crime.

Significantly, this would encourage independent research into the purported links between high levels of HIV and crime in general, as well as improved awareness related to AIDS in prison settings. It would strengthen and scale up programs. There is a need to develop strategies to prevent the undermining of the proper functioning of judicial and court systems, particularly in settings where the separation of powers and state building are not yet consolidated. This should be complemented by a process to develop an agenda for AIDS and governance, including AIDS governance within public sector institutions (especially as there has developed so little consensus on what "good" AIDS governance entails).

The fourth area is the relationship between AIDS and uniformed services. New research needs to explore the relationships between uniformed services and their host environments, whether at home or on overseas deployment. This should include the integration of prevention, diagnosis, treatment, and care services for households and families of military and other uniformed service personnel, paying particular attention to gender issues. There has been a particular research silence on the impact of AIDS in police services, so a comparative study of HIV/AIDS and police forces in a range of countries to assess the availability of services for these forces would be timely. To facilitate this, detailed ethnographic studies of uniformed service behaviours in peacekeeping operations are required.

This context is compounded by the rising threat of tuberculosis, especially multidrug-resistant tuberculosis in high-AIDS prevalence areas. This can only add to the weight of the problem, and the incremental effect of parallel epidemics should be explicated. At the behavioural level, research is needed regarding the relationship between sexual risk taking and training with the aim of exploring the hypothesis that risk taking in combat training results in sexual risk-taking behaviour among military personnel. Institutionally there also needs to be more examination of the question of how HIV/AIDS is being addressed in the context of security sector reforms, rule of law, and sexual violence in relation to concentrations of uniformed service populations.

Conclusion

In addressing these issues, analysts should be wary of notions invoking any so-called "tyranny of best practice". AIDS is not a monolithic epidemic; it has a variety of impacts in different localities. Thus "intervention can move away from a 'one size fits all' approach into much smarter and more targeted policies and programmes" (Netherlands Ministry of Foreign Affairs 2005). That said, the global AIDS pandemic offers an enormous opportunity for societal and intellectual learning – in that way it can go beyond an assemblage of tragic anecdotes and become a truly transformational social agent.

But in order to get there, one must heed this chapter's most basic lesson: the securitization of AIDS needs to be done in a conscious and nuanced manner. Securitization comes with significant normative and ideological baggage, and it has become fashionable to securitize everything from the "war on terror" to global water scarcity and famine. Securitization has significant implications as an enabling tool – it can determine who is demonized, who "the enemy" is, who is excluded or included in decision making, who the saviours are, what are the myths regarding guilt and exculpation, as well as serve a multitude of industries.

Yes, securitization can be remarkably effective for public health interventions in particular, for mobilizing money, creating institutions, galvanizing a sense of crisis, and implementing short-term, rapid responses. However, given the long-wave reality of the global AIDS "crisis" and the multilateral consensus regarding a global human rights-based response, such securitization and a focus on quick fixes may actually blind those in power to the more systemic and temporal realities of the pandemic. The proactive, long-term changes required in gender relations, sustainable behaviour change and memetic cultural adaptation may not be served by the knee-jerk reactivity of AIDS securitization.

References

Altman, Dennis (1999). "AIDS and Questions of Global Governance". *Pacifica Review* 11(2): 195–211.

Altman, Dennis (2003). "AIDS and Security". *International Relations* 17(4): 417–27.

Altman, Dennis and Kent Buse (2012). "Thinking Politically about HIV: Political Analysis and Action in Response to AIDS". *Contemporary Politics* 18(2): 127–40. doi: 10.1080/13569775.2012.674334.

Barnett, Tony (2006). "A Long-Wave Event. HIV/AIDS, Politics, Governance, and "Security": Sundering the Intergenerational Bond?" *International Affairs* 82(2): 297–313.

Barnett, Tony and Gwyn Prins (2006). "HIV/AIDS and Security: Fact, Fiction, and Evidence: A Report to UNAIDS". *International Affairs* 82(2): 359–68.

Behrman, Greg (2004). *The Invisible People: How the United States Has Slept through the Global AIDS Pandemic, the Greatest Humanitarian Catastrophe of Our Time*. New York: Free Press.

Benatar, Solomon (2005). "The HIV/AIDS Pandemic: A Sign of Instability in a Complex Global System". In *Ethics and AIDS in Africa: The Challenge to Our Thinking*, Anton A. van Niekerk and Loretta M. Kopelman, eds. Claremont, South Africa: David Philip Publishers, pp. 71–83.

Buzan, Barry and Ole Wæver (2003). *Regions and Powers: The Structure of International Security*. Cambridge: Cambridge University Press.

Carment, David (2003). "Assessing State Failure: Implications for Theory and Policy". *Third World Quarterly* 24(3): 407–27.

Cook, Alethia H. (2010). "Securitization of Disease in the United States: Globalization, Public Policy, and Pandemics". *Risks, Hazards and Crisis in Public Policy* 1(1): 10–30.

Davies, Sara (2013). "Securitizing Infectious Disease". *International Affairs* 84(2): 295–313.

de Waal, Alex (2003). "Human Rights Organizations and the Political Imagination: How the West and Africa Have Diverged". *Journal of Human Rights* 2(4): 475–94.

de Waal, Alex (2006). *AIDS and Power: Why There Is No Political Crisis – Yet*. New York: Zed Books.

Eizenstat, Stuart E., John Edward Porter, and Jeremy Weinstein (2005). "Rebuilding Weak States". *Foreign Affairs* 84(134): 134–46.

Elbe, Stefan (2006). "Should HIV/AIDS Be Securitized? The Ethical Dilemmas of Linking HIV/AIDS and Security". *International Studies Quarterly* 50(1): 119–44.

Elbe, Stefan (2009). *Virus Alert: Security, Governmentality, and the AIDS Pandemic*. New York: Columbia University Press.

Fidler, David P. (2007). "A Pathology of Public Health Securitism: Approaching Pandemics as Security Threats". In *Governing Global Health: Challenge,*

Response, Innovation, Andrew F. Cooper, John J. Kirton, and Ted Schrecker, eds. Aldershot: Ashgate, pp. 41–64.

Fidler, David P. and Laurence O. Gostin (2006). "The New International Health Regulations: An Historic Development for International Law and Public Health". *Journal of Law, Medicine, and Ethics* 34(1): 85–94.

Fourie, Pieter (2007). "The Relationship between the AIDS Pandemic and State Fragility". *Global Change, Peace, and Security* 19(3): 281–300.

Fourie, Pieter and Melissa Meyer (2010). *The Politics of Aids Denialism: South Africa's Failure to Respond.* Farnham: Ashgate.

Fourie, Pieter and Martin Schönteich (2001). "Africa's New Security Threat". *African Security Review* 10(4): 29–42.

Garrett, Laurie (2005). "Lessons of HIV/AIDS". *Foreign Affairs* 84(51): 51–64.

Garrett, Laurie (2007). "The Challenge of Global Health". *Foreign Affairs* 86(1): 14–38. http://www.foreignaffairs.com/articles/62268/laurie-garrett/the-challenge-of-global-health (July 2013).

High-Level Panel on Threats, Challenges, and Change (2004). "A More Secure World: Our Shared Responsibility". United Nations, New York. http://www.un.org/secureworld/ (July 2013).

Ingram, Alan (2007). "HIV/AIDS, Security and the Geopolitics of US–Nigerian Relations". *Review of International Political Economy* 14(3): 510–34.

Kelle, Alexander (2007). "Securitization of International Public Health: Implications for Global Health Governance and the Biological Weapons Prohibition Regime". *Global Governance* 13(2007): 217–35.

King, Nicholas (2002). "Security, Disease, Commerce: Ideologies of Postcolonial Global Health". *Social Studies of Science* 32(5–6): 763–89.

Krasner, Stephen and Carlos Pascual (2005). "Addressing State Failure". *Foreign Affairs* 84(4): 153–63.

McInnes, Colin (2006). "HIV/AIDS and Security". *International Affairs* 82(2): 315–26.

Netherlands Ministry of Foreign Affairs (2005). "AIDS, Security, and Conflict Initiative". Summary of briefing, Netherlands Mission, New York, June 3.

Nye, Joseph S. (2000). *Understanding International Conflicts*. 3rd ed. New York: Longman.

O'Keefe, Michael (2012). "Lessons from the Rise and Fall of the Military AIDS Hypothesis: Politics, Evidence, and Persuasion". *Contemporary Politics* 18(2): 239–53. doi: 10.1080/13569775.2012.674340.

Ostergard, Robert L. and Crystal Barcelo (2005). "Personalist Regimes and the Insecurity Dilemma: Prioritizing AIDS as a National Security Threat in Uganda". In *The African State and the AIDS Crisis*, Amy Stephenson Patterson, ed. Aldershot: Ashgate, pp. 155–79.

Patrick, Stewart (2006). "Weak States and Global Threats: Fact or Fiction?" *Washington Quarterly* 29(2): 27–33. http://www.cgdev.org/files/7034_file_06spring_patrickTWQ.pdf (July 2013).

Patrick, Stewart and Kaysie Brown (2006). “Fragile States and U.S. Foreign Assistance: Show Me the Money”. Working Paper 96, Centre for Global Development, Washington DC. http://www.cgdev.org/publication/fragile-states-and-us-foreign-assistance-show-me-money-working-paper-96 (July 2013).

Pirages, Dennis C. (2007). “Nature, Disease, and Globalization: An Evolutionary Perspective”. *International Studies Review* 9(4): 616–28.

Poku, Nana K., Neil Renwick, and Joao Gomes Porto (2007). “Human Security and Development in Africa”. *International Affairs* 83(6): 1155–70.

Shaw, Timothy M., Sandra J. MacLean, and David R. Black (2006). “Introduction: A Decade of Human Security: What Prospects for Global Governance and New Multilateralisms?”. In *Human Security: Global Governance and New Multilateralisms*, Sandra J. MacLean, David R. Black, and Timothy M. Shaw, eds. Aldershot: Ashgate, pp. 3–18.

Sontag, Susan (2002). *Illness as Metaphor and Aids and Its Metaphors*. London: Penguin Classics.

UNAIDS (2012). “Global Report: UNAIDS Report on the Global AIDS Epidemic 2012”. Geneva. http://www.unaids.org/en/media/unaids/contentassets/documents/epidemiology/2012/gr2012/20121120_UNAIDS_Global_Report_2012_en.pdf (June 2013).

United States (2002). “The National Security Strategy of the United States”. Washington DC, September 17. http://nssarchive.us/NSSR/2002.pdf (January 2014).

United States National Intelligence Council (2005). “Mapping Sub-Saharan Africa’s Future”. Discussion paper CR2005-02. http://www.au.af.mil/au/awc/awcgate/nic/africa_future.pdf (July 2013).

Vallings, Claire and Magui Moreno-Torres (2005). “Drivers of Fragility: What Makes States Fragile?”. PRDE Working Paper 7, Department for International Development, London. http://purl.umn.edu/12824 (July 2013).

van den Assum, Laetitia (2005). “Towards a UNAIDS Framework Agenda for AIDS and Security”. Unpublished report produced for UNAIDS.

Woodward, Susan L. (2004). “Fragile States: Exploring the Concept”. Paper presented to the “States and Security” Learning Group at the Peace and Social Justice meeting of the Ford Foundation, November 29, Rio de Janeiro. http://statesandsecurity.org/_pdfs/Fragile%20States_Exploring%20the%20Concept.pdf (July 2013).

World Health Organization (2007). “The World Health Report 2007 – A Safer Future: Global Public Health Security in the 21st Century”. Geneva. http://www.who.int/whr/2007/en (October 2012).

Zacher, Mark (2007). “The Transformation in Global Health Collaboration since the 1990s”. In *Governing Global Health: Challenge, Response, Innovation*, Andrew F. Cooper, John J. Kirton, and Ted Schrecker, eds. Aldershot: Ashgate, pp. 15–27.

Chapter 5

Assessing African Health Governance amid Global Biopolitics

Siphamandla Zondi

While global health standards have gradually been improving over the last five decades, the health situation in the world remains precarious, with occasional outbreaks of violent epidemics such as avian and swine influenza as well as the increasing incidence of lifestyle illnesses such as diabetes and hypertension. Several infectious diseases that were overcome and put under control in the 1980s are re-emerging, causing much morbidity and mortality, and threatening to erode the health gains of the past few decades. HIV and AIDS emerged in the mid 1980s and a few years later became a pandemic with a global reach. Although the outbreak of an unusual infection called avian influenza (H1N5) killed a small number of people between 2003 and 2009, it caused alarm all over the world (World Health Organization [WHO] 2013a). The outbreak of the swine influenza (H1N1) in Mexico in April 2009 forced the world to be on high alert because of the deadly nature of the virus, which by the end of May had killed about 115 people, mostly in the Americas (WHO 2009b). These examples reveal the soft underbelly of global health regimes underpinned by the effects of globalization, in spreading pathogens between countries and continents, in perpetuating conditions of underdevelopment and marginalization on the periphery such as in Africa.

With globalization, many improvements have been registered in the area of health. There is better and more accurate health information available. There is a general global consensus about shared health problems and the need for collective action. There is much more funding for health programs than was the case in the 1990s. There is a larger pool of basic and skilled health professionals. Medical research has also improved with the help of generous support from the pharmaceutical industry and governments. The arsenal of health technology and pharmacopoeia at the disposal of health workers today is remarkably large. Nonetheless, the countries on the periphery have experienced the globalization of marginality, underdevelopment, inequality, and poverty. The attendant weakening of the state and its sovereignty, including in the area of health policy, while opening up space for a variety of actors including nongovernmental organizations (NGOs) to boost health responses, has resulted in weak health governance at national and regional levels.

This chapter argues that the solution of complex health situations at both global and African levels requires Africa to overcome its internal governance deficit; moreover, the continent will benefit from a significant transformation of global governance, in general, and health governance, in particular, which is the structural condition that help to perpetuate and complicate health problems. Health governance in this context means mechanisms, processes, leadership, and institutions through which people's health needs and rights are met. These conditions or capacities include health systems or capacities such health leadership, disease control and information management systems, acquisition of essential technologies, inter-sectoral coordination including private and public sectors, synergy between primary and secondary health care, infrastructure development, alignment between health and economic policies, and health insurance and social security. This chapter argues that the relationship between Africa's health sovereignty and globalization is a complex one with both benefits and disadvantages. Therefore, the challenge for Africa is to harness the advantages such as technology, flow of information, advances in science, access to capital, and the role of the private sector while addressing the historical distortions that globalization reinforces.

The Problem Is Not Funding

For a long time many thought healthcare failures were due to inadequate funds. However, there is now no serious shortage of funds for public health in general, even as there may be insufficient resources for dealing with sudden and seasonal crises such as Ebola and *E. coli* epidemics in Central Africa in 2009 and 2011. Health spending as a component of total government expenditure has increased dramatically across the world. Massive funds have been injected into the health system (private and public) in the last decade to respond to the global health burden. Billions of US dollars now go into programs designed to combat HIV and AIDS, malaria, and tuberculosis in the developed world by governments as well as private philanthropists such as Bill and Melinda Gates and George Soros. This surge in health funding is a direct consequence of the AIDS epidemic, which exposed the health inequities between the developed and developing world. But it is also because the world has realized the economic and human costs of the persistence of illness.

The recent resurgence of infectious epidemics shocked the world in the same way that world citizens have been shaken into action by images of starving mothers and infants during famines in Africa. Western governments reacted with outrage and dramatically improved health funding across the board. The Clinton administration in the US increased its funding for health-related programs in African countries ten-fold from around $87 million in 1996 to $865 million in 1999 (Garrett 2007, 17). The Bush administration in turn doubled its health aid with a large share going into HIV and AIDS programs. In May 2009, the

Obama administration announced the new Global Health Initiative, making $63 billion available for a comprehensive health program. Recent assessments of this initiative suggest that while the intentions to expand foreign health assistance balancing preventive and curative health care are noble, these remain unfulfilled, and the funds pledged were recycled from the Bush initiative. The Bill and Melinda Gates Foundation alone gave some $6.6 billion between 2003 and 2006 for global health programs. Between 2007 and 2010, the figure was $6.9 billion, with almost a billion added. There was a decline of more than half a billion (below average) in annual global health expenditure in 2010, slightly compensated by a rise of $200 million in annual spending in 2011. The bulk of these funds went into fighting tuberculosis, HIV, AIDS and other sexually transmitted diseases.[1] Health spending by member countries of the Organisation for Economic Co-operation and Development (OECD) also increased in the same period.

This is part of long-term trend that saw health expenditure rise from an average increase of 6.6 per cent in 1980 to 9 per cent by 2008. Health expenditure actually increased by an average of 7 per cent between 2000 and 2003 before declining to 3 per cent in 2005–08. However, the World Health Report for 2010 published by the World Health Organization (WHO) suggests that this average increase, which continued to 2010, fell below the increase in destitution, with 150 million people unable to pay out-of-pocket health expenses and falling government revenues resulting in declining health spend as a percentage of total public expenditure (WHO 2010). Drug spending by both private and public sectors also registered substantial growth in the same period. Although there is not enough funding to meet the rising need, especially as the social costs of the 2008 global economic crisis become apparent, the global health regime has sufficient funding to drive a much-improved provision of health care, especially for countries that cannot raise their own funds.

In 2002, a new and autonomous global funding mechanism, the Global Fund to Fight AIDS, Tuberculosis, and Malaria, was created. It received donations from governments, donor agencies, and private philanthropists to spend on health programs, especially those designed to fight HIV and AIDS, tuberculosis, malaria, and other infectious diseases.

According the Global Fund's grant portfolio, more than $26.7 billion had been approved to 151 countries through 1,000 programs by 2013, the bulk of which went to Africa.[2] This is a dramatic rise from $15.6 billion in 140 countries in 2008. By 2013, the fund was responsible for providing antiretroviral drugs to more than 4.2 million HIV-infected people and medical care for 6.3 million AIDS orphans. It had also provided almost 90 per cent of all international financing for tuberculosis, supporting programs that had detected and treated 9.7 million

1 Figures tallied from the annual reports of the Gates Foundation for 2003–11 at http://www.gatesfoundation.org/Who-We-Are/Resources-and-Media/Annual-Reports.

2 See the Grant Portfolio of the Global Fund to Fight AIDS, Tuberculosis, and Malaria at http://portfolio.theglobalfund.org/en/Home/Index.

cases of tuberculosis between 2002 and 2012. By 2012, the Global Fund had provided 310 million insecticide-treated bed nets and financing for treating 260 million cases (Global Fund 2013). It had contributed 21 per cent of global funding for HIV and AIDS programs, 82 per cent of funds to combat tuberculosis, and 50 per cent of funds to combat malaria (Global Fund 2012).

The Global Fund's research suggests that this investment has produced some positive results. Malaria infection and deaths in Ethiopia, Niger and Zambia have declined remarkably. HIV and AIDS awareness is reported to have increased, with the effect that infection rates are beginning to decline in Botswana, Democratic Republic of Congo, and Zimbabwe. Access to Directly Observed Treatment – Short Course (DOTS) in Ethiopia and Lesotho has expanded remarkably, thus reinforcing the prevention of unnecessary deaths.[3] But the Global Fund itself notes that outcomes do not neatly match the size of the investment made (Global Fund 2004). The reason is that money is being poured into countries with weak health governance. Improved governance should contribute to enhancing health outcomes.

Until the global economic crisis, the increase in health expenditure by countries in general and international finance institutions had been increasingly yearly.[4] This plus the write-offs of debts of poor countries, most of them in Africa, because they were hard hit by a deadly combination of infectious diseases and poverty made available a few more resources for the fight against health problems such as HIV and AIDS. The World Bank started to focus its funding on promotion of healthy behaviour in order to minimize what it saw as the long-term costs of the persistence of risky behaviour, especially among young people. The *World Development Report 2007* noted that there was a major problem that undermined improved funding, as health systems were ill prepared and incapable of responding to an increased burden (World Bank 2007, 122–5). Funders had created programs that in turn led to greater numbers of people visiting health centres. But they found that the facilities were ill suited to cope. As a result, many sick people were turned away from hospitals because they were already filled to capacity with HIV-infected people.

In the same period, world health activists shocked by health inequities mobilized to pressure pharmaceutical companies to reduce the costs of life-saving drugs used to treat HIV and AIDS, malaria, tuberculosis, and cholera. Then came the 13th International AIDS Conference in Durban, South Africa, in 2000. It also galvanized the public and private sector into releasing even more funds into the health system. And then, four years later, the main resolution of the 2004 International AIDS Conference in Bangkok, Thailand, came down to two issues: more courageous political leadership and increased funding for AIDS programs (*Vax* 2004). Nelson

3 Information drawn from "Country Successes" pamphlets produced by the Global Fund to Fight AIDS, Tuberculosis, and Malaria in 2010.

4 See the World Health Statistics produced by WHO at http://www.who.int/gho/publications/world_health_statistics/en/index.html.

Mandela used this platform to mobilize even greater involvement of the private sector in health funding, especially in response to AIDS, malaria, and tuberculosis. In fact, there has been so much focus on raising funds for global health responses at these conferences that many lament the neglect of other equally important issues of content and strategies (see Nduru 2004).

So much money streamed in after the 2004 conference that the concern was no longer money, but how it was to be spent. Peter Piot, executive director of UNAIDS, said so many billions of US dollars became available for health programs to fight AIDS, malaria, and tuberculosis that the world needed to shift its focus to "how to make the money work to save lives" (Sternberg 2004). Others were worried that science and policy took a back seat as the conference focused on raising funds.

The emergence of the avian influenza, which threatened to become a global epidemic in 2006, stimulated even more health spending. The pledges increased, with the health ministers of the G8 countries meeting in April 2006 with stakeholders such as the WHO, UNAIDS, and the World Bank as well as ministers from China, Brazil, India, Mexico, and South Africa. They made concrete commitments on epidemiological surveillance, disease control, and health awareness generally (*Medical News Today* 2006). The major industrialized countries had come to a realization that with the shift in global power balance, serious decisions to respond to embedded global health inequities would need the participation of major powers from the south. When the G8 leaders met in St. Petersburg at their summit in July, they issued a declaration on infectious diseases supported by financial pledges (G8 2006).

The poor countries are not passive recipients of global generosity, but have themselves increased health funding across the board. This is partly because of the end of structural adjustment programs that discouraged social spending and partly due to a change in attitude to social services. In the 1990s, African countries spent on average less than 3 per cent of their budgets on health. A World Bank study of public expenditure on health care found that by 1996 a typical African country had a low per capita gross domestic product (less than $400) and spent on average a mere $6 per capita on public health (World Bank 2000). As a result, on average countries recorded low immunization coverage, mediocre access to contraception, and fewer than 45 per cent of deliveries supervised by trained health professionals. Countries typically reported very high levels of child and adult mortality from infectious diseases, high rates of general morbidity, and a decline in life expectancy. The study noted the effect of a relatively weak bureaucracy and high levels of corruption. It did not make much of the latter observations except to note them, suggesting a failure to recognize the effect of weak health governance on health outcomes. While many of the issues raised by this study became a major focus of rising World Bank investments, the trend of African governments spending little on health care continued (Garrett 2007).

Thus the problem can no longer be ascribed simply to a lack of funding or poor resourcing of the fight against disease, but to the ability to make effective and efficient use of the funds that become available. Donors lament the inability of governments in poor countries to spend the funds allocated efficiently. They observe that much funding to combat infectious diseases is drained by high personnel costs and general wastage. There is even suspicion that corruption is rife in donor-funded national health programs. Often neglected is the impact of a culture of donor dependence, including the tendency for donors to use their own consultants, implementation agencies, and weak domestic ownership of donor-funded programs. This has led to a view of donor support as a form of development based in binary terms of developed and underdeveloped places and people whereby the latter "catch up" with the former (Escobar 1995).

Africa is the epicentre of the global health challenge epitomized by a complicated disease environment that requires sophisticated response regimes. Global health failures such as weak health systems, inadequate health delivery mechanisms, weak disease surveillance, and poor coordination arise in their worst form in Africa.[5] Generally, the developing world bears the brunt of these failures with a higher incidence of both re-emerging and stubborn old infections. Africa is particularly vulnerable to the new global infections, although global control mechanisms have succeeded in preventing the spread of these new infections to Africa. Were the bird and swine influenzas to spread into Africa, the effect in numbers of deaths and the scale of trauma would be much greater than in the West, Asia, and Latin America. The global disease incidence and the particularly precarious situation in Africa continue, notwithstanding improved ammunition against disease from the laboratory and the ability of health authorities to communicate quickly and relatively easily the world over. There has also been an improvement in the application of social policy, resulting in better socioeconomic conditions in most parts of the world.

Health Governance and Underdevelopment in a Time of Globalization

Understanding Africa's health challenge requires grasping how disease incidence nests in the failure of development and the ubiquity of poverty. Increasingly Africa's health problem is a major element of the growing global health challenge. International health becomes global health when the causes and consequences of ill health are oblivious of the territorial boundaries of states. At this point, health issues are beyond the capacity of individual states to manage and control. States cannot deal effectively with the determinants of ill health. This globalization of health challenges is facilitated largely by the integration of states into the global system through easier and faster international travel and communication. It has led to frequent contact between populations through frequent migration and technological connectivity. While increased international migration presents a logistical nightmare for public health systems the world over, the global

5 These are major indicators of failure in the global health system according to the *World Health Report 2008* (WHO 2008a).

movement of vulnerable groups such as the sickly, refugees, and trafficked individuals present even more complicated problems for public health officials (Lee et al. 2002). Globalization has become a consistent factor in both the cause (health determinants) and effect (health status) of the health burden globally and in Africa. It is thus essential to scrutinize globalization in the social, political, economic, technological, and ecological spheres of human endeavour as part of the broader understanding of the causes and effects of health conditions in every part of the world.

The dichotomy between developed and developing countries or between poor and wealthier areas within countries has become blurred by increased interaction between them in response to transnational challenges, a number of which are in the area of health. Global power distribution has become a useful prism through which to explain the unequal distribution of the health burden in the world and Africa's particularly bad health situation. The patterns of political economy that predispose some areas more than others to higher incidence of infectious diseases have much to do with the impact of the economic dimension of globalization. This means that health responses should be sufficiently comprehensive to respond to ill health, the conditions that reproduce it, and the factors that help weaken the capacity of the African state to appropriately deal with health problems. In this sense, both the internal and external factors that undermine health governance become crucial (Cornia and Mwabu 1997; Woodward et al. 2001; Garrett 2007).

Due to the impact of globalization, the traditional ways of explaining health problems at national, regional, and global levels have become somewhat obsolete. Common policies, programs, and institutions designed to combat illness the traditional way have become inadequate. One factor often missed is that the darker side of globalization has undermined state capacity to address health problems effectively and meet basic health needs. Health challenges have become so complicated that old governance tools have become somewhat obsolete. This implies that globalization and attendant health challenges are undermining existing governance mechanisms.

While globalization has also had positive impacts, such as demands for innovation in state policy and institutional responses to health challenges, and the embrace of technologies in all levels of health care from primary to tertiary, it weakens the very capacity of states and institutions to respond and promote healthy living. The globalization of cultures, ideas, and thoughts (cognitive globalization) has resulted in lifestyle choices that complicate the cause and effect of ill health. Diet and lifestyle have become major determinants of health globally and increasingly on the African continent (Lee 2001). The incidence of cardiovascular disease remains a big problem in high-income countries notwithstanding behavioural changes. It is a rising health problem in Africa, further complicating the continent's poor health status due to the ubiquity of communicable diseases.

Cognitive globalization brings new attitudes and ideas about the management of health that change the very manner of making and implementing health policies and programs. Health policy choices are increasingly conditioned by the imperatives of global transformation, including the demands and whims of capital and faceless market forces. This dimension of globalization is bequeathing a value system that leads to choices made in the health sector that undermine the fight against disease. The notions of managerial efficiency, value for money, and technological panaceas undermine the critical importance of primary health care and promote highly expensive, hospital-based health care. The innovations taking place in global health responses include new invasive treatment technologies and a plethora of new drugs that are themselves of limited effect because they take place within an environment of highly inequitable distribution of values and norms. Donor programs generally exclude African medical ideas, tools, and technologies because western medical thought, which has over centuries been inculcated in others too as part of what Edward Saïd calls Orientalism, sees western medicine as superior and most effective. African medicine and therapies are viewed as inferior where western medicine is caught up in what Slavoj Žižek (1999) describes as a western identity that in the eighteenth century moved from self-mastery – "I think therefore I am" – to validating itself by seeking domination over others – "I conquer therefore I am".[6] A browse through funded programs, which are well recorded in donor annual reports and government documents, reveals this mission to spread only one source of medical ideas and innovations (western biomedicine) such that it is hard to know if alternatives including western social medicine, eastern therapies, and indigenous African medical therapies continue to flourish in public health. As a result, major advances in western medical therapies including the construction of forensic laboratories, the training of health specialists to provide tertiary health care, access to new drugs, new disease control measures in major African hospitals, and the growth of equipped mobile clinics, are transforming the African health landscape.[7] Often, on close analysis, Africans have appropriated these new medicines into a range of therapies to choose from at any given time.[8]

The western values that dominate the broader global system take precedent over any other in the area of health care as well. For instance, western modernity emphasizes pathogens over environmental factors and individuals over communities, whereas African medical thought patterns are influenced by values of group identity and, therefore, promote the treatment of groups rather than the individual and espouse eclectic therapies rather than the displacement of older ways by "modern" ones.[9] These forces have relative control over the world order being fashioned and can veto any ideas or values that may clash with their own dogma.

6 See Žižek's (1999) discussion of the making of a western self-identity that would evolve into a tendency to "thingify" others.

7 Information on the kinds of improvements is drawn from personal communication with Lydia Mugabe, director of the WHO's regional office in Pretoria, September 19, 2012.

8 This has been the case since Africans' contact with western medicine. See Siphamandla Zondi (2012).

9 For lucid analyses of medicine as a tool of western modernity and superiority during and after imperialism, see Roy MacLeod and Milton Lewis (1988). On western medicine as

In this climate, there is very little room for innovation, variation, and adaptation of responses to local conditions and knowledge. There is no room for alternative ideas and responses outside the control of the forces that propel globalization.

This affects both the cause and effect of globalized health. Africa is worst positioned in this power structure due to historical reasons pertaining to the manner in which the continent was integrated into the global order under colonial rule. The idea of health as a human right espoused at Alma Ata in 1978 is fast giving way to health as a tradable commodity whose enjoyment by individuals is being regulated in the marketplace. This is increasingly affecting the very definition of the health burden (as measurable and quantifiable in a cost-effectiveness analysis) and values that in turn are used to determine the allocation of resources.

As Wolfgang Reinicke (1998, 1–2) said, "without a greater effort to understand the origin and nature of the current global transformation and its implications for public policy, we will continue to respond to events rather than act to shape the future course of world politics. Such passivity will leave our societies vulnerable to the risks that change will undoubtedly bring, while forgoing the gains that more active policymaking could realize" (quoted in Lee 2001, 13). This means progressive change will come from conscious public policy interventions designed both to cushion societies from the adverse effects of globalization and to expand opportunities for susceptible people to acquire new means of survival and progress. In this sense, therefore, public policy is crucial for the defence of the vulnerable in society against the impact of a changing global political economy. Public policy includes policy instruments and structures designed to create chances for a better life for all.

When limited to national public policies, however, such a response would not be sufficient to transform Africa's health status and bring about true health sovereignty, for, as Ramon Grosfoguel (2009) shows, "development projects that focus on policy changes at the level of the nation-state are obsolete in today's world-economy and they lead to development illusions. A system of domination and exploitation that operates on a world-scale, such as the capitalist world-system, cannot have a national solution, and inversely, a global problem cannot be solved at the nation-state level – it requires global decolonial solutions".

Africa's Share of the Global Health Burden

Africa's health conundrum largely epitomizes the worst of the global health problem in all its forms. The health challenges currently facing the world and Africa can be categorized as problems of disease incidence (demand-side issues) and challenges facing the health systems themselves (supply-side questions). These fundamental but distinct challenges are mutually reinforcing, making

a colonial tool, see Megan Vaughan (1991). On African medical thought patterns, see John M. Janzen (1978).

effective responses to the health problems extremely complex. They are mutually reinforcing because an astronomical increase in the incidence of ill health in the context where health systems are not adequately developed complicates and deepens ill health. This in turn tends to weaken the capacity of health systems to prevent and treat illnesses. Demand-side issues will be difficult to overcome without sorting out the supply-side problems, the problems of capacity, and the effectiveness of the health governance system.

Death due to illness is frequent the world over. Many more people die of sickness, mostly preventable and curable diseases, than violence and accidents. As Table 5.1 indicates, WHO's (2013b) global disease burden statistics indicate that sickness caused 49.6 million deaths of a total of 54.6 million in 2011. Mortality from all causes in people under the age of 50 shows that children under the age of five lead with 6.9 million deaths, followed by the 30–49 age group at 6.1 million, the 15–29 age group at 3 million deaths, and the 5–14 age group at 1.4 million deaths. The 49.6 million deaths from disease suggests that diseases accounted for 91 per cent of all mortality globally. The largest number of disease-caused deaths was 22.9 million among people over the age of 70, followed by 17.4 million deaths among people aged 15–29, 12.4 million among those aged 50–69, 10.9 million among those aged 5–14, and 6.6 million among those under the age of five. The least affected group was age 30–49 where only 4.9 million deaths were recorded.

Table 5.1 Deaths by Age and Cause for 2011

	0–59 months	5–14 years	15–29 years	30–49 years	50–69 years	70+ years	Total
All causes	6,941,242	1,396,854	2,961,733	6,123,412	13,414,301	23,753,872	54,591,414
Communicable diseases	5,764,612	782,288	936,716	1,883,899	1,590,567	2,425,697	13,383,778
Non-communicable diseases	852,562	308,493	806,004	2,976,835	10,845,596	20,447,405	36,236,895
Injuries	324,068	306,073	1,219,013	1,262,678	978,138	880,769	4,970,740

Source: Adapted from World Health Organization (2013b).

Death is thus experienced differently from age group to age group. The fact that the 70+ age group died from illness in the largest numbers is perhaps not unusual given the susceptibility of this age group to the degeneration of body resistance that come with age. But that so many millions of infants and children died from disease prematurely is unusual and unnecessary. This can only be ascribed to failures in global health systems. Children under five die mainly from infectious diseases. Some 1.9 million children died from communicable conditions such as respiratory and diarrheal infections in 2011 (WHO 2013b). Most of these deaths happen in Africa. Malaria deaths occur mostly in Africa. HIV and AIDS and measles are also important causes of death among children and in the 30–44 age group.

The global disease incidence statistics also show that a very large proportion of death caused by disease arises from the incidence of communicable or infectious diseases that should have long been eliminated by vaccines and effective curatives that have existed for decades now. In 2010–11, 33 per cent of disease-caused deaths were due to communicable diseases. That is, 17.9 million deaths were as a result of infectious illnesses such as tuberculosis, cholera, and malaria. While the leading causes of deaths in the world in general tended to be noncommunicable illnesses such as cancer and cardiovascular conditions, in Africa many more people continue to die from communicable diseases than sicknesses of lifestyle.[10]

HIV/AIDS

Like smallpox in the seventeenth century and tuberculosis in the nineteenth century, the incidence and spread of HIV and AIDS illustrate well how globalization has not only introduced a lethal virus to "virgin" populations least prepared to cope with such a virus, but has also led to millions of deaths. HIV/AIDS is the sixth leading cause of death in the world (WHO 2013c). Although the estimated number of deaths from HIV globally fell from 2.3 million in 2006 to 1.7 million in 2011 and the number of new infections decreased from 2.8 million to 2.5 million in the same period, the number of people living with HIV continues to grow (UNAIDS 2012a). These are people on whom families rely for income and factories and farms depend for labour. They are the main consumers of products and services that world economies produce. Some 16.7 million women and 3.3 million children were living with the virus in 2011 (UNAIDS 2012c). An estimated 330,000 children were infected by HIV in 2011 alone.

In 2011, Africa alone accounted for more than 23.5 million people living with HIV in the world (UNAIDS 2012a). The exact figure is not certain because UNAIDS and other international organizations subscribe to the ideology that distinguishes between North Africa and Africa south of the Sahara. An excessively large number of new infections (more than 1.8 million of 2.5 million) happened in Africa. African children have the overwhelming share of children living with

10 See, for example, Angola Press Agency (2012).

AIDS at more than 3.1 million of 3.3 million globally. Of the 1.7 million people who died from AIDS-related causes in the world in 2011, about 1.2 million died in Africa. More than 90 per cent of children who acquired HIV in 2011 live in Africa (UNAIDS 2012b). The northern part of Africa has lower averages compared to other parts of the continent.

HIV and AIDS prevalence increased constantly throughout the world from 2001 to 2011 (UNAIDS 2012a). Africa remains the most affected region, representing 69 per cent of the global burden (UNAIDS 2012b). The rate at which HIV and AIDS incidence happened in Africa was faster than in the rest of the world. As a result, the number of people infected has been consistently higher in Africa than in the rest of the world. In 1990 around 5 million of 8 million people living with HIV in the world were in Africa (UNAIDS 2008). Africa carried this disproportionate share of the global HIV burden.

However, a number of AIDS epidemics hit various parts of Africa at different times, with varying impacts.[11] National adult HIV prevalence rate in countries in Central, North, and West Africa have remained below 2 per cent for the past decade and a half.[12] By 2007, the rate exceeded 5 per cent in Cameroon, the Central African Republic, Gabon, Malawi, Mozambique, Uganda, and Tanzania, causing alarm among health observers.

Although it is the most recent of the regional epidemics, Southern Africa's AIDS epidemic grew stronger and faster than in other regions of the continent. This is partly due to relatively developed transport and communications infrastructure, high levels of regional migration, and high inequalities (Iliffe 2006, ch. 5). In this region, HIV prevalence peaked at close to 20 per cent in 2006–07 and marginally declined from 2008. Seven countries in particular have been affected worst by the epidemic: Botswana, Lesotho, Namibia, Swaziland, South Africa, Zambia, and Zimbabwe.[13] All indications are that all AIDS epidemics in Africa have now begun to stabilize. But this means that southern Africa's epidemic is stabilizing at very high levels. While new evidence suggests that the rate of new infections is falling, the number of previously infected people and AIDS sufferers in this region is so high that the AIDS burden will remain high for some time. In South Africa alone, some 5.6 million people live with HIV, suggesting that this country will be dealing with the grave impact of AIDS for, at least, another decade or so (UNAIDS 2013). Worse, small and vulnerable countries such as Lesotho and Mozambique have reported an increase in the number of pregnant women infected with HIV (UNAIDS 2008, 32–42). Southern Africa will remain the epicentre of

11 For a succinct analysis of the evolution and the regional spread of the African AIDS epidemic, see John Iliffe (2006).

12 See briefs on West and Central Africa published by UNAIDS at http://www.unaids.org/en/regionscountries/regions/westandcentralafrica.

13 See the 2005–12 editions of the "HIV and AIDS Epidemiological Surveillance Reports for the WHO African Region" published by WHO.

the global AIDS epidemic long after the HIV prevalence rates have either reached a plateau or declined.

In East Africa, where the AIDS epidemic peaked in the 1980s and infection rates started to decline by the mid 1990s, the risky sexual behaviour that predisposed this region to high HIV infection rates in the first place are re-emerging, raising fears of a resurgence of HIV in countries such as Uganda. In this country, prevalence rates declined dramatically during the 1990s from around 15 per cent to 5.4 per cent. UNAIDS and WHO are keeping a close watch on the impact that the rise of risky behaviour will have on infection and prevalence rates in the region. They are keen to avoid the reversal of some of the greatest strides made by the global action against AIDS in East Africa. AIDS experts are also trying to draw lessons about sustained HIV control in an environment where conditions that predispose people to risky behaviour are ubiquitous (UNAIDS 2008, 42). Such lessons would apply almost immediately in Southern Africa, where similar conditions exist.

Women bear the brunt of the lethal African AIDS epidemic. While this gender profile of AIDS epidemics is a world-wide phenomenon, it is particularly acute in Africa. The gap between men and women is highest in South Africa where HIV prevalence among women in 2011 was 11.9 per cent in contrast to 5.3 per cent among men (UNAIDS 2013). This means that for every South African man infected by HIV, there are at least two women. Similar gender patterns are found in Tanzania, Uganda, Mozambique, Zimbabwe, and Zambia: six of the 10 countries with the highest prevalence of HIV among women are in Southern Africa. This gender profile suggests that the patriarchal social ideology that conspires to give men disproportionate power over women is a major factor influencing HIV prevalence in parts of Africa, especially Southern Africa.

An Enduring Malaria Epidemic

Malaria in Africa today is a classic example of how with globalization an endemic disease becomes a virulent epidemic and how with globalization stronger and stronger medical therapies have become available. Africa has the highest concentration of malaria-endemic countries in the world: 43 of 106 countries classified as malaria-endemic are in Africa (WHO 2012). Table 5.2 indicates that African countries accounted for an average of 79.5 per cent of all malaria cases in 2010. Malaria killed some 596,000 people in Africa alone in 2010, which amounted to 90 per cent of all malaria deaths in the world that year (WHO 2012). Of those deaths, 86 per cent were among children under the age of five years. The largest cumulative number of deaths was recorded in Nigeria, followed by Democratic Republic of the Congo, Burkina Faso, and Mozambique. In 2008, only ten African countries recorded numbers of deaths that are lower than a thousand (WHO 2008b). Most of these are small and island states with small populations.

Table 5.2 Malaria Cases, 2006, 2010

	2006	2010
Africa	85.83	79.45
Americas	1.09	0.50
Eastern Mediterranean	3.28	4.75
Europe	0.0016	0.0001
South East Asia	8.50	14.61
Western Pacific	0.89	0.78

Source: Based on World Health Organization (2008b, 2012).

While effective prevention and treatment methods exist, they are not adequately accessible in areas that are in greatest need. Moreover, it is not known whether these methods are used as they should be. This challenge is most acute in the African countries where the bulk of malaria incidence and deaths happens. In a number of countries the problem is a shortage of funds needed to acquire and supply treated bed nets, chemicals for vector control, antimalarial drugs, and diagnostic equipment. In some cases, the problem is supply-side constraints relating to weak distribution systems, inefficient public health systems, poor coordination within governments, and weak transport/communication systems.

Worse, vectors and pathogens are increasingly resistant to insecticides and antimalarial drugs. This undermines malaria control programs that WHO has helped develop in all malaria-endemic countries. If resistance spreads, the global Roll-Back Malaria campaign will come to nothing. Prevention has reduced the risk for millions of Africans, while treatment is one of the generally effective tools against deaths from malaria.

The impact of malaria incidence on the economy is generally underestimated, even though the economies of Southern Europe grew rapidly after the eradication of malaria in the 1980s. When malaria incidence decreased from the 1960s, economies grew in tandem (MicrobiologyBytes 2009). The total cost of preventing and treating malaria increased from an estimated $800 million in the late 1980s to well over $1.8 billion by 2008. The wealth gap between countries affected by malaria and those that are malaria-free is widening. The economic burden of malaria is $12 billion per year in direct losses, with a loss of 1.3 per cent of growth in gross domestic product per year for Africa. Malaria has a deleterious effect on productivity and business in general (Bloom et al. 2006). The costs of preventing and treating malaria drain the public purse. This includes government spending on the purchase of treated mosquito nets and insecticides, the maintenance and upgrade of public health facilities to deal with the malaria burden, and health education and training. In some countries malaria accounts for up 40 per cent of total annual public expenditure, as much as 50 per cent of all inpatient admissions, and up to 50 per cent of outpatient visits (Roll Back Malaria undated).

Historically, countries with a high prevalence of malaria have lower economic growth rates. In these cases, malaria control adds to the costs of doing business. Besides the direct costs such as medical insurance contributions and the acquisition of nets and drugs, there are indirect costs such as loss of productivity due to frequent sickness among workers, loss of workdays, and absenteeism. Anxiety among business leaders and workers in malaria-prone countries is generally high.

Malaria also affects the wealth of individuals and households. Acquisition of treated nets, doctors' fees, hospital fees, purchase of antimalarial drugs, transport for health care, and support for patients are some of the major health costs that affect individuals and households in countries with malaria. The cost of a course of treatment ranges from $0.90 to $1.40 per adult or $0.30 to $0.40 per child (Roll Back Malaria 2012). There are also indirect costs such as the loss of able-bodied members of families who provide much-needed labour for subsistence-based household economies. The death of a breadwinner robs an African family of income potential over a long period.

Complicating the social and economic costs of malaria is the fact that diseases nest in poverty and underdevelopment in Africa. Poverty renders many Africans vulnerable to malaria due to their inability to acquire preventive material or access health centres. It affects the poorest of the poor most acutely. They are unable to break the cycle of poverty because of the social and economic costs of the disease. For this reason, malaria is often described as a disease of poverty and a cause of poverty. Like poverty, malaria causes enduring scars in the social fabric due to emotional strain and pain suffered by those that survive vicious attacks or that survive the death of loved ones.

A major effect of the ubiquity of malaria in Africa is the loss of human resources deemed critical for the economy and health care. This is more than simply the loss of earnings. An even deeper challenge is the sickness and death of people with scarce skills in countries already suffering from low human resource capacities. Incessant malaria and other forms of infectious sickness is one of the reasons that scarce skills migrate from rural areas and then out of Africa to healthier working areas in the West, Asia and in America. Health workers bear the brunt of the prevalence of malaria and other sickness, forcing them to flee in search of better employment elsewhere. This adds to the brain drain and high rates of emigration, especially among health professionals. These experts find it hard to practice their professions with success where there is a shortage of basic health equipment and sanitary services and where there are low salaries.[14]

14 Personal communication with African nurses in Cambridge and London, March 21–24, 2004.

Cholera and Other Diarrheal Diseases

Diarrheal diseases are another form of disease of contact. They are a major cause of illness in the world, especially among infants and children. They affect many more individuals than it is generally thought. In 2010, an estimated 1,445,800 people died of diarrheal diseases, of whom 666,022 were under the age of five (Institute for Health Metrics and Evaluation [IHME] 2013). Deaths from diarrheal diseases at 1.4 million were higher than deaths from major killers such as measles (106,161 deaths), malaria (675,951 deaths), tetanus (47,709 deaths), diphtheria (2,269 deaths), pertussis (79,032 deaths), meningitis (204,691 deaths), and hepatitis (31,474 deaths) (IHME 2013). Children are followed by the elderly over the age of 70 years at a distant 301,491 deaths. Cholera, which was first introduced into eastern and southern Africa by imperial trade ships in the seventeenth and eighteenth centuries, is a major cause of death in this category of diseases. It remains endemic in many parts of Africa partly due to poor environmental and sanitary control.

Diarrheal diseases are closely associated with deep levels of poverty, or the poor living conditions to which the poor are subjected, such as poor nutrition, unclean water, and poor ablution services. They are treatable and preventable. But many people die in Africa from this due to poor access to the essential and basic medicines used for their treatment. The 1.4 million deaths from these illnesses are completely preventable and avoidable. This had led some to argue that in fact sufferers die in these large numbers because the world's political economy has condemned them to poverty.

These diseases are also abetted by the failure of health governance in that health systems remain weak in the absence of adequate skilled personnel and medical technologies, ineffective disease management, and poor political decision making. They break out and persist because states have weak public health systems. They flourish in conditions where primary health facilities are inaccessible and health information is erratic. They also tend to break out in countries where general political governance is weak, such as countries in political crisis. The cholera epidemic that broke out in Zimbabwe in August 2008 is a case in point. Human contact with the cholera pathogen led to 98,424 people getting infected, including 4,276 deaths, by May 2009 (WHO 2009a). Almost all were poor people who had no option but to drink infected water for survival. This outbreak can be blamed on the collapse of the Zimbabwean economy and governance that began when the ruling party lost a constitutional referendum in 2001. Over time the state haemorrhaged, the economy collapsed, and poverty skyrocketed. So the cholera virus, which could have easily been contained, found a fertile ground in this convergence of political and economic failure. The epidemic spilled over to neighbouring countries, affecting mainly the poor of the northern parts of South Africa, western Mozambique, and north-eastern Botswana.

Disease is Poverty and Poverty is Disease

Persistent health problems in the developing world and Africa, in particular, are nested in more complex challenges of poverty and underdevelopment. Poverty is in many cases itself symptomatic not just of economic failures and social disintegration, but also of bad governance. As a result, policy failures and weak institutional mechanisms have negative impacts on both poverty and disease patterns in Africa.

Africa's disease burden is constituted mainly by the following conditions: HIV and AIDS, tuberculosis and respiratory diseases, malaria, and cholera and other diarrheal diseases. All can be prevented using the existing drugs, therapies and prevention tools, but they continue to kill millions of people unnecessarily. To an extent, this can be blamed on inadequate access to drugs and therapies, which itself is partly an artefact of lack of equity in global health governance. But it is also an outcome of weak health governance in Africa.

The "disease of governance" that is partly to blame for Africa's health burden includes poor institutional capacity to manage healthcare systems, poor and ineffective leadership in general, weak coordination, and rampant corruption. This denies the poor adequate access to available health measures. The very poor, who are most susceptible to preventable conditions, are the least able to access existing medicines. This is a problem of public health governance as much as it is a matter of resources. The poor are generally not vaccinated against common illnesses because states plan poorly and have limited resources. Big pharmaceutical companies driven by a need to make exorbitant profit sometimes constrain access to basic medicines by setting excessively high prices for essential drugs. Tariffs and taxes that exporting and importing countries impose on tradable commodities such as medications also disadvantage the poor. Questionable political priorities and decisions such as spending scarce resources on the purchase of arms in peace times instead of public health militate against the fight against disease. Increasingly, the needy depend on donor programs and NGO initiatives for basic health care, a situation that absolves governments from their responsibility to provide decent health care. Many African countries have the bulk of their health care provided through or by non-state actors including NGOs, funded by mostly western donor countries (Mhone 2003).

Africa's health conundrum is broadly about the manner in which transformations that accompany globalization have increased the global burden of disease with Africa as both the epicentre of the problem of a complex interplay between poverty and disease. Until recently, the world thought this could be overcome by simply pumping more funds into health programs designed to combat specific health challenges in isolation of complex health of systems. Consequently, billions of dollars have come into the system helping to guarantee access to some health care for the poor but failing to help fix the main problem, namely system failure. This is because funds have been dumped into a leaking bucket or dysfunctional governance systems. Very little of this funding and technical support has gone into rebuilding health system, reskilling health professionals, improving management of health facilities, and enhancing health policy and planning.

Reinicke's judgement above is all the more applicable to Africa's health sector where incorrect actions by Africans and donors have rendered hundreds of millions of Africans vulnerable to all manner of illness. What undermines African responses to the spectre of disease is not just the size of domestic funds that are invested or the scale of programmatic interventions, but also the inadequate appreciation at the policy-making levels of the negative and positive effects of globalization in poor countries. As a result, except in a few countries, African governments respond to diseases as if they were purely medical phenomena or matters of pathogens to be cured through drugs rather than outcomes of deeper systematic problems. In many cases, authorities focus their energies on combating sickness that has already broken out. There is generally failure to recognize the potential effects of comprehensive social policy and economic transformation, both of which are necessary for the eradication of poverty and underdevelopment in which diseases thrive.

The health governance conundrum also has to do with how globalization and its permutations on the African continent have weakened the capacity of the public sector to respond effectively and comprehensively to complex health challenges. The transformation of Africa's political economy has the effect of eroding health governance by promoting the commodification of public services and forcing governments in donor-dependent countries to allow significant space for markets in health care. So the African experience suggests that with globalization governments share decision-making power in health governance with external countries (donors), the third sector (NGOs), and market forces. This limits the amount of power of national and regional public institutions in the provision of public health. The African development literature is replete with examples of this deleterious effect of neo-liberal interventions in African countries, the darker side of western global hegemony (see Obadina 2008).

The imposition of structural adjustment programs on debt-ridden African countries by the World Bank and International Monetary Fund helped perpetuate globalization and liberalization. The public sector was weakened to allow market forces to take over areas of public policy such as the provision of safe drinking water, health services, education, and social protection. In the notorious report entitled *Accelerated Development for Africa: An Agenda for Africa*, the World Bank (1981) ascribed the economic development crisis in Africa to the existence of strong, corrupt, and inefficient states. The panacea proposed was not just to stabilize inflation rates and liberalize trade, but, more importantly, to roll back the state from areas of public policy (Mhone 2003). The ultimate goal was to create a managerial state that would leave room for market forces to sort out the social and economic crises that affected the continent.

The World Bank-driven agenda had a much more direct bearing on the health sector in Africa. The economic structural adjustment programs (ESAPs) trimmed both the size and spending ability of the African state in an effort to create a lean and mean state. There were huge cuts in social spending, which had up to that point shielded the poor from the effects of globalization and policy blunders of the African state. As a result, health expenditures declined markedly in most African countries since they were subjected to ESAPs.

Thus the public sector's capacity to deliver essential services such as health was sacrificed and control over elements of public policy was usurped by donors. The African state became even more dependent on the generosity of others in the globalized world, mainly donor countries, agencies, and NGOs. In many respects donor countries, agencies, and NGOs also took over control of much public policy in many African countries. They came to define health priorities and imposed response programs, rendering the public sector mere implementers of ideas from elsewhere. The overwhelming portion of all health policy responses and funding in most African countries comes from donors.

At the level of civil society, western-style NGOs and social movements provided basic health care among the poor who were denied decent health by market forces because they could not afford medical aid or drugs. But, in the process, they displaced other forms of public action. Although these institutions generally have radical agendas and constantly confront power, they also do not necessarily seek to relocate this power in public institutions in African countries. In fact, they have become active in weakening the state on the African continent, partly because many states have undemocratic credentials. Issa Shivji (2006) argues that NGOs have noble motivations, but they emerged out of the womb of the post-World War II neo-liberal agenda that has undermined development and governance in Africa. They evolved from metropolitan civil society of the colonial era, a civil society that was critical of the excesses of colonialism, while it was not fundamentally anticolonial in paradigm or ideological terms. While this segment of civil society desired the end of colonialism, it did not have an unequivocal interest in building a capable and efficient African state to lead the national project. For this reason, this civil society has not promoted a comprehensive increase in the delivery of essential services such as health care for the benefit of the poor in society. Instead it has focused on individual issues such as HIV and AIDS because of the hype that surrounds them. There is very limited NGO advocacy in favour of comprehensive health reform in Africa. The decline in funding for NGO will worsen this.

Current Health Governance Actors

The nature and conduct of the African state are on their own major factors in the deterioration of health standards on the continent, adding to the effects of the neo-liberal agenda. The very weaknesses of the state and the development crisis led to the ascendancy of the neo-liberal solutions on the African continent in the first place (Dibua 1998; Founou-Tchuigou 1996; Onimode 1988). Georges Nzongola-Ntalaja (1987, x) posits that decolonization suggested that there would be "transformation of the inherited structures of the state and the economy in order to make them capable of serving the interests of the African workers and peasants". But in Africa, the petit bourgeoisie that led the national movements at independence simply captured the colonial state and deployed it in its existing form for the delivery of public goods to newly independent societies. In the process, the reinforcement of the state and nation building took precedence over democratization and equitable distribution of the benefits of independence.

Amilcar Cabral (1966), a radical African philosopher, concluded in the 1960s that the new African leaders were more interested in inheriting rather than in transforming the colonial state. The inheritor state, he argued, was ill suited to the task of bringing about social and economic transformation in pursuit of a better life for all. Cabral concluded that the post-colonial state surrendered to external forces (from capital to aid agencies) the moral duty to uplift their populations, build economies, and overcome poverty. The post-colonial state replicated the mistakes of its predecessor in a number of ways, including the bureaucratization of public administration and the neglect of social and economic services. To this day the African state in general has deep-seated capacity weaknesses that stem from the failure of the independence leaders to transform the state in order to enable it to meet the aspirations of Africans. The problems of health care are inextricably linked to this general flaw in post-colonial African governance. The state that was designed to exclude and marginalize was not transformed for an emancipatory agenda offering a better life for all.

The African Union (AU) and regional economic communities such as the Southern African Development Community share a portion of the blame for failing to drive real transformation of healthcare systems and for allowing the commodification and privatization of health as a citizen's right. They have reflected the sum total of the distortions that African countries typify. Without such an AU-inspired concerted framework for action and response, donors cannot be blamed for implementing narrow and poorly coordinated health programs. Africa remains unwilling or ill prepared to define for itself first the causes and effects of its heavy health burden and what ought to be ways in which health for all can be realized on the continent. African countries continue to put narrow national interests, mainly budget support, above the need for comprehensive responses that include collective action on health governance and practical African solutions to Africa's health problems. Aid dependence is not only addictive, but it tends to weaken initiative and agency on the part of beneficiary countries. Notwithstanding advances in the discussions on aid effectiveness, there is yet to be a change in paradigm toward self-reliance or a change of behaviour from paternalism and dependence toward partnership.

There has generally been a failure of leadership in the bureaucracy, the private healthcare sector and at political levels. Leaders have failed to respond energetically to the need to strengthen health systems and to improve institutional effectiveness and healthcare management. There is a generally poor appreciation among political leadership of the critical importance of social policy in general.

African leaders are preoccupied with political/security issues, many of which are urgent, but sometimes they are attended to because of concerns about regime security. This manifests itself in poor responses to economic problems since the end of colonial rule. African governments have thought and acted politically even on matters that required economic or social logic. Even when a handful of African hegemons steamrolled an economic agenda in the Abuja Treaty of 1991 and, more recently, the New Partnership for Africa's Development (NEPAD), the momentum at leadership level has been short-lived. This has allowed social decline or crisis including the incidence of curable infectious epidemics to worsen. Under these conditions, Africa could not benefit optimally from the surge in global health funding and general global interest in Africa's health challenges, even if one removes the factor of the coloniality (asymmetry) of global power.

In April 2007, African ministers of health gathered in an AU executive council meeting in Johannesburg, South Africa, acknowledged that part of the problem was the failure of African governments to organize themselves better to engage global actors on the basis of a collective agenda. Under the theme "Strengthening of Health Systems for Equity and Development", they concluded that until health governance was improved by strengthening health systems and stemming the brain drain, Africa's health challenges would persist, notwithstanding the political will and resources to respond (AU Conference of Ministers of Health 2007). This implied that African states failed millions of people that have died unnecessarily from diseases that could have been prevented and treated if systems functioned well and leadership was exercised.

The World Health Reports of both 2008 and 2010 identified weak health systems, therefore governance, as a primary factor behind the worsening global health standards (WHO 2008a, 2010). Other factors identified were growing inequality, changing values and expectations, and new challenges that come with more globalized, urbanized, and aging world. Thus, WHO accepts that the global health burden is an outcome of the very manner in which power, statehood, and peoplehood are organized in the world, the world system in which its member states are members either to their advantage or to their disadvantage, being either at the centre or periphery of it.

The challenge for Africa is, in this regard, the failure of African leadership and countries to understand these factors. Instead they have been quick to adopt the system's solutions that tend to perpetrate Africa's disadvantage or peripheralization. This includes hasty decentralization and devolution, economic structural adjustment, focusing on secondary and tertiary health care before primary health care, privatization of health care, and fast introduction of user-fees. These policy reforms, which formed part of the Washington consensus and donor agenda that came to dominate policy thinking in Africa after the 1970s, have led to fragmentation of the health system and growth in the unequal access to health. These interventions were fundamentally flawed for they presupposed that African countries had essential capacities, infrastructure, capital circulation, and sufficient basic community development. States still arising from colonial rule were expected to operate like European states that had been in existence for centuries.

At their 2007 meeting, AU health ministers (2007) committed the continent to an integrated, well-coordinated, harmonized, and comprehensive response. They undertook to develop an African health strategy in collaboration with the AU, regional economic communities, civil society organizations, and the private sector. They committed to engage development partners and United Nations agencies in the process so that they understood what Africa planned to do to overcome its health challenges. They planned to "address all the elements of the health workforce crisis in Africa, including achieving improved performance and effective deployment, tackling migration, scaling up production, securing sustainable financing, enhancing governance, stewardship and partnership, among others". They also decided that the health strategy would not work unless Africa also developed comprehensive social protection systems for the poor and vulnerable people with a special focus on ensuring universal access to medical care and good nutrition.

These undertakings were further affirmed by a larger gathering of African leaders at the International Conference on Primary Health Care and Health Systems in Africa (2008) in Ouagadougou, Burkina Faso, in April 2008. The conference further resolved to strengthen inter-sectoral coordination, integrated planning, enhanced health information and exchange, and greater emphasis on awareness and behavioural change. It also recognized the importance of strengthening these key elements of health governance. Most importantly, the conference noted that these interventions would fail unless there was an equally energetic focus on health determinants such as social cohesion, economic development, food security, gender equality, environmental degradation, peace, and governance. The meeting committed every African country to progressively increase health expenditure to 15 per cent of its overall national budget.

A weak AU commission and poor linkages between it and regional economic communities means that these grandiose undertakings depend largely on the interconnectedness of national initiatives, which exist only unevenly across the continent. Under these conditions, there has not emerged a strong institutional champion for the strategy. Such a champion would have led the engagement of donors that fund the bulk of health programs and therefore determine what gets done on the ground to act in support of the African strategy. The champion would have also pushed for domesticization of the continental common position on health for all by ensuring that country plans mesh with the continental blueprint. Instead, donor programs and national plans have continued without a conscious alignment with the African strategy. As a consequence, there is no visible transformation of health governance including linkages with donors and linkages with nation-states, inter-sectoral coordination, strengthening of health systems, and so forth.

The global economic crisis has the impact of reducing the amount of resources available for health expenditure. In the preface to the 2010 World Health Report, WHO director general Margaret Chan suggested that countries should have to improve the efficiency of governance systems in order to ensure universal health care and that a country's level of development should not excuse it from this (WHO 2010). The report makes the point that until health governance improves, no amount of funding would solve global health problems. The tendency of countries and funders to throw money at problems is tantamount to wasteful expenditure. This is very true of Africa as well.

Conclusion

African leaders have allowed it to be assumed that Africa's problem is its natural susceptibility to disease. This perception allows the stereotyping of Africa in the form last seen in the early colonial period when Africa was seen as a dark and sick continent, a death trap for all its visitors. This is because the continent is the epicentre of the rise of infectious epidemics such as HIV and AIDS, malaria, and tuberculosis as well as the growing problem of lifestyle illnesses such as heart disease. Tens of millions in Africa suffer disadvantage due to ubiquitous sickness.

African leaders and world powers have failed Africa by allowing Africa's health systems to weaken. There has been insufficient focus by both on strengthening health systems or capacities such health leadership, disease control and information management systems, acquisition of essential technologies, coordination, synergy between primary and secondary health care, infrastructure development, alignment between health and economic policies, health insurance and social security, and so forth. For this reason, new infections immediately become pandemic killers of high proportions. This means Africa is least prepared to realize the goals of Alma Ata 30 years on.

The health conundrum is primarily an artefact of a complex interaction between the costs of globalization on health governance globally and in Africa, and Africa's deficit of leadership, institutions, and capacities. On this basis, Africa's health sovereignty, especially as epitomized by its ability to rely on itself for building healthy states and to own its health policy agenda, remains elusive. African leaders in government, intergovernmental organizations, business, and civil society, have long realized this, but they have generally failed to take concrete measures to redefine Africa's place in global health governance. Until African health governance is sorted out, there is no hope of Africa winning the war against illness and unnecessary death.

References

African Union Conference of Ministers of Health (2007). "Johannesburg Declaration of the 3rd Ordinary Session of the African Union Conference of Ministers of Health". Johannesburg, April 9–13. http://www.africa-union.org/root/UA/Conferences/2007/avril/SA/9-13%20avr/doc/en/SA/DECLARATION_OF_JOHGANNESBURG.pdf (September 2013).

Angola Press Agency (2012). "Africa: Communicable Diseases Leading Causes of Deaths in the Continent – WHO Official". *All Africa*, November 12. http://allafrica.com/stories/201211200297.html (January 2014).

Bloom, David, Lakshmi Reddy Bloom, and Mark Weston (2006). "Business and Malaria: A Neglected Threat?", World Economic Forum, Davos. http://www.weforum.org/pdf/MalariaReport.pdf (July 2013).

Cabral, Amilcar (1966). "The Weapon of Theory". Address delivered to the first Tricontinental Conference of the Peoples of Asia, Africa and Latin America, Havana, January. http://www.marxists.org/subject/africa/cabral/1966/weapon-theory.htm (September 2013).

Cornia, Giovanni Andrea and Germano Mwabu (1997). "Health Status and Health Policy in Sub-Saharan Africa: A Long-Term Perspective" Working Paper 1997/141, United Nations University World Institute for Development Economics Research. http://www.wider.unu.edu/publications/working-papers/previous/en_GB/wp-141 (July 2013).

Dibua, J.I. (1998). "Journey to Nowhere: Neo-liberalism and Africa's Development Crisis". *Comparative Studies of South Asia, Africa, and the Middle East* 18(2): 119–30.

Escobar, Arturo (1995). *Encountering Development: The Making and Unmaking of the Third World*. Princeton: Princeton University Press.

Founou-Tchuigou, Bernard (1996). "Africa Confronted with the Ravages of Neo-liberalism". *Africa Development* 21(2–3): 5–24.

G8 (2006). "Fight against Infectious Disease". St. Petersburg, July 16. http://www.g8.utoronto.ca/summit/2006stpetersburg/infdis.html (September 2013).

Garrett, Laurie (2007). "The Challenge of Global Health". *Foreign Affairs* 86(1): 14–38. http://www.foreignaffairs.com/articles/62268/laurie-garrett/the-challenge-of-global-health (January 2014).

Global Fund to Fight AIDS, Tuberculosis, and Malaria (2004). "Report of the Executive Director". Ninth board meeting, Arusha, Geneva, November 18–19. http://www.theglobalfund.org/documents/board/09/BM09_03ExecutiveDirector_Report_en (September 2013).

Global Fund to Fight AIDS, Tuberculosis, and Malaria (2012). "Strategic Investments for Impact: Global Fund Results Report 2012". Geneva. http://www.theglobalfund.org/documents/publications/progress_reports/Publication_2012Results_Report_en/ (September 2013).

Global Fund to Fight AIDS, Tuberculosis, and Malaria (2013). "Fighting AIDS, Tuberculosis, and Malaria". Geneva. http://www.theglobalfund.org/en/about/diseases/ (September 2013).

Grosfoguel, Ramón (2009). "A Decolonial Approach to Political-Economy: Transmodernity, Border Thinking, and Global Coloniality". *Kult* 6 (Special Issue): 10–38. http://postkolonial.dk/artikler/GROSFOGUEL.pdf (January 2014).

Iliffe, John (2006). *The African AIDS Epidemic: A History*. Athens, OH: Ohio University Press.

Institute for Health Metrics and Evaluation (2013). "GBD Data". Database, Seattle WA. http://www.healthmetricsandevaluation.org/search-gbd-data (September 2013).

International Conference on Primary Health Care and Health Systems in Africa (2008). "Ouagadougou Declaration on Primary Health Care and Health Systems in Africa: Achieving Better Health for Africa in the New Millennium". Ouagadougou, April 28–30. http://www.who.int/management/OuagadougouDeclarationEN.pdf (September 2013).

Janzen, John M. (1978). *The Quest for Therapy in Lower Zaire*. Berkeley: University of California Press.

Lee, Kelley (2001). "Globalization: A New Agenda for Health?" In *International Cooperation and Health*, Martin McKee, Paul Adrian Garner, and Robin Stott, eds. Vol. 1. Oxford: Oxford University Press, pp. 19–28.

Lee, Kelley, Suzanne Fustukian, and Kent Buse (2002). "An Introduction to Global Health Policy". In *Health Policy in a Globalising World*, Kelley Lee, Kent Buse, and Suzanne Fustukian, eds. Cambridge: Cambridge University Press, pp. 3–17.

MacLeod, Roy and Milton Lewis, eds. (1988). *Disease, Medicine, and Empire: Perspectives on Western Medicine and the Experience of European Expansion*. London: Routledge.

Medical News Today (2006). "Canadian Health Minister Clement Notes Progress At G8 Health Ministers Meeting". April 30. http://www.medicalnewstoday.com/releases/42487.php (September 2013).

Mhone, Guy (2003). "The Challenges of Governance, Public Sector Reform, and Public Administration in Africa: Some Research Issues". *DPMN Bulletin* 10(3). http://www.dpmf.org/images/challenges-governance-guy.html (July 2013).

MicrobiologyBytes (2009). "Malaria". April 8. http://www.microbiologybytes.com/introduction/Malaria.html (September 2013).

Nduru, Moyiga (2004). "The Mandela Charm Glistens AIDS Conference". *Common Dreams*, July 15. http://www.commondreams.org/headlines04/0715-03.htm (January 2014).

Nzongola-Ntalaja, Georges (1987). *Revolution and Counter-Revolution in Africa: Essays in Contemporary Politics*. London: Zed Books.

Obadina, Tunde (2008). "The Myth of Neo-colonialism". *Africa Economic Analysis*. http://www.africaeconomicanalysis.org/articles/55/1/Myths-about-globalisation/Page1.html (September 2013).

Onimode, Bade (1988). *A Political Economy of the African Crisis*. London: Zed Books.

Reinicke, Wolfgang H. (1998). *Global Public Policy: Governing without Government*. Washington DC: Brookings Institution.

Roll Back Malaria (2012). "Key Malaria Facts". http://www.rollbackmalaria.org/keyfacts.html (September 2013).

Roll Back Malaria (undated). "Economic Costs of Malaria". Geneva. http://www.rbm.who.int/cmc_upload/0/000/015/363/RBMInfosheet_10.pdf (September 2013).

Shivji, Issa G. (2006). "The Silences in the NGO Discourse: The Role and Future of NGOs in Africa". Special Report 14, Pambazuka News, Oxford. http://www.pambazuka.org/en/publications/pz_sr_14.pdf (July 2013).

Sternberg, Steve (2004). "AIDS Discussion Focuses on Funds". *USA Today*, July 15. http://usatoday30.usatoday.com/news/health/2004-07-15-aids-conference_x.htm (September 2013).

UNAIDS (2008). "2008 Report on the Global AIDS Epidemic". Geneva. http://www.unaids.org/en/dataanalysis/knowyourepidemic/epidemiologypublications/2008reportontheglobalaidsepidemic/ (July 2013).

UNAIDS (2012a). "Global Fact Sheet: World AIDS Day 2012". Geneva. http://www.unaids.org/en/media/unaids/contentassets/documents/epidemiology/2012/gr2012/20121120_FactSheet_Global_en.pdf (September 2013).

UNAIDS (2012b). "Regional Fact Sheet 2012: Sub-Saharan Africa". Geneva. http://www.unaids.org/en/media/unaids/contentassets/documents/epidemiology/2012/gr2012/2012_FS_regional_ssa_en.pdf (September 2013).

UNAIDS (2012c). "UNAIDS Global Report 2012: Epidemiology Slides". Geneva. http://www.unaids.org/en/resources/campaigns/20121120_globalreport2012/epislides/ (September 2013).

UNAIDS (2013). "AIDSinfo". Database, Geneva. http://www.unaids.org/en/dataanalysis/datatools/aidsinfo/ (September 2013).

Vaughan, Megan (1991). *Curing Their Ills: Colonial Power and African Illness*. Stanford: Stanford University Press.

Vax (2004). "A Tale of Two Timeframes: Short- and Long-Term Agendas for the Response to AIDS". *Vax: The Bulletin on AIDS Vaccine Research* 2(7): 1–2. http://www.vaxreport.org/Back-Issues/Documents/IAVI_VAX_AUG_2004_ENG.pdf (January 2014).

Woodward, David, Nick Drager, Robert Beaglehole, et al. (2001). "Globalization and Health: A Framework for Analysis and Action". *World Health Bulletin* 79(9): 875–81. http://www.who.int/bulletin/archives/79%289%29875.pdf (July 2013).

World Bank (1981). "Accelerated Development in Sub-Saharan Africa: An Agenda for Action". Washington DC. http://go.worldbank.org/6W8EDJW0T0 (September 2013).

World Bank (2000). "Health Expenditures, Services, and Outcomes in Africa". *Findings: Africa Region*, April, no. 157. https://openknowledge.worldbank.org/bitstream/handle/10986/9459/548070BRI0Box31570Apr0200001PUBLIC1.pdf (September 2013).

World Bank (2007). "World Development Report 2007: Development and the Next Generation". Washington DC. http://go.worldbank.org/Q42ZSKGOP0 (September 2013).

World Health Organization (2008a). "The World Health Report 2008 – Primary Health Care (Now More Than Ever)". Geneva. http://www.who.int/whr/2008/en (October 2012).

World Health Organization (2008b). "World Malaria Report 2008". Geneva. http://whqlibdoc.who.int/publications/2008/9789241563697_eng.pdf (September 2013).

World Health Organization (2009a). "Cholera in Zimbabwe: Update 4". Geneva, June 9. http://www.who.int/csr/don/2009_06_09/en/index.html (September 2013).

World Health Organization (2009b). "Influenza A(H1N1): Update 42". Geneva, June 1. http://www.who.int/csr/don/2009_06_01a/en/index.html (September 2013).

World Health Organization (2010). "The World Health Report 2010 – Health Systems: The Path to Universal Coverage". Geneva. http://www.who.int/whr/2010/en/ (September 2013).

World Health Organization (2012). "World Malaria Report 2012". Geneva. http://www.who.int/malaria/publications/world_malaria_report_2012/report/en/index.html (September 2013).

World Health Organization (2013a). "Cumulative Number of Confirmed Human Cases for Avian Influenza A(H5N1). Reported to WHO, 2003–2013". Geneva, August 29. http://www.who.int/influenza/human_animal_interface/EN_GIP_20130829CumulativeNumberH5N1cases.pdf (September 2013).

World Health Organization (2013b). "Global Health Estimates Summary Tables: Deaths by Cause, Age, and Sex". Geneva, June. http://www.who.int/entity/healthinfo/global_burden_disease/GHE_DthGlobal_2000_2011.xls (September 2013).

World Health Organization (2013c). "The Top 10 Causes of Death". Geneva, July. http://who.int/mediacentre/factsheets/fs310/en/ (September 2013).

Žižek, Slavoj (1999). *The Ticklish Subject: The Absent Centre of Political Ontology*. London: Verso.

Zondi, Siphamandla (2012). *Public Health and African Initiative in South Africa: Aspects of the History of Public Health*. Saarbrucken: Lambert Academic Publishing.

Chapter 6

Conceptual Events: Bridging the Epistemological Divide among Stakeholders

Dennis G. Willms

Suffering is felt by more people in this world than anyone wishes to know. It is experienced in the current "climate" of moral uncertainty, climate change, civil unrest (in so many regions in Africa), and the contingencies and despair that characterize lives in motion, crossing borders, all in search of a better day, a more complete future for their children.

Scholars or academics of one sort or the other continue to wonder and search for arguments that would set this imbalance straight. The world is at a crossroads of policy formations and conceptual reorganization. Whether this be a challenge-response-innovation model of major relevance or some iteration of the same that points to a better direction, the world wants a necessary and appropriate set of actions.

And yet the so-called structural violence of current systems encourages cynicism and its own form of suffering – perhaps less experienced physically, but emotive and intellectual nonetheless.

Truth to tell, the world is in the process of examining morally reasoning notions of "health sovereignty" and "health governance" in the context of external control, agency, and power. Paul Farmer (1999) calls this situation – locally and globally – the experience of "structural violence".

So how can proper and good sovereignty concerns be addressed? What is the best approach to handling these contingencies and challenges?

In short, in addressing the health concerns of vulnerable populations moving across borders and within fragile nation-states, the first step might be to ask where this sovereignty should lie. What methods or processes should be engendered and engaged to address any number of current or emergent health concerns – whether they be new pathogens crossing borders, climate change, or any other health-related threat? How should these problems be addressed (Ritvo et al. 2005; Willms and Werner 2009)? What methods or processes could or should be implemented or used?

The next step might be to stretch this concern: Who is in control when governments – supposedly in control – are not acting, implementing, or making available the health resources required to address today's health concerns? Why is it acceptable that others (nongovernmental organizations [NGOs], for example) feel compelled to step in to offer their support in the absence of government responsibility? And how might these stakeholders work together to keep themselves accountable?

Many people are concerned about the access of individuals in vulnerable circumstances to the health care, food, shelter, and protection they need. Yet where is the voice of those individuals? How could they contribute and be mobilized for action?

The methodological innovation required – in response to the challenge-response-innovation model – is to resurrect an indigenous process of community participation that was tested and experienced to work in the past. African leaders in years past relied on the *pitso, palaver*, and *ubuntu* participation (in community) to creatively respond to concerns (Malunga 2009).

Innovation here is simply a resurrection of indigenous forms and processes for community action. The proposed method is quite simply a revitalization of original and indigenous forms and processes of community action. Everyone has a voice in this instance, every leader a position and station of respect and acknowledgement. Everyone is accountable and a stakeholder in advancing a better day.

There is a long list of concerns confronting Africans today. The consequences of climate change are compelling and troubling, as are the challenges of HIV/AIDS, poverty, vulnerable children and orphans, migration, and conflict.

This chapter argues for addressing these concerns through an innovative, participatory method called conceptual events. And yet it is not really that innovative: it simply builds on what was experienced and formed in an enduring African life of reflection and action – over many hundreds of years.

The participatory process of conceptual events transcends specific problems. It could be utilized to address any number of health- and development-related concerns in Africa and elsewhere.

This chapter describes the use of this method to address the problem of HIV/AIDS. The method applies to all other concerns, and is not specific to HIV/AIDS. Critical issues related to health sovereignty and governance can be examined through the lens of HIV/AIDS discourse, but it is germane to any health and development concern affecting everyone – in Africa and in anyone's backyard.

The Method: Conceptual Events

Epidemiological studies, clinical studies, and social scientific assessments have identified, described, and interpreted risk for HIV/AIDS. These types of assessment are now part and parcel of a collective commitment to address the underlying disparities and related problems that impinge on individual agency, cause undue suffering, and function as determinants of risk for HIV/AIDS: problems such as poverty, gender inequality, ethnic strife, and marginalization. Investing more energy and resources where human lives are compromised has become an ethical and global imperative that at a foundational level, if solved, would to some extent ameliorate the problem of HIV transmission.

Yet to be successful, cross-cultural or cross-sectoral communication on urgent issues such as HIV/AIDS must be creative and transcend personal histories and individual views of the world. It must be fundamentally cooperative. The collective thinking that can arise from deliberate, sustained communication of this type is based on the accumulated and integrated wisdom of multiple disciplines, cultures, experiences, and truth paradigms. This process is inherently trans-disciplinary in nature.

These intervention dialogues are known as conceptual events: facilitated, creative, problem-based forums that "*intentionally* nudge persons with differing truth perspectives (or paradigms) to construct a shared, ethically compelling framework for understanding the problem and the behavioural and social solution" (Willms et al. 2004, 26; see also Suwanwela and Neufeld 2001, 253). Conceptual events held in Zimbabwe, Malawi, and Uganda have served as interventions that deliberately bring together individuals who are affected by HIV/AIDS and who share the goal of addressing the problem and finding life-sustaining solutions. More significantly, however, these individuals exhibit profound differences in their understanding of the fundamental "truths that govern their lives", in how they perceive determinants of health and illness in the context of HIV/AIDS, and in their behavioural responses to evidence of risk (Willms 2009).

The conceptual event – as social-cultural process – is an intervention based on participatory action research methods and principles. Authentic participation by all relevant stakeholders is contingent upon an agreement to reason together as equals (a strategy of moral equivalence) and to reconcile or bridge their epistemological and cultural differences through "cycles of dialogue, reflection and action or praxis" (Willms et al. 2004, 26).

To engage in such a process it is critical and essential that trust between the stakeholders is established. Through sharing personal stories and experiences, and reflecting upon what is "wrong" in their practices, participants in the conceptual event move into a space of vulnerability, wherein a trusting relationship evolves and a shared critical consciousness emerges. When all participating stakeholders agree to reason together as equals because of the trust that they have experienced and engendered together, all the critical components of the conceptual event converge. Even when the outcome is only vaguely understood, there is a sense of mutual benefit because of the trust that has been nurtured, and where there is the potential advance of a "way out" of the difficulty confronted.

In short, a challenge is presented ("what are we to do about the problem of water shortage in this 'dry corridor'?"), a response engendered ("we need to rethink access issues to water – in a manner that is collaborative and cooperative"), and an innovation introduced ("perhaps we can calmly rethink the nature of the concern – get, for example, environmental and scientific assessments of what we are faced with, and then plan accordingly") through a process of community reflection and action that bridges the cultural and epistemological divide between those in control (government and even NGOs) and those who can find a proper and ethical "way out of this mess". The innovation, in this instance, is simply a process of reflection and action through conceptual events.

These events are much more than focus groups – simply eliciting information for an external researcher. These are process instances of bringing all stakeholders to the table, reflecting on a challenge or concern, wondering and reasoning through the options and responses, and creatively (innovatively) digging deep within African indigenous lore and culture to construct a solution.

Ubuntu meets conceptual event; process aligns with purpose; an innovative solution is engineered and implemented.

The Results: African Case Studies of Conceptual Events

"Dialogue for Life": Men and Women in Zimbabwe Reconcile Notions of Sexual Risk

In Zimbabwe, men and women from a high-density suburb outside Harare were brought together for a conceptual event called "Dialogue for Life". The goal of this intervention was to determine what differences existed between men and women in their experiences and understandings of sexual risk and, in the process, to stimulate the construction of shared understanding of both HIV risk and the behavioural solutions that would safeguard against it.

"Dialogue for Life" lasted for five days. Participants in this event met in a retreat setting. The 15 men and 15 women, who were all from the same district, but who were not sexual partners, initially met separately.

The women spoke about men. They expressed their concerns about male infidelity, risk taking, and gender relations. The stories they told were videotaped, and by the end of the second day, they created a short documentary video that revealed the highlights of their deliberations and the things they wanted to say to the men in their lives.

The same procedure occurred independently with the men. They talked about their sexual relations, their understanding of HIV/AIDS, and in the process (with facilitation), came to identify the "logic" of risk taking. They also produced a short documentary video based on their storytelling.

When the men and women came together as a group, both documentaries (which they had produced independently) were shown in a plenary session. The results were astonishing. The women in particular were shocked by some of the statements men made about them – as women, wives, and sexual partners. For example, men would say that when they saw an attractive woman, their eyes physiologically triggered a reaction in their body that they could not control; they were compelled to have sex with that woman. This cultural "logic" challenges behavioural intervention strategies since it is less about reason and more about emotion: "risk reality, risk situation, and risk event" (Willms and Sewakambo undated). Women, on the other hand, talked about the need to be more careful because of the financial imperatives of managing their homes and feeling that they were the sole support for their dependent children. Theirs was a more nurturing logic and less individually inclined.

Following these visual, narrative disclosures between men and women, there was a need to come to terms with the differences between men's and women's views and feelings through the construction of a shared story of concerns and decisions on how to proceed. The critical reflection that followed was both humbling and energizing for all participants, since at the end of this series of conceptual events, the men and women jointly produced a "Declaration of Sexual Health and Well-Being" – a manifesto of how they would live as sexual persons, so as to protect themselves, their partners, their children and their families.

This conceptual event generated understandings that transcended the divide between stakeholders – in this instance, the surprising discrepancy between men and women who came from the same place, the same culture, and the same socioeconomic situation.

An HIV/AIDS Intervention with Zimbabwean Traditional Healers

Zimbabwe health personnel presented the problem of how to convince traditional healers (*n'gangas*) that their methods of scarification elevated HIV risks. The urgent challenge for the Ministry of Health was how to communicate the reality of HIV (that there is a virus that causes AIDS) and HIV transmission.

At the time of this conceptual event, the *n'gangas* did not have a name for HIV/AIDS. Rather, they saw "it" as a manifestation of other indigenous diseases resulting from moral indiscretion. They believed that whatever this disease was, their *mudzima*, or ancestral spirits, would protect them whenever they engaged in their therapeutic practice. In short, there was an epistemological divide that had to be bridged with cross-cultural communication.

Ministry of Health personnel originally employed traditional educational strategies for communicating HIV/AIDS constructs. They did this in didactic lectures – one-way communications that had little impact on the healers. As they walked out of these sessions, the *n'gangas* were heard to say: "This does not apply to us … our *mudzima* protect us".[1]

In this context, a series of conceptual events brought together a multidisciplinary team of Zimbabwean health scientists with traditional healers. A participatory process was begun. This process was designed to establish relationships of trust among the healers, researchers, and Ministry of Health personnel, and to establish a negotiated space for reconciling issues of power, agency, and control. First, the participants all came to a point where they were able to admit that no one had a cure for HIV/AIDS – neither the scientists nor the traditional healers. Second, the

1 From field notes. See also Dennis Willms, Nancy Johnson, Alfred Chingono, et al. (2001).

facilitators came to realize that the healers were daily consulting their *mudzima* (in dreams and other consultations) and that these ancestral spirits (the "dead half" of the moral equation) had an equal voice in events.[2] They were equal to the healers themselves.

The conceptual events, which lasted four days, were framed by the components of a ritual-healing event. Participants parsed out the processes of entering the "surgery" (traditional healing hut), invoking the spirits, diagnosis, treatment, and payment to the spirits, as they navigated between scientific truths (about the virus and modes of HIV transmission) and traditional constructs of illness (what HIV is like in traditional terms). Through this participatory process, the healers eventually came to accept that it might be necessary to consult with their spirits about "this one" (this disease of HIV/AIDS). Perhaps there were safer ways to treat patients such as scarifying with new razors, they came to realize, and extracting the "dirt" (*tsvina*) with a tennis ball cut in half (instead of using their bare hands). These approaches were eventually adopted.

Conceptual Event Forums with Malawian Faith Leaders

Malawians are fervently religious. Whether Christian, Muslim, or African traditional religionist, faith leaders in Malawi are powerful, persuasive, and poised to present health messages to their religious adherents that reflect the urgency of the HIV/AIDS problem. In short, they are well positioned to be agents of behavioural change within their communities. Increasingly, the government of Malawi, as well as the donor community, has recognized the critical role faith leaders play in Malawian culture.

However, faiths in Malawi have typically been isolated from each other, conversing minimally with one another about HIV/AIDS. Catholics do not easily converse with Presbyterians, nor do Baptists with Lutherans, let alone Christians (in general) with Muslims, independents, or adherents of African traditional religions. In addition, many faith leaders continue to promote a theology that is replete with languages of sin, blame, immorality, and fault. These languages fail to "break the silence" about the risk realities of the disease or diminish the experiences of stigma and discrimination.[3] Also, these faith leaders have generally discouraged condom use because they believe it inadvertently encourages infidelity and adultery and creates an unnatural reproductive barrier (Spittal et al. 1997).

Conceptual events have successfully brought the leadership of these groups together in dialogue to construct an ecumenical theology of HIV/AIDS and to construct preventive, supportive care, and educational programs that reflect these new theological understandings. Since 2000, numerous conceptual events have been organized in the process of tackling the thorny and contentious issues that

---

2 The author's colleague Christopher Justice came up with the term "dead half" to describe the actions of ancestral spirits on the living.

3 S. Macdonald, personal communication, 2007.

divide the faith groups: condoms (their use/non-use), access to antiretroviral treatment, faith community/government relations, advocacy, marketing messages to the public, and the construction of an ecumenical theology of HIV/AIDS. These events have been very effective in bridging diverse realities and truth paradigms and in constructing a shared solution.

As a result of many conceptual events, a new theology of HIV/AIDS is being successfully implemented. It expresses hope, compassion, and acceptance and reduces the stigma and discrimination associated with the disease. This theological approach accepts condoms as a prevention method in cases where it can protect the lives of innocent people. The faith leaders together drafted, ratified, and signed a declaration called "Our Faiths and HIV: Expressions of Hope and Compassion for the People of Malawi", exemplifying their commitment to continue tackling contentious issues surrounding HIV/AIDS and to implement the new theology within their communities.

Uganda

Lyantonde District in Uganda was considered in the mid 1980s to be the epicentre of the AIDS epidemic in Africa. In the trucking and trading town of Lyantonde, the people had lost all hope, and fatalist attitudes toward life and becoming HIV-positive prevailed (Spittal et al. 1997). The HIV/AIDS epidemic had destroyed this community, the social fabric had unravelled, and, for the youth, there was no escaping the negative influences in the home, school, and social environment. Guidance for these youth was no longer available – relatives had given up or died or moved away. Extreme gender disparities frequently put girls and young women at risk. There was little opportunity for schooling, and there were few options for employment or obtaining goods.

Since then, however, attitudes have changed, and there is a sense of renewed hope. The traditional "aunt" and "uncle" mentoring institutions (*ssengas* and *kojjas*) have been revitalized, a community development centre has been built, and a library has been established. A vocational school is currently being completed (phase 1) planned for orphans and vulnerable children, and a micro-credit program has been implemented. All of these projects have emerged out of conceptual events held on development topics of critical concern to the community. These conceptual events were organized by a local/international NGO called the Salama SHIELD Foundation, which has worked in Uganda since the mid 1980s.[4]

4 *Salama* is Kiswahili for "peace" or "safety"; SHIELD is an acronym for sustaining health initiatives, enabling local development.

Conclusion

In Zimbabwe, Malawi, and Uganda, conceptual events resulted in the achievement of a shared understanding of risk for HIV, or a shared moral calculus, within a particular social reality (Farmer 1992). The events achieved solidarity between stakeholders by drawing attention to an overriding moral imperative to alleviate human suffering through collective action. The conceptual events also resulted in the construction of conceptual frameworks that transcended individual truths and world views, and that at the same time did not compromise or alter these scientific, spiritual, and moral perspectives but, somehow, strengthened them. These conceptual frameworks, or moral algorithms, provided a platform from which culturally appropriate and compelling solutions were designed and implemented.

At these conceptual events, emotive and moral aspects of the participants' shared humanity became the impetus to action. Out of these events, there emerged an ethical imperative to act on the issues at hand and to form a moral community made up of people who felt that their common humanity transcended their commitment to any particular group or groups to which they happened to belong. This intentionally created, moral community enhanced the participants' sense of ownership over the decisions that were made, allowing for the generation of pragmatic, sustainable solutions.

Critical to the success of each of the conceptual events was the underlying moral imperative to reduce immense human suffering. This imperative allowed a variety of stakeholders to truly own a problem and collectively enter a vulnerable space to solve that problem.

Whether the problem is HIV/AIDS, water scarcity, the impact of climate change on health and food security, or any other "development" concern, conceptual events can potentially bring diverse perspectives and groups together in the search for solutions. As characterized in the case studies, these local initiatives work as a method of searching for resolution of seemingly intractable problems; there is no reason why the methodology could not also be implored at policy and government levels if properly facilitated.

Yet these events take time. In each of the cases described in this chapter, the conceptual events were ongoing over a number of years: trust had to be established first (in a development culture where persons and communities have distrusted researchers and NGOs for not staying the course). Yet funders are wary of long-term studies or programs: one-off programs are funded, but not usually longer-term initiatives that are required to replace a mind-set of dependence in the development world with independence and respect for the agency and voice of all affected by the programs. The Uganda programme has lasted almost 20 years, Malawi was seven years, Zimbabwe was six. It took that amount of time, and funding, to get to the achievements made together as stakeholders.

The intervention method of conceptual events can be a crucial step toward genuine collaboration. While not a perfect solution, this method or process provides a common ground of understanding and an equitable and ethical language of purpose for all stakeholders.

The stories of scientists and of indigenous persons must converge for a larger purpose. Real solutions are required in the ongoing struggle among all stakeholders for meaning and resolution – in the epistemological divide that opens up when scientific truths clash with indigenous truths (about viruses and the causes of disease, for example).

To bring people to action, a dynamic process of movement between spaces of individual and group vulnerability is needed with all stakeholders. This is a form of "quiet liberation". In this process, one's sense of being in this world and experience of this world meets the sciences. In this process, vulnerable communities are engaged, mutual trust is garnered, and the moral imperative for true dialogue is acknowledged and acted upon.

Ultimately, it is in the spaces of individual and group vulnerability where innovative, creative, and effective solutions for underlying, fundamentally human problems can be addressed and resolved, where problems can be defined and then represented in numerical, narrative, or even visual ways, and where shared evidence and knowledge experience are then translated into action.

References

Farmer, Paul (1992). *AIDS and Accusation: Haiti and the Geography of Blame*. 1st edn. Berkeley CA: University of California Press.

Farmer, Paul (1999). *Infections and Inequalities: The Modern Plagues*. Berkeley: University of California Press.

Malunga, Chiku (2009). *Understanding Organizational Leadership through Ubuntu*. London: Adonis and Abbey Publishers.

Ritvo, Paul, Kumanan Wilson, Dennis Willms, et al. (2005). "Vaccines in the Public Eye". *Nature Medicine Supplement* 11(4): 520–24. http://www.canprep.ca/publications/ritvovaccines.pdf (September 2013).

Spittal, Patricia, Janette Nakuti, Nelson Sewakambo, et al. (1997). "'We Are Dying and Getting Finished!': Linking an Ethnographic Research Design to an HIV/AIDS Participatory Approach in Uganda". In *Nurtured by Knowledge: Learning to Do Participatory Action-Research*, Susan E. Smith and Dennis Willms, eds. New York: Apex Press, pp. 86–110.

Suwanwela, Charas and Victor Neufeld (2001). "Health Research for Development: Realities and Challenges". In *Forging Links for Health Research: Perspectives from the Council on Health Research for Development*, Victor Neufeld and Nancy Johnson, eds. Ottawa: International Development Research Centre, pp. 241–66.

Willms, Dennis (2009). "Understanding Must Precede Behavioural Change". *Waterloo Record*, April 1.

Willms, Dennis, Maria-Ines Arratia, and Patrick Makondesa (2004). "Malawi Faith Communities Responding to HIV/AIDS: Preliminary Findings of a Knowledge Translation and Participatory-Action Research (PAR) Project". *African Journal of AIDS Research* 3(1): 23–32.

Willms, Dennis, Nancy Johnson, Alfred Chingono, et al. (2001). "AIDS Prevention in the *Matare* and the Community: A Training Strategy for Traditional Healers in Zimbabwe". In *Applying Health Social Science: The Best Practice in the Developing World*, Nick Higginbotham, Roberto Briceño-León, and Nancy Johnson, eds. London: Zed Books.

Willms, Dennis and Nelson Sewakambo (undated). "Title". Plattsville ON: Salama SHIELD Foundation. Unpublished.

Willms, Dennis and Karolina Werner (2009). "Climate Change and Conflict in Africa". In *Climate Change in Africa: Adaptation, Mitigation, and Governance Challenges*, Hany Besada and Nelson Sewankambo, eds. Waterloo ON: Centre for International Governance Innovation, pp. 26–30.

PART III
Global Governance Responses

Chapter 7
Doing Things Differently: World Bank Health Governance Innovations in Sub-Saharan Africa

Oscar F. Picazo

This chapter discusses the role of the World Bank as an international development institution in fostering new forms of capital financing arrangements to assist African countries responding to transnational disease challenges. The World Bank has traditionally provided development assistance to individual countries. While this model remains its main function, the World Bank is increasingly exploring other approaches that do not particularly focus on individual countries' health needs but use a regional, transnational perspective to address problems of externality and scale.

The chapter starts with an introduction of the World Bank's role in health in sub-Saharan Africa and its increasing financing in the control of four diseases for which there are clear cross-border dimensions: HIV/AIDS, tuberculosis, malaria, and avian influenza. The World Bank has begun using innovative instruments to take account of the cross-border and regional dimensions of disease transmission. Although these instruments are still in the early stages of use, they are beginning to show promising results.

Two themes are explored, showcasing ways in which the transnational approach has been used. The first theme addresses cross-border disease transmission (e.g., in HIV/AIDS, malaria, and avian influenza) that warrants new funding modalities and governance structures to arrest infections across sovereign territories. The second theme deals with the diseconomies of scale that some countries in Africa suffer from due to their small geography, small population size, and small economy. These require new operating norms on regional cooperation so that greater economies can be achieved in international procurements of key inputs, health worker training, disease surveillance, laboratory referral, and the implementation of health interventions.

The World Bank's Role in Sub-Saharan African Health

The World Bank continues to be a major financier of health and other social services in Africa. In absolute terms, annual lending to this sector in sub-Saharan

Africa rose by 16 per cent from $590.3 million in 2005 to $687.3 million in 2007, after a visible decline in lending in the earlier part of the decade. However, while lending to health has modestly recovered in recent years, its share of total World Bank lending in the region began to decline. Two factors account for this relative decline. First, the period saw the massive infusion of grant resources from global disease initiatives into the region. Second, as these grant resources became increasingly available for health and the fight for HIV/AIDS, the World Bank moved more aggressively into the infrastructure arena, which required major investments to address deficits in power, telecommunications, and the like.

Still, the World Bank's role in supporting sub-Saharan African health sectors is extensive. Many projects focus on health systems strengthening. Most of these support the sector-wide programs in the country, as is the case in Tanzania, Malawi, Mozambique, Lesotho, and Ghana. These projects fund the procurement of civil works, goods, and technical assistance determined by the government, in consultation with cooperating donors, in an annual joint planning exercise, usually as part of the sector's Medium-Term Expenditure Framework. These projects typically focus on financing key health interventions defined in "essential" or "basic health packages". Program performance is formally assessed in the annual joint reviews. Policy dialogue with the host government often occurs during implementation support missions, most of which are now arranged with other cooperating donor-partners.

HIV/AIDS

In the early 2000s, concern was raised within the World Bank about the HIV/AIDS and malaria epidemics that continued unabated in sub-Saharan Africa, as well as the prospect of an avian human influenza pandemic. To reduce the impact of these scourges, the World Bank decided to focus some of its investments on these diseases. In 2000, it approved the Multi-Country HIV/AIDS Program (MAP) with an initial $500 million in credits from the interest-free International Development Association (IDA). In 2001, the World Bank approved another $500 million in grant funds from IDA resources. By 2013 about $2 billion had been committed from IDA in 33 countries and four regional projects (World Bank 2013e).

The estimated impact of this funding is immense: about 173 million people reached with information and education; about 7 million people tested for HIV/AIDS; about 1.5 million women enrolled in prevention of mother-to-child transmission of HIV/AIDS programs; about 288,000 people living with HIV/AIDS treated for opportunistic infections; some 3,000 sites providing antiretroviral treatment (ART) in 26 countries; and about 1.8 million orphans and vulnerable children receiving support.

The World Bank's (2008) "The World Bank's Commitment to HIV/AIDS in Africa: Our Agenda for Action, 2007–2011" calls on the institution to be the financier of last resort, but financier of first resort to cover program gaps; to use evidence-based and prioritized national HIV/AIDS strategies integrated in national development planning (national epidemiological profiles); to scale up targeted multisectoral and civil society response, particularly among vulnerable groups; to deliver effective results through increased country monitoring-and-evaluation capacity including strengthening surveillance systems; and to harmonize donor collaboration and knowledge sharing.

Tuberculosis

The justification for World Bank involvement in tuberculosis is clear. The disease is a major public health problem, with sub-Saharan Africa countries having the highest rates of infection and the worst treatment outcomes. Tuberculosis control in the region is distinguished from other continents by the high prevalence of tuberculosis/HIV co-infection, with each disease accelerating the other's progression. Multidrug-resistant tuberculosis (MDR) is becoming an increasing threat to health and development gains, particularly in Southern Africa. The economic justification for tuberculosis control is also strong. A recent World Bank report found that the economic cost of tuberculosis-related deaths (including HIV co-infection) in sub-Saharan Africa would be about $52 billion annually through 2015 in the absence of effective treatment.

Malaria

The World Bank launched the Booster Program for Malaria Control in Africa in 2005. Commitments for malaria control in Africa have increased from $2 million at the start of the program in 2005 to $763 million by 2011 (World Bank 2013a). The program had three objectives. The first was to contribute to the implementation of national strategic and operational plans for malaria control as developed by the affected countries themselves. The second was to finance through these national plans a combination of activities including distribution of long-lasting insecticide-treated bed nets, indoor residual house spraying where appropriate, intermittent preventive treatment for pregnant women, and treatment with artemisinin-based combination therapies. The third objective was to assist client countries to accelerate progress toward the achievement of the Abuja targets by 2008, which call for at least 60 per cent utilization of effective malaria prevention and treatment.

By 2011, the Malaria Booster Program supported 21 projects in 18 countries. It has a very flexible project approach. The design of each project is adapted to the country context and lending instrument, e.g., stand-alone operation (as in Benin, Nigeria, and Zambia), embedded in an existing project such as nutrition, child survival, or HIV/AIDS (as in Burkina Faso, Eritrea, Ghana, Kenya, and Senegal), or part of a sector-wide program (as in Malawi and Niger). The malaria projects in the Democratic Republic of Congo and Ethiopia piggyback on broader social protection and social rehabilitation projects. In their potential impact, these projects cover a total population of 240 million, of whom 42 million are children under five years of age and 10 million are pregnant women.

Avian Influenza

The highly pathogenic avian influenza broke out in Asia in 2003, Europe in 2005, and Africa in 2006. Avian influenza hit Nigeria in 2006, and outbreaks were also reported in Egypt, Sudan, Cameroon, Burkina Faso, Côte d'Ivoire, Djibouti, Ghana, Niger, Togo, and Benin through 2007. All countries in sub-Saharan Africa are considered high risk. The large potential economic, social, and public health costs of this epidemic, especially when the virus crosses species into humans (thus becoming a human influenza epidemic), required a drastic global response.

To address this problem, the World Bank created the Avian Influenza Task Force. It produced in 2005 a framework document for grants and loans of $500 million for the Global Program for Avian Influenza. The World Bank subsequently created the Avian and Human Influenza Facility (AHIF), with seed money from multilateral donors, to manage the grant support to countries.

In 2006, the World Bank created the Africa Region Avian and Human Influenza Task Force, with members from the sustainable development and human development networks (World Bank 2011b). This was a clear case of intersectoral collaboration. This cross-sectoral task force prepared the region's avian and human influenza program with three objectives: to strengthen the veterinary services in African countries, particularly in mounting emergency and medium-term responses to outbreaks, to improve the capacities of African health systems to respond to a potential pandemic, and to support country efforts in developing coordinated national response programs to avian and human influenza.

The World Bank's activities in the control of avian influenza have been highly strategic. IDA financed ongoing projects in Nigeria ($50 million) and Niger ($4.5 million) (World Bank 2009). Out of the $9 million AHIF allocation, some $4.4 million grants were also given to Zambia, Malawi, Cameroon, and the Republic of Congo. In addition, around $400,000 went for preoperational activities or rapid assessments of animal and human influenza. About $7.5 million was obtained to finance the early work of the ALive Partnership for Livestock Development, Poverty Alleviation and Sustainable Growth, whose secretariat was originally hosted by the World Bank but was transferred to the African Union-InterAfrican Bureau of Animal Resources in Nairobi in 2009 (ALive Partnership for Livestock Development 2013). Rapid assessments were completed in 16 sub-Saharan countries by 2009. Following these assessments, integrated national action programs were prepared.

Cross-Border Disease Transmission

The cross-border transmission of infection, both animal and human, is increasingly appreciated by national policymakers and development partners alike. Human migration and the increasing trade in goods and services contribute to this increased infection risk. Sub-Saharan Africa is particularly prone to over-land transmission of disease because it is a large geographic landmass, with people and goods flowing increasingly across borders. Indeed, the persistence of HIV/AIDS in Southern Africa has been seen by many analysts as originating from cross-border and within-border labour mobility initially to meet the staffing demands of the mines and increasingly as a reflection of the opening up of South Africa after apartheid. Increasing trade between countries and the rising volume of cargo movement from seaports to countries inland also increase the risk of cross-border disease transmission. In this light, the cross-border impact of disease transmission is merely a negative externality that must be dealt with on a supra-national basis.

Malaria Control in Contiguous Countries

On their own, several contiguous states have taken up the issue of cross-border disease transmission and have designed projects that use flexible means of managing and patrolling borders so that they can better deal with controlling infections. A classic example is the malaria control component of the Lubombo Spatial Development Initiative (LSDI), a tri-country effort intended to spur agro-economic development in the areas bordered by south-eastern Swaziland, the South African province of KwaZulu-Natal, and southern Mozambique. LSDI is the brainchild of South Africa's Department of Environmental Affairs and Tourism, which planned to turn the area into an economic zone. A major constraint in this area, however, was the high burden of malaria. The Medical Research Council of South Africa and its collaborating institutions in the other two countries thus designed a malaria control component of LSDI, and, in 1999, the relevant ministers of the three countries signed the Malaria Protocol of LSDI, which defined the terms of cooperation for disease control in the area. The malaria control component of the LSDI was managed by the Regional Malaria Control Commission, a core group of public health experts and scientists from the three countries. The project provided effective treatment interventions on malaria and indoor residual spraying with insecticides.

As the malaria interventions progressed, the LSDI project managers realized that more intensive control interventions were needed in southern Mozambique reaching up to Maputo Province and then to Gaza Province, which both border South Africa. The Mozambican, South African, and Swazi governments understood the well-documented negative effect of malaria on the tourism and investment potential of this region. They immediately agreed on a full-blown control program crisscrossing their borders. Prevalence studies have shown that malaria cases have dramatically declined at LSDI and at Maputo and Gaza provinces.[1] The key LSDI target of reducing malaria incidence from 250/1,000 population to less than 20/1,000 population was achieved. LSDI has therefore demonstrated the virtue of a transnational strategy in dealing with a major public health problem.

Following the success of the LSDI, the World Bank's Malaria Booster Program was launched to support regional multi-country initiatives, in addition to country-specific malaria projects. From 2006 to 2013, the World Bank committed $110 million to the Senegal River Basin regional malaria project, which benefited Guinea, Mali, Mauritania, and Senegal. The Booster Program also considered sub-regional integration initiatives for Zambia-Mozambique-Malawi; Kenya-Uganda-Tanzania, centred on the Victoria Lake Region; Rwanda-Burundi; and the Democratic Republic of Congo-Nigeria-eastern border countries.

HIV/AIDS Control along Transport Corridors

The World Bank's $16.6 million HIV/AIDS Project for the Abidjan-Lagos Transport Corridor was launched in 2003 to provide HIV/AIDS information and services to transport workers and their clients. The project, which ended in 2007, was based on a declaration of agreement at the level of heads of state of the five countries using the transport corridor, namely Côte d'Ivoire, Ghana, Togo, Benin, and Nigeria (Brushett and Osika 2005). Participating states set up a representative institutional structure to manage the project; these countries contributed to the upkeep of the project through annual payments.

The Southern African HIV/AIDS Transport Corridor Project was another regional project supported by the World Bank from 2003 to 2007 (World Bank 2013d). The corridor, which includes Malawi, Zambia, Zimbabwe, Mozambique, and South Africa, is the world's most heavily affected region. The project supported the coordination, monitoring, and evaluation of HIV/AIDS interventions in the long-haul transport sector, as well as in communities located along the transport corridor.

There are other important transport corridors where transnational HIV/AIDS interventions are needed (Brushett and Osika 2005). In a few of these corridors, interventions are already underway or planned; the rest are for future development.

- Bamako-Ouagadougou-Tema corridor
- Bamako-Ouagadougou-Niamey corridor
- Cotonou-Niamey corridor
- Dakar-Bamako corridor
- Lome-Ouagadougou-Bamako-Niamey corridor

---

1 See the Lubombo Spatial Development Initiative website at http://www.malaria.org.za/lsdi/home.html.

- Abidjan-Ouagadougou corridor
- Abidjan-Bamako corridor
- Djibouti-Addis Ababa corridor
- Mombasa-Kampala-Kigali-Bujumbara-Goma corridor
- Dar Es Salaam-Kigali-Bujumbara-Goma corridor
- Dar Es Salaam-Lusaka-Lilongwe-Blantyre corridor
- Durban-Lusaka-Lubumbashi corridor
- Beira-Harare-Lusaka-Lilongwe-Blantyre corridor
- Maputo-Johannesburg corridor
- Nacala-Lilongwe-Blantyre corridor

HIV/AIDS Control among Refugees and other Mobile Groups

The World Bank has used the same transnational approach in dealing with the regional dimension of disease transmission. In addition to the national HIV/AIDS projects, its Multisectoral AIDS Projects (MAP) has also embarked on regional initiatives in Africa. The Great Lakes Initiative on HIV/AIDS Support Project (GLIA) was a $20 million initiative approved in 2005 to add value to national HIV/AIDS efforts and to support interventions for mobile groups including refugees, internally displaced people, and rebel returnees (World Bank 2013c). It provided seed capital for the formation of a regional institution, wholly owned by its member-states of Burundi, Democratic Republic of Congo, Kenya, Rwanda, Tanzania, and Uganda. It involved UNAIDS as well as the United Nations High Commission for Refugees as an implementing partner.

Africa-Wide Onchocerciasis Control

The World Bank is also involved in the prevention and treatment of onchocerciasis, the disease caused by filarial worms, mainly as a partner in the African Program for Onchocerciasis Control launched by the World Health Organization (WHO). The principal strategy of this regional control program is the establishment of sustainable community-directed treatment with ivermectin (Mectizan) to ensure that a high proportion of the at-risk population receives the drug at least once a year. Merck provides the drug through its Mectizan Donation Program. The World Bank has statutory responsibility under the onchocerciasis fund agreement for donor coordination, mobilizing donor financing, and managing the program's trust fund. Program activities include assessment of disease distribution, surveillance, vector control, training and distribution of ivermectin, capacity building, advocacy and information campaigns, and research. The program originally focused on the 11 countries in West Africa affected by the disease. It was later expanded to 19 other African countries (outside the West Africa control area), with an estimated population of 109 million, of whom 50 million are at risk of contracting onchocerciasis (WHO 2013a).

Diseconomies of Scale in Small Countries

A second, less appreciated, rationale for regionalization is the diseconomies of scale constraining small countries (such as Botswana, Lesotho, Namibia, and Swaziland in Southern Africa, and Burundi, Rwanda, and Uganda in East Africa) to develop full-fledged health systems. A small economy or a small population base makes it very uneconomical to develop critical services such as medical research, policy development, standard setting, health regulation, disease surveillance, laboratory referral, medical and dental education, and in-service training. A small country – or even a medium-sized country if it is poor – is severely constrained in establishing the necessary institutions to deal with these needs for budgetary reasons and due to the scarcity of requisite technical skills in-country. An appropriate solution would be to regionalize some of these functions so that sunk costs or even administrative costs can be shared.

Regionalizing Laboratory Networks

The World Bank explored the possibility of regionalizing certain critical health services to help smaller countries access such services, which they otherwise would find difficult to have. One case is reference laboratories for tuberculosis. Taking a regional approach to the global public good of controlling drug-resistant tuberculosis, the World Bank designed a regional health and tuberculosis support project that aims at increasing the number of supranational reference labs to support national labs at the country level in diagnosing extensively drug-resistant tuberculosis (XDR-TB), providing training, quality assurance, technical assistance, and support to drug-resistance surveys. An emerging regional dimension in Southern Africa is the spread of drug-resistant forms across borders, mainly through miners. This regional approach supports the emerging close cooperation on lab strengthening in Africa, being coordinated by WHO's Global Laboratory Initiative.

In 2010, the World Bank (2013b) approved a $63.66 million East Africa Public Health Laboratory Networking Project to establish a network of high-quality public laboratories focusing on diagnostic services in Kenya, Tanzania, Rwanda, and Uganda. The laboratories are particularly useful among vulnerable population living in cross-border areas across the four contiguous countries. The project is a realization of the countries' leadership in the need to respond to tuberculosis not only as a national but as a continental concern.

These labs serve as "surveillance sites to monitor hot spots for disease transmission" and "make optimal use of internet and mobile communications to improve public health" (World Bank 2010a). They also support the use of new diagnostic technologies for monitoring drug resistance. The regional approach used in this project reflects East African countries' move toward a common market that will allow greater mobility of workers and, with it, the increased risk of disease transmission throughout the countries in the region.

By banding together in a regional laboratory network, the countries can more easily identify cases, diagnose them, and treat them, even without having to transport people back to their home countries. The regional approach not only makes it more cost-effective to deal with patients, but also expedites the process of obtaining accurate and up-to-date diagnosis, a problem often encountered in a system where each country operates a lab independently of each other.

Under this project, each country serves as a centre of excellence for a key thematic area, which also promotes regional collaboration. Specialization can take place, which is otherwise difficult to achieve if national labs operate independently. Thus, Rwanda can take the lead in information and communication technology and performance-based financing, Kenya can serve as a centre for integrated disease surveillance and response and operations research, Uganda can lead on laboratory networking and accreditation, and Tanzania can develop high-quality training programs and allow other countries' use of its state-of-the-art National Health Laboratory Quality Assurance and Training Centre. Such specialization would not be possible under a status quo where each country would have to do everything itself.

In 2012, Burundi also joined the East Africa Network of Public Health Laboratories with a $15 million grant from the World Bank.

Regional Drug Procurement

Regional procurement of essential health commodities (drugs) to achieve larger market size – and therefore economic power – needs to be explored in sub-Saharan Africa. High-prevalence HIV/AIDS countries should consider alternative options for ART and commodity security through several instruments.

One such instrument is international partnerships in joint drug procurement and production. Joint procurement could be arranged among countries, international organizations, and drug companies. However, since technology and global prices are so quick to change, there are risks in that the partnership may restrict a country from making other arrangements if drug prices fall, or if better, new-generation drugs become available. The performance of the drugs in use is also relevant, as drug resistance can render them increasingly irrelevant. Given this, African countries should stay alert and should periodically reassess affordability.

A second instrument is regional partnerships in joint or pool drug procurement and production. Countries in the Southern Africa Development Community (SADC) are at the epicentre of the global AIDS pandemic. Although some members are small – Botswana, Lesotho, Namibia, and Swaziland have high prevalence rates but low populations of about 2 million each – a joint regional program would increase the size of the market for antiretroviral drugs. For purchasing countries, pool procurement lowers drug prices by increasing the purchase volume, reduces market and distribution costs, and improves production planning thanks to better demand forecasting. For suppliers, increased purchase volume creates economies of scale and lowers operational costs. While pooled procurement looks like a win-win approach, the key constraints are the unharmonized drug regimens, procurement rules, and import policies. In 2012, the SADC health ministers approved a strategy for pooled procurement strategy, which had been identified as an immediate priority (South African Regional Programme on access to Medicines and Diagnostics 2012)

A third instrument is bilateral negotiations with countries that produce generic or inexpensive branded drugs, such as Brazil, India, South Africa, and Thailand. South-South cooperation has been increasing, including with regard to HIV/AIDS treatment assistance to Africa. In 2007, Brazil provided locally manufactured antiretroviral drugs to 11 developing countries, including five in Africa (United Nations General Assembly 2007). Brazil was also coordinating an international HIV/AIDS technical cooperation network to facilitate the transfer of technologies for the production of antiretroviral drugs.

A fourth instrument is access to up-to-date comparative ART technologies/regimens, drug prices, and suppliers in the international market. This remains a challenge for treatment program managers. The bewildering array of products and producers makes such access to critical information extremely hard. Providing such information is a public good that a regional body like SADC could perform, with technical assistance from a specialized pharmaceutical agency or consulting firm.

Conclusions

The potential for expanding and strengthening health services using a transnational or regional perspective is large. But this is a new way of doing things for the World Bank, and current projects need to be documented and evaluated. What can be concluded from the experiences so far?

First, while it seemed initially that regionalization of health services to ease problems of diseconomies of scale would be a daunting political and management challenge, the case of the East Africa Regional Public Health Laboratory Network showed that the immediate impact on sovereignty was minor. Indeed, the additional costs of designing a regional project seemed small relative to the potential benefits. There were four key elements: harmonization and use of regional health service standards, including standardized training and laboratory certification requirements; peer review assessments of participating laboratories in the network; agreeing on a joint regional framework for cross-border epidemiological surveillance, including sharing population and epidemiological data and statistics on services; and common planning and programming so that joint outputs are met. What seemed to have expedited the process of different countries' agreeing to these common key elements was the fact that they are all members of the WHO Regional Office for Africa (WHO/AFRO). This made cross-country standardization much easier, since they already follow WHO/AFRO technical guidelines.

Second, while working within the framework of existing institutions is called for, it may be necessary to create new institutions to cater to the regional dimension and requirements of transnational projects. This was particularly seen in the case of regional HIV/AIDS projects that were designed along transnational transport corridors. Despite strong national interests, national leaders and managers often underestimate the actual processing and time needed to define and allocate the respective roles and responsibilities of participating countries, the justification of these roles and responsibilities especially in terms of equity in sharing the costs and benefits that each partner should have, and the legal framework within which any new institution can work (Brushett and Osika 2005).

In the case of the regional tuberculosis networks, new forms of institutions could also emerge. For instance, Tanzania's national training and quality assurance centre may evolve into a regional one supplying trainees and receiving resources (tuition, matriculation, fees) from participating countries. A regional research consortium on laboratory management could also emerge. Regional laboratory planning may become an annual or bi-annual activity. These are possibilities that the participating countries in the East Africa laboratory network must sort out.

Third, national programs (in transport or tourism and health) are not geared to addressing health problems in cross-border areas, nor do they have units (in the ministries of health, transport, tourism, labour, or economic development) to deal with them specifically. In the case of the LSDI malaria regional program, the tourism ministry in the largest country in the partnership (South Africa) did much of the initial technical and organizational spadework, since the two other partners (Swaziland and Mozambique) are institutionally weaker. This arrangement could work if the strong partner is seen by the others as acting solely for altruistic reasons, but it may be difficult if there is a level of distrust.

Fourth, a few regional initiatives with large potential have not moved apace, specifically on regional drug procurement. Little documentation exists on the reasons behind the lack of progress on this front in sub-Saharan Africa. But it may be due to its technical difficulty, lack of regional leadership, or the scarcity of good examples or their diffusion. SADC was at one point interested in exploring this area, but its health unit seems to be saddled with other more urgent tasks.

Finally, the World Bank has supported such regional initiatives using existing lending and grant instruments, so the type of financing instrument does not seem to be the binding constraint in propagating these transnational models. In recent years, the World Bank has also been open to crafting new innovative instruments if necessary (such as learning and innovation loans, adaptable program loans, loans blended with grants, and performance-based financing).

References

ALive Partnership for Livestock Development, Poverty Alleviation and Sustainable Growth (2013). "About ALive". http://www.alive-online.org/web/page/521/sectionid/339/pagelevel/2/interior.asp (September 2013).

Brushett, Stephen and John Stephen Osika (2005). "Lessons Learned to Date from HIV/AIDS Transport Corridor Projects". World Bank Global HIV/AIDS Program Discussion Paper, August, World Bank, Washington DC. http://siteresources.worldbank.org/INTHIVAIDS/Resources/375798-1103037153392/Transport.pdf (September 2013).

South African Regional Programme on access to Medicines and Diagnostics (2012). "SADC Pooled Procurement Strategy for Essential Medicines and Health Commodities 2013–2017". http://www.sarpam.net/archives/2103 (September 2013).

United Nations General Assembly (2007). "The State of South-South Cooperation". A/62/296, August 23, New York. http://daccess-dds-ny.un.org/doc/UNDOC/GEN/N07/488/80/PDF/N0748880.pdf (September 2013).

World Bank (2008). "The World Bank's Commitment to HIV/AIDS in Africa: Our Agenda for Action, 2007–2011". Washington DC. http://siteresources.worldbank.org/INTAFRREGTOPHIVAIDS/Resources/WB_HIV-AIDS-AFA_2007-2011_Advance_Copy.pdf (September 2013).

World Bank (2009). "World Bank: Avian and Human Influenza Operations (Status as of December 31, 2008)". Washington DC. http://siteresources.worldbank.org/EXTAVIANFLU/Resources/3124440-1208294248389/WB_AHI_Matrix_Apr09.pdf (September 2013).

World Bank (2010). "Cross-country Laboratory Network to Raise East Africa's Defenses Against Disease". Washington DC. http://go.worldbank.org/4WZODJ72I0 (September 2013).

World Bank (2011). "Towards One Health: Interim Lessons from the Global Program on Avian and Human Pandemic Influenza". Washington DC. http://siteresources.worldbank.org/EXTARD/Resources/336681-1242670845332/TowardsOneHealth.pdf (September 2013).

World Bank (2013a). "Booster Program for Malaria Control in Africa". Washington DC. http://go.worldbank.org/H31FEKFWE0 (September 2013).

World Bank (2013b). "East Africa Public Health Laboratory Networking Project". Warsaw. http://www.worldbank.org/projects/P111556/east-africa-public-health-laboratory-networking-project?lang=en (September 2013).

World Bank (2013c). "Great Lakes Initiative on HIV/AIDS (GLIA) Support". Washington DC. http://www.worldbank.org/projects/P080413/great-lakes-initiative-hivaids-glia-support?lang=en (September 2013).

World Bank (2013d). "HIV/AIDS Project for Abidjan-Lagos Transport Corridor". Washington DC. http://www.worldbank.org/projects/P074850/hivaids-project-abidjan-lagos-transport-corridor?lang=en&tab=overview (September 2013).

World Bank (2013e). "Meeting the Challenge: The World Bank and HIV/AIDS". Washington DC. http://www.worldbank.org/en/results/2013/04/03/hivaids-sector-results-profile (September 2013).

World Health Organization (2013). "African Programme for Onchocerciasis Control (APOC)". Geneva. http://www.who.int/blindness/partnerships/APOC/en/ (September 2013).

Chapter 8

Can the World Trade Organization Be Trusted? The Impact of Trade Law and Politics in Global Health Governance

Rangarirai Machemedze

Since 1948, the World Health Organization (WHO) has been responsible for "providing leadership on global health matters, shaping the health research agenda, setting norms and standards, articulating evidence-based policy options, providing technical support to countries and monitoring and assessing health trends" (World Trade Organization 1994). This has been the vision of the United Nations system since it established the organization. However, with globalization and the creation of new institutions at global and regional levels, health matters have become a shared responsibility, with a number of institutions assuming different roles and duties. Today several organizations are involved in health policy and health-related matters. Their involvement is assumed not to dilute the role of WHO but rather to contribute to the realization of its objectives. But the question arises: is this the case with the current global health players, including the World Trade Organization (WTO)? It administers trade agreements that require countries to change their domestic laws, thereby affecting many policy issues including health and its related social and economic determinants.

This chapter examines the impact of WTO agreements on the governance of health issues at the global as well as the regional level in Southern Africa. It starts by examining trade before the WTO under the 1948 General Agreement on Trade and Tariffs (GATT) to locate how issues have gradually been placed on the WTO agenda. After covering the definitional issues concerning GATT, the establishment of the WTO, and the expansion of the WTO agenda, the chapter explores governance issues at the WTO, particularly with regard to decision making and the principles guiding the organization. This examination helps to see whether the WTO can be trusted, given the way decisions are made. The chapter then analyses specific agreements that have a direct impact on health, particularly the General Agreement on Trade in Services (GATS) and the Agreement on Trade-Related Aspects of Intellectual Property (TRIPS), and what these mean for universal access of health services by the general populace of developing countries. The chapter concludes with policy options that developing countries may consider to achieve universal equitable access to health services and to have health governance to achieve the proper balance between international policies and domestic regulations.

The Neo-liberal Inheritance and WHO Governance

The dominant economic paradigm that most developing countries, particularly in Africa, have been following in the past two decades is neo-liberalism. It holds that free trade and liberalization of the economy are a panacea, not only for the developed world but also to promote development in the developing world (Tandon 2003). This ideology has been at the core of the Bretton Woods institutions, supposed to promote development in poorer countries and help extricate these countries from the vicious cycle of poverty, disease, and underdevelopment. Yet more than 20 years of implementing neo-liberal policies have not resulted in the envisaged improved living standards of people and reduced general poverty. Many more people have been impoverished.

In Africa, both urban and rural citizens are confronted by health crises of vast proportions. HIV/AIDS, malaria, and tuberculosis are the most frequently mentioned. All require access to affordable medication and other medical services. Yet the provision of drugs and access to health services are no longer the preserve of governments and local authorities. They have been left to the dictates and vagaries of the market through international organizations such as the WTO. Access to basic services and the cost of those services, particularly those affecting the economic, environmental, and social determinants of health including nutrition, have become issues in the international trade domain. No government can unilaterally deal with them outside international influences and events under current international trade law.

The dramatic events in the global economy in 2008 brought to the fore the failure of an ideology and the urgency needed to fix the problems that have been mounting since 2000. The beginning of 2008 witnessed an unprecedented rise in energy prices that have a strong causal link with the rise in food prices globally and the riots that rocked countries from Haiti to South Africa. The global economy went into recession in the United States, the European Union (including France and the United Kingdom, with Portugal, Italy, Greece, and Spain suffering the most), and Japan (*Economist* 2008). The financial meltdown coupled with the earlier food and energy price rises fuelled global economic instability. These are all products of a failing ideology.

Market fundamentalism will not solve the world's problems, let alone the crises afflicting developing countries. Further liberalization in services, particularly financial services, will compound the problems facing developing countries in other sectors such as health (Raja 2010). Most African countries have introduced market-based reforms in their financial sectors. While normally liberalization was expected to encourage financial deepening, with a positive effect on savings mobilization and credit allocation, for most of Africa, ratios of money and credit to gross domestic product have not increased (World Bank 2005). This means resources that were supposed to be available for other sectors such as health and education have not been realized through financial liberalization.

In addition, as if to respond to the challenges of the global economic crisis, at the World Health Assembly and the WHO Executive Board meeting in 2011, WHO members agreed to major reforms of the organization and endorsed an agenda of reforms as set out in the director general's report. These reforms aim to achieve three major objectives:

1. Improved health outcomes, with WHO meeting the expectations of its Member States and partners in addressing agreed global health priorities, focused on the actions and areas where the Organization has a unique function or comparative advantage, and financed in a way that facilitates this focus.
2. Greater coherence in global health, with WHO playing a leading role in enabling the many different actors to play an active and effective role in contributing to the health of all peoples.
3. An Organization that pursues excellence; one that is effective, efficient, responsive, objective, transparent and accountable (WHO 2013f).

WHO governance matters have produced interesting observations from different players following the increase in the number of actors in global health issues (Stuckler et al. 2011). It is not only actors outside the UN system but also different agencies within the system that make immense contributions. This complex architecture has led to concern about the lack of effective coordination across UN policies and the inadequate machinery for monitoring implementation of the hundreds of multilateral treaties, which, although sectoral in character, also impinge on global public health. Moreover, WHO (2011d) has noted that the number of global health partnerships has increased steadily in recent years: there are now more than 100 private global foundations.

The multiplicity of these actors raises the issue of where control and leadership of the vision, mandates, and functioning of those partnerships lie. It is therefore fundamental for health sovereignty to remain within the ambit of the public institutions that carry the mandate from the people to govern them.

From GATT to the WTO

Before the twentieth century many governments conducted trade as an issue between one government and another on bilateral terms. In the post-1900 period, ideas promoted by the leading industrializing countries because of their own needs resulted in the rapid expansion of communication technologies. Later came the economic crisis in Europe before the Second World War, and the concept that trade relations were better conducted in the context of international rules (Munyuki et al. 2005). The thinking was that governments represented merchants well, being better placed to agree on what measures were necessary to promote international trade and, at the same time, create law and order in the commercial jungle. This was the framework of the proposed but aborted International Trade Organization (ITO) and later the GATT, agreed to in 1948. As Anne Krueger (1998, 3) wrote, the ITO

> was envisaged as a third pillar—along with the IMF [International Monetary Fund] and the International Bank for Reconstruction and Development (later the World Bank)—of the postwar world economic order ... there was a significant divide between those who anticipated a postwar return to depression as in the 1930s, and those who expected a return to "normal" economic conditions. The former group pushed for a number of provisions in the ITO Charter that effectively permitted signatories to undertake virtually any trade policy they desired if it was done to pursue domestic "employment objectives". There were sufficient objections to this in the U.S. Congress that the ITO Charter was not submitted for ratification, and other major countries did not ratify the charter, pending US action.
>
> While work was progressing on the ITO Charter, the United States undertook an initiative for a first multilateral round of trade negotiations. In order to make the round meaningful, the GATT was formulated and accepted. At the time it was anticipated that the GATT articles would become part of the charter of the ITO, but in the absence of the ITO, the GATT articles became the basis for governance in the international trading system.

The GATT focused mainly on trade in goods and the reduction of tariffs. It had provisions for strong government intervention and institutionalized flexibility such as the ability to enact measures to protect small, new, and vulnerable industries. It required foreign investors to employ domestic workers and leadership and to purchase local products and services.

The establishment of the WTO represented a paradigm shift in global trade and trade-related policies (United Nations Development Programme 2003). It expanded global trade policies to cover the majority of economic activities of its members, apart from security matters such as police and military activities. The WTO, alongside the Bretton Woods twins, actively played the umpire role to reduce and clip the wings of governments and domestic policy interventions to the advantage of foreign traders and investors with new rights. Furthermore, the WTO proposed a system of continuous rounds of trade negotiations in order to promote irreversible steady and deeper liberalization of world trade and domestic trade policies (see Table 8.1).

Table 8.1 GATT and WTO Trade Rounds

Name of round or meeting	Period and number of parties	Subjects and modalities	Outcome
Geneva I	1947 23 countries	Tariffs	Signing of GATT; concessions on 15,000 tariff lines
Annecy	1949 33 countries	Tariffs	5,000 tariff concessions
Torquay	1950 34 countries	Tariffs	8,700 tariff concessions
Geneva II	1956 22 countries	Tariffs	Modest reductions
Dillon Round	1960 45 countries	Tariffs	4,400 concessions exchanged
Kennedy Round	1963–1967 48 countries	Tariffs, antidumping	Average tariffs reduced by 35 per cent; 33,000 tariff lines bound; agreement on antidumping
Tokyo Round	1973–1979 99 countries	Tariffs, antidumping, government procurement, import licensing, product standards, safeguards, special and differential treatment of developing countries	Average tariffs reductions; voluntary codes of conduct
Uruguay Round	1986–1994 103 countries in 1986; 117 by 1993	Tariffs, services, intellectual property, trade-related investment measures, dispute settlement, transparency and surveillance	Average tariffs reductions by one third on average; agriculture, textiles and clothing subjected to rules; creation of WTO; agreements on services and TRIPS
Doha Round	2001–? 142 countries in 2001; 159 as of March 2013	Tariffs, trade facilitation, rules, services	

Source: Based on World Trade Organization (2007, 198).
Note: GATT = General Agreement on Tariffs and Trade; TRIPS = trade-related aspects of intellectual property; WTO = World Trade Organization.

The policy space that the advanced countries had enjoyed for their own development before the GATT, and even under the GATT regime, is now severely eroded, and no longer available to developing countries for their industrial and employment reconstruction. When advanced countries were developing, they did so behind walls of protectionism, cushioning their infant industries from foreign competition until such time as they had fostered their competitiveness. Developing countries today face the challenge of foreign competition, especially in sectors where they are still developing their industries because of the role of the WTO.[1]

WTO member states have remained locked in heated negotiations to define the modalities of trade since the Doha Round was initiated in 2001. The Doha Round has exposed serious and sharp differences between the developing and developed countries. Although dubbed a development round, many developing and even developed countries are not satisfied with the process and the progress regarding development. Major issues exposing these differences include subsidies and tariff reduction in agriculture and non-agricultural market access, implementation of former promises on behalf of industrialized countries, special and differential treatment, and other interests of developing countries. WTO agreements contain provisions for special and differential treatment that give developing countries special rights in recognizing special needs because of the nature of those economies and the fact that those countries are at different levels of development. The trade ministers at the ministerial conference in Doha mandated the Committee on Trade and Development to examine these provisions in all the agreements. As a result, they are an integral part of all negotiations.

Negotiations at the WTO have been about market access of goods and services including health services. The dominant trading countries (including the US, EU, Japan, and Canada) use their control of global production and marketing to seek markets in developing and emerging economies for their own goods and services (Kaubab 2005). Market access is also sought for sectors traditionally regarded as public, strategic, or domestic (such as essential services). Liberalization is not only limited to trade in goods but also includes essential services such as health, education, water supply, and sewage reticulation.

Pressure on developing countries to open up their economies also comes directly from major trading powers through various bilateral investment treaties and regional trade agreements. The US enacted the *African Growth and Opportunity Act,* which allows textile products from Africa to enter American territory free of duties and

---

1 For example, Lesotho became a major textile manufacturer in Africa between 2000 and 2003. At one point Lesotho accounted for 31 per cent of textiles exported to the United States. The IMF pinpointed the textile and clothing industry as the key engine of growth in Lesotho's economy. However, by December 2004, six textile factories had shut down, resulting in the loss of more than 6,000 jobs; some estimates put the job losses as high as 22,000. The decrease in demand was blamed on the WTO's trade liberalization agenda and the expiry of the Multi-Fibre Agreement (MFA), which regulated the textile trade, and the resulting increase in Chinese imports.

quotas. It put in place conditionalities for the African countries to qualify and calls for them to adhere to the Washington consensus principles, remove all barriers to trade, and refrain from activities that undermine US security in the war on terrorism.

The EU is also negotiating free trade agreements with African countries, referred to as economic partnership agreements (EPAs) under the auspices of the Cotonou Partnership Agreement.[2] Since 2002 when EPA negotiations were launched formally in Brussels, the negotiating parties (African, Caribbean, and Pacific [ACP] countries on one hand and the EU on the other hand) had been given a deadline by the WTO of December 31, 2007, to bring their trade relations into conformity with the institution's norms (Equinet and Southern and Eastern African Trade Information and Negotiations Institute (SEATINI) 2007). A new trade pact should have been signed and operational by January 1, 2008. However, technical and political hurdles have stood in the way of concluding a full EPA. Consequently, most of the countries have only initialled interim EPAs that cover trade in goods with the EU and provide for negotiations on other issues, including services and intellectual property. Negotiations took place amid serious divisions between the EU and the Eastern and Southern African countries, especially on what development means.

These trade pacts, together with the policies of the IMF and World Bank, force developing countries under the sanctions-bearing authority of the WTO that can discipline countries through the Dispute Settlement Body. There seems to be a fight between the major trading partners (EU, US, and most recently China) for markets in developing countries. And Africa remains the sleeping giant that can provide the market for mass-produced goods and services (see Table 8.2).

2 From about 1975 to 2000, trade and other economic relations between the EU and ACP countries were governed by the Lomé convention. The Lomé trade regime provided preferential access to the EU market for ACP countries, covering a wide range of export products subject to certain restrictions relating to the so-called "sensitive" products and rules of origin. The EU's future trade policy towards the ACP group beyond the Lomé trade regime was articulated in various proposals leading to the ACP-EU Cotonou Partnership Agreement signed in the Benin Republic in 2000. This 20-year agreement is meant to be a comprehensive arrangement governing aid and trade relations between the EU and ACP countries. It indicates the commitment of the parties to negotiate EPAs compatible with the WTO, starting in 2002. Negotiations are continuing.

Table 8.2 World Trade Organization Dispute Settlement Body

It is expected that differences arise in the context of international trade. WTO statutes make room for dispute resolution via the Dispute Settlement Body. This body is made up of members of the General Council, usually the ambassadors of WTO members in Geneva, where the WTO is based.

It is expected that differences arise in the context of international trade. WTO statutes make room for dispute resolution via the Dispute Settlement Body. This body is made up of members of the General Council, usually the ambassadors of WTO members in Geneva, where the WTO is based.

The Dispute Settlement Body uses a consultation process as the first step in conflict resolution; thereafter, in the absence of an agreement, member states take each other through the argumentative phase. More than 460 claims have been brought before the WTO since its inception in 1995, compared to the 300 cases brought before the GATT between 1947 and 1994. there have thus been many more disputes, and the figure will continue to rise. Ironically, the WTO sees this trend as indicative of growing confidence in the system.

Benin and Chad attempted to use the dispute settlement procedure, although rather than initiate a complaint they piggy-backed onto a claim brought by Brazil against the US's use of subsidies in cotton production. The African countries derived nothing of substance from this adventure, because the WTO ruled that as third parties they only had procedural rights. Benin and Chad had claimed that US cotton subsidies were ruining their economies by depressing world cotton farmers. The WTO unfortunately accepted the evidence produced by Benin and Chad of farmers' suffering caused by these subsidies as proof that Brazilian farmers were suffering. So the involvement of Benin and Chad only added substance to the Brazilian cotton producers' claims of injury. Whether the WTO was correct on this ruling remains a question for further work.

Source: Based on Elijah Munyuki, Rangarirai Machemedze, and Helene Bank (2005).

Trade Agreements and the Governance of Health

Health is fundamental to the development of a state. A healthy state is a productive state. The current state of the health sector in Southern African countries is deplorable. The sector is confronted by challenges ranging from inadequate infrastructure (hospitals, clinics, and bedding), underfunded services, inadequate health workers due to migration to high income countries and generally low annual intake of trainees, expensive and unavailable drugs, and the transfer of health service provision from governments and local authorities into the hands of the private sector (see Table 8.3). While these challenges broadly represent common problems in almost all countries, the last two problems are serious ones that affect access to universal equitable health services. They are compounded by the global trade policies signed on to by African governments, namely the WTO agreements as shown below.

Table 8.3 Medical Institutions in Zimbabwe, 1991–96

	1991	1992	1993	1994	1995	1996
Central hospital	4	6	6	6	6	5
General hospital	7	7	7	7	7	7
Maternity hospital	–	6	3	3	3	3
District hospital	41	37	37	37	37	34
Rural hospital	58	57	58	58	58	59
Private hospital	14	175	204	204	204	209
Special facilities	6	10	11	11	11	13
Church-related hospital/clinic	97	120	126	126	126	128
State clinic	–	377	370	370	370	349
Provincial clinic	–	452	451	451	451	497
Municipal clinic	–	102	105	105	105	102
Number of beds	18,612	16,574	16,231	16,886	18,160	22,975
Number of maternity beds	–	3,206	2,888	2,980	3,763	4,120
Number of beds per 10,000 people	19	19	18	18	18	23

Source: Elijah Munyuki and Shorai Jasi (2009).
Note: This table shows a remarkable growth in private hospital facilities from 1991 to 1996. The rapid expansion of private sector healthcare facilities is in sharp contrast with the static and negative performance in the public health sector institutions. It could be argued that the cuts in public expenditure, which were part of the structural reform program, play a role in the decline of public health facilities.

The WTO's agreements are premised on an architecture different from that of the IMF, World Bank, or UN organizations. Its agreements are legally binding, making it one of the most powerful institutions. Acceding to WTO agreements means a country must domesticate or change its national laws in order to comply.

Balancing trade rules and the need to ensure access to public health services has always been challenging in the current global economic architecture. Table 8.4 illustrates the differing nature of trade policy objectives on the one hand and public health policy objectives on the other. With objectives at such variance, achieving health sovereignty becomes more important and should be a priority for any country's plans for development.

Table 8.4 Trade Policy Objectives versus Health Policy Objectives

Trade Policy Objectives	Health Policy Objectives
Economic growth and capital	Improved population health
Efficient allocation of resources	Equitable allocation of resources
Eliminate barriers to free trade	Control risks to health
International specialisation	Universal access to health services

Source: Equinet (2007).

General Agreement on Trade in Services

The GATS, which came into force in 1995, lays down rules to conduct and remove barriers to international trade in services (SEATINI and Equinet 2004). It applies to all services including transport, health, education, banking, insurance, and telecommunications. It is governed by the principles of most favoured nation and national treatment.

The removal of barriers to trade in services means that countries agree to liberalize their services sector and allow in foreign competitors, hence the proliferation of private health institutions in Southern Africa. WTO members are under no legal obligation to make commitments under the GATS agreement. Nevertheless, when a country commits health and health-related services under GATS, it makes specific obligations to liberalize the sector. Health services could have been spared from liberalization by the agreement, as it excludes services supplied in the exercise of governmental authority – either on a commercial basis or in competition with one or more service suppliers. Most health and health-related services in developing countries are provided by governments and local authorities, and, as such, should be excluded from the GATS mandate. The agreement, however, is not explicit enough on governmental services (especially public services) since it says services provided on a commercial basis or in competition with other service suppliers are covered by GATS (WTO 1994). This means any transactions that involve buying and selling services (including use of user fees) even at subsidized rates will be covered by GATS. Increasingly, most health services are provided by private entities as well (in competition with government in some cases) and therefore this exemption does not apply.

Moreover, social services including health have been liberalized under IMF/ World Bank structural adjustment programs (SAPs). Some countries (such as Malawi and Zambia) committed to liberalize their health sectors under GATS, perhaps to increase competition in the sector and hence improve service delivery. In practical terms, the results could be different. This alone highlights the tradability, openness to competition, and commercialization of the services sector. Hence health services are part of GATS (Kategekwa 2008).

Modes of Trade

The health sector is one of the fastest growing service sectors in the global economy. This is evidenced by the increased delivery of services across countries.

The GATS defines the modes through which services are supplied across countries. Table 8.5 below elucidates these cross border activities.

Table 8.5 GATS Modes of Supply

Mode	Meaning	Example
1: Cross-border trade (article I.2a)	trade takes place from the territory of country A into that of B	tele-medical advice; passing of information by means of post or e-mail
2: Consumption abroad (article I.2b)	services consumed by nationals of country A in country B where the service is supplied; services are supplied to the consumer outside the country of residence	consumers who cross borders to obtain medical treatment that might be less expensive or better than that available domestically; tourism
3 : Commercial presence (article I.2c)	service supplier of country A crosses the border to establish presence and provide a service in country B	establishment of a private hospital by a European company in an African country
4: Movement of natural persons (article I.2d)	persons from country A stay temporarily in country B in order to supply a service	doctors and other medical specialists who practise abroad temporarily

Source: SEATINI (2004).

Impact of GATS on Health Governance

Under the WTO services negotiations, developing countries have been under pressure to liberalize their services sector including health. Moreover, most governments find it increasingly difficult to provide health services due to supply side constraints.

Where governments have liberalized the health sector especially under SAPs, the results have been disastrous. User fees and price increases in health services through cost-recovery programs resulted in a decline in the use of medical services in most developing countries, particularly in Kenya, Ghana, and Zimbabwe (SEATINI and Equinet 2004). In South Africa at the end of the 1990s the Kwazulu-Natal provincial government took steps towards privatization by charging rural residents for water. Thousands of poor households could not afford it and began using nearby rivers and stagnant ponds. Cholera broke out in August 2000 and by the following April 181 people had died (WHO 2001a). Critics argue that healthcare services tend to be of better quality in privately controlled clinics and hospitals than in their government counterparts. Those who can afford private health care will be forced to leave the country to seek it elsewhere. But because of prevailing poverty in Southern African countries and the costs of privately delivered health services, very few people can afford health care, as illustrated by the South African case.

GATS has many implications for health governance. The privatization of basic health services means the transfer of control of basic services from national governments to private providers, especially big national and international corporations. GATS takes away what little access the poor women, men, and children have to basic services and resources, and separates those who can pay for services from those who cannot. It leads to deepening poverty and increased discrimination and social exclusion of women and marginalized communities, as well as the destruction of the environment. The privatization of basic services is an abdication of responsibility by all levels of governments and a surrender to national and international corporations and private providers that do not recognize social responsibility or accountability to people and communities.

However, proponents of privatization argue that there are numerous benefits of placing health service delivery in the hands of private enterprise. These benefits include the provision of high-quality health care, including specialized services, with the best trained health personnel. They also argue that competition from private hospitals enhances quality and reduces costs.

Trade-Related Aspects of Intellectual Property Rights

The TRIPS Agreement was brought under the WTO under pressure by industrialized countries (Correa 2000). The scope and coverage of the agreement make it the most comprehensive international instrument on intellectual property rights. The agreement sets out minimum standards in the field of intellectual property and covers five broad areas: how basic principles of the trading system and other international intellectual property agreements should be applied, how to give adequate protection to intellectual property rights, how countries should enforce those rights adequately in their own territories, how to settle disputes on intellectual property between members of the WTO, and special transitional arrangements during the period when the new system is being introduced (WTO 2013). Members must comply with these standards by modifying their national regulations.

Intellectual property rights were brought onto the WTO agenda because of two major technological revolutions in the industrialized countries, namely information technology and biotechnology (Machemedze 2003). With developed countries having a huge competitive edge over developing countries in these technologies, they wanted to secure economic incentives as rewards for their innovations and the time they spend on research and development (R&D). This created serious problems, especially for developing countries that are afflicted by diseases and other health-related crises. Pharmaceutical companies, through the TRIPS Agreement, have patented drugs and other medicines essential for public health, leading to high economic and social costs especially for African countries, notably on antiretroviral drugs. Patent protection of pharmaceutical products and process inventions is granted for a minimum period of 20 years (WTO 2013). As soon as the agreement comes into force in a member, unauthorized copies of patented drugs are prohibited. Countries that break this rule will incur trade sanctions through the Dispute Settlement Body (Mugambe 2002).

While the need to increase access to medicines in poor countries was accepted, the means of doing so was disputed. Consequently, the Declaration on the TRIPS Agreement and Public Health was issued at the WTO ministerial conference in Doha in 2001.

The Doha Declaration on the TRIPS Agreement and Public Health

The Doha Declaration was considered a milestone in the move toward balancing drug companies' need for economic rewards with developing countries' need for increased access to medicines. The declaration gave countries the authority to use the flexibilities provided in the TRIPS Agreement in the interest of public health. These included giving transition periods for laws to comply with the TRIPS Agreement; providing for compulsory licensing or the right to grant a license, without permission from the license/patent holder, on various grounds including public health; providing for parallel importation or the right to import products patented in one country from another country where the price is lower; and providing for early testing (known as the Bolar provision) allowing generic producers to obtain health authority approvals before a patent expires, so cheaper generic drugs can be made available more quickly at that time (WHO 2001b).

Although the declaration was a positive step toward ensuring access to drugs by poor countries, a number of constraints and technical hurdles arose. For example, paragraph 6 of the declaration recognized that while developing countries have the right to issue compulsory licences, they faced difficulties due to their lack of manufacturing capacity in the pharmaceutical industry. The WTO's TRIPS Council was mandated to find an expeditious solution by late 2002. It was not easy to do so, however, as sharp differences emanated, especially between the EU and the US on one hand and developing countries on the other. But a solution was found in 2003. In 2005 WTO members agreed to permanently amend the TRIPS Agreement once two-thirds of them had agreed. As of December 31, 2013, 49 members (including the EU) of the 159 members had formally accepted the amendment of the TRIPS Agreement.

Other constraints include insufficient technical and infrastructural capacities for medicines regulations, bilateral, and other pressure not to use the TRIPS flexibilities for public health purposes, difficulties in regulating anti-competitive practices and abuse of patent rights, and difficulties in accessing pricing and patent status information.

Impact on Health Governance

As WHO (2013e) states, "health sovereignty is the exercise of a state's sovereign power to protect and promote health and provide health services". Besides the conventional problems that countries face in meeting health standards for their citizens, their capacity to provide health services is also eroded by trade policies imposed by other countries.

The TRIPS Agreement usurps the power of governments to provide health services, especially drugs, and puts it in the hands of individual transnational corporations that have the R&D capacity to manufacture drugs. The TRIPS Agreement has facilitated and exacerbated public health crises in developing countries, particularly because of the high prices, scarcity, and the commodification of drugs.

A classic example of the challenge of intellectual property regarding access to medicines is the recent case reported in South Africa where the Innovative Pharmaceutical Association of South Africa is working on a plan to challenge the draft national policy gazetted by the South African government in September 2013. The draft provides for the "compulsory licensing of crucial drugs at the lower of two typical rates of payment" (allowing "the state to assign the right to make a drug to a third party with only limited compensation to the owner"), the parallel importation of drugs, and the ability of "holders of intellectual property to protect their own rights rather than rely on state institutions" (De Wet 2014).

Despite such challenges as presented by the South African case, developing countries should implement laws to use TRIPS flexibilities to their full advantage, protect indigenous knowledge, resist "WTO plus" obligations in bilateral or regional agreements, monitor drug prices, and consider the local or regional production of drugs. In their trade negotiations, developing countries should demand the capacity to develop and enhance pharmaceutical drug production, including technology transfer from developed countries.

Conclusion

Social progress has slowed since the days of SAPs and privatization policies under the IMF, World Bank and the WTO. The attainment of the Millennium Development Goals and universal access to treatment requires an investment in rights and quality public services. This goal is proving difficult to achieve as the health sector in most Southern African countries is collapsing. This situation calls for further negotiation on WTO rules with a view of rebalancing them to allow millions of people in developing countries access to affordable health services.

The protests at WTO meetings in Seattle in 1999, Cancun in 2002 and Hong Kong in 2005 were a manifestation of the global problems associated with a trading regime that had not yet fully taken into account the development dimension of trade as a means to achieving development and not an end in itself. Thus the WTO incited social movements to protest because of the sheer impact it had in causing misery and displacement of people. As this chapter has shown, health governance under the WTO is left to the dictates and vagaries of the market with GATS and the TRIPS Agreement restricting access to health services by most people in developing countries. Under such circumstances, the WTO cannot be trusted to deliver on health as governments or local authorities would do.

However, if governments can implement the flexibilities contained within GATS and the TRIPS Agreement, then this damage may be minimized the damage. A long-term solution lies with the reform of the WTO itself by balancing the rules and ensuring that all countries are adequately represented and protected. The reform process should also consider the structural problems that exist in Southern African countries that must be addressed before economies can be opened up.

References

Correa, Carlos M. (2000). *Intellectual Property Rights, the WTO, and Developing Countries: The TRIPS Agreement and Policy Options.* London: Zed Books.

De Wet, Phillip (2014). "Big Pharma's 'Satanic' Plot Is Genocide, Mtsoaledi Rages". Mail and Guardian, January 17. http://mg.co.za/article/2014-01-16-motsoaledi-big-pharmas-satanic-plot-is-genocide (January 2014).

Economist (2008). "Redisigning Global Finance". November 13. http://www.economist.com/node/12599261 (October 2013).

Equinet (2007). "Reclaiming the Resources for Health: A Regional Analysis of Equity in Health in East and Southern Africa". Harare. http://www.equinetafrica.

org/bibl/docs/EQUINET%20Reclaiming%20the%20Resources%20for%20 Health%20in%20ESA.pdf (October 2013).

Equinet and Southern and Eastern African Trade Information and Negotiations Institute (SEATINI) (2007). "Trade and Health in East and Southern Africa". Policy Series No. 18, July, Equinet, Harare. http://www.equinetafrica.org/bibl/docs/POLBRIEF18%20trade.pdf (October 2013).

Kategekwa, Joy (2008). "Liberalization of Trade in Health Services: Balancing Mode 4 Interests with Obligations to Provide Universal Access to Basic Services". July, South Centre. http://www.southcentre.int/wp-content/uploads/2013/05/RP16_Liberalization-of-Trade-in-Health-Services_EN.pdf (October 2013).

Kaubab, Rashid (2005). *Benchmarking Development for Hong Kong and Beyond: Strengthening Africa in World Trade*. Harare: Southern and Eastern African Trade Information and Negotiations Institute (SEATINI).

Krueger, Anne O. (1998). "Introduction". In *The WTO as an International Organization*, Anne O. Krueger, ed. Chicago: University of Chicago Press.

Machemedze, Rangarirai (2003). "Trade Related Aspects of Intellectual Property Rights (TRIPs Agreement)". Fact Sheet. http://www.seatini.org/publications/factsheets/trips.htm (October 2013).

Mugambe, Lydia (2002). The Exceptions to Patent Rights under the WTO-TRIPS Agreement: Where Is the Right to Health Guaranteed?, LLM thesis, Community Law Centre, University of the Western Cape, Cape Town.

Munyuki, Elijah and Shorai Jasi (2009). "Capital Flows in the Health Care Sector in Zimbabwe: Trends and Implications for the Health System". Discussion Paper 79, August, Equinet, Harare. http://www.equinetafrica.org/bibl/docs/DIS79pppMUNYUKI.pdf (October 2013).

Munyuki, Elijah, Rangarirai Machemedze, and Helene Bank (2005). "WTO Systems and Processes: Making People Understand the Impact". Issue 1, Occasional Paper Series, Southern African People's Solidarity Network.

Raja, Kanaga (2010). "Trade: Concerns over Financial Crisis Surface at TNC Meeting". October 22, Third World Network. http://www.twnside.org.sg/title2/wto.info/twninfo20081010.htm (October 2013).

Southern and Eastern African Trade Information and Negotiations Institute (SEATINI) and Equinet (2004). "The WTO Global Agreement on Trade in Services (GATS) and Health Equity in Southern Africa". Policy Paper No. 12, February. http://www.equinetafrica.org/bibl/docs/POL12trade.pdf (October 2013).

Stuckler, David, Sanjay Basu, and Martin McKee (2011). "Global Health Philanthropy and Institutional Relationships: How Should Conflicts of Interest Be Addressed?" *PLoS Medicine* 8(4). doi: 10.1371/journal.pmed.1001020.

Tandon, Yash (2003). "Are There Alternatives To Neo-Liberalism? Yes There Are". Southern African and Eastern African Trade Information and Negotiations Institute (SEATINI). http://www.seatini.org/publications/epas/AlternativesToNeoliberalism.htm (October 2013).

United Nations Development Programme (2003). *Making Global Trade Work for People*. New York: Earthscan.

World Bank (2005). "Meeting the Challenge of Africa's Development: A World Bank Group Action Plan". Washington DC. http://siteresources.worldbank.org/INTAFRICA/Resources/aap_final.pdf (October 2013).

World Health Organization (2001a). "Cholera in South Africa". Geneva, April 17. http://www.who.int/csr/don/2001_04_17/en/index.html (October 2013).

World Health Organization (2001b). "Globalization, TRIPS, and Access to Pharmaceuticals". WHO Policy Perspectives on Medicines, No. 3, Geneva. http://apps.who.int/medicinedocs/en/d/Js2240e/ (October 2013).

World Health Organization (2011). "WHO Reform for a Healthy Future". July 20, Geneva. http://www.who.int/dg/reform/en_who_reform_overview.pdf (October 2013).

World Health Organization (2013a). "Trade, Foreign Policy, Diplomacy, and Health: Sovereignty". Geneva. http://www.who.int/trade/glossary/story082/en/index.html (October 2013).

World Health Organization (2013b). "WHO Reform". Geneva. http://www.who.int/about/who_reform/en/ (October 2013).

World Trade Organization (1994). *The Results of the Uruguay Round of Multilateral Trade Negotiations: The Legal Texts*. Geneva: General Agreement on Tariffs and Trade.

World Trade Organization (2007). "World Trade Report 2007". Geneva. http://www.wto.org/english/res_e/booksp_e/anrep_e/world_trade_report07_e.pdf (October 2013).

World Trade Organization (2013). "Intellectual Property: Protection and Enforcement". Geneva. http://www.wto.org/english/thewto_e/whatis_e/tif_e/agrm7_e.htm (October 2013).

Chapter 9

G8 Health Governance for Africa

John J. Kirton, Jenilee Guebert and Julia Kulik[1]

The Challenge

Africa's health challenges are unlike those of any other region in many critical ways. Africans face the highest maternal, newborn, and child mortality rates in the world (World Health Organization [WHO] 2013g). HIV/AIDS affects more than half of the population in several countries. Of all the deaths from malaria in 2012, 90 per cent were in Africa, mostly among children under the age of five (WHO 2013h). Many people lack easy access to clean water and adequate sanitation. The limited health systems and health workers in Africa cannot cope with the burden. There are only 2.5 physicians, nine nurses and midwives, and fewer than one dentist or pharmacist per 10,000 people (WHO 2013g).

Health challenges in Africa are disproportionately high due to the multiple movements spurred by globalization. These include the transborder spread of infectious diseases, particularly the big three of HIV/AIDS, tuberculosis, and malaria (Besada 2009). They also include the migration of already scarce health workers, and inadequate and ineffective health systems (Cooper et al. 2013). They extend to the growing burden of noncommunicable diseases (NCDs). Famine, lack of clean water, inadequate sanitation, limited education, corruption, climate change, and stifled economic growth compound these health challenges.

The Group of Eight (G8) major market democracies has increasingly addressed these issues at its annual summit, with varying degrees of success (Cooper 2013). Its leaders have long looked outward from health challenges in their own countries to focus on those in developing countries, in Africa above all. Infectious diseases, struggling health systems, and the social determinants of health in developing countries, as opposed to the NCDs and the particular pandemics that have significantly affected their own citizens, have usually been G8 members' primary concern. Until very recently, G8 summits have become a central global forum for governing health, Africa, and the combination of the two. Since the G8 first addressed malnutrition in developing countries in 1979 and famine and disease in Africa more specifically in 1985, the issues of health

1 This chapter draws and builds on the early analysis of G8 health governance presented in John Kirton and Jenevieve Mannell (2007) in *Governing Global Health: Challenge, Response, Innovation*, edited by Andrew F. Cooper, John J. Kirton, and Ted Schrecker. The authors gratefully acknowledge the contribution of Jenevieve Mannell.

and of Africa have increasingly overlapped and received growing G8 attention, particularly since 2000 when the Global Fund to Fight HIV/AIDS, Tuberculosis, and Malaria was conceived.

In the twenty-first century, Africa has regularly been a high priority on the G8's health agenda. At the 2000 Okinawa Summit, African leaders were invited to participate on the margins of the summit for the first time (Kirton and Takase 2002). At the 2001 Genoa Summit, where the Global Fund was born, African leaders attended the summit itself. At the 2002 Kananaskis Summit, health in Africa was a key theme, as leaders gave African development priority placement and highlighted many of the health challenges that the region faced. The 2005 Gleneagles Summit, following the Kananaskis model, put African development as a top priority and highlighted the big three infectious diseases. At the 2006 St. Petersburg Summit, health was chosen, for the first time ever, as a priority theme. And at the 2010 summit, the Muskoka Initiative for Maternal, Newborn and Child Health was launched as the signature deliverable. Only from 2011 to 2013 did the G8's direct attention to Africa's health decline and almost disappear, as the related issues of nutrition, food, and agriculture assumed centre stage on the G8's African agenda.

G8 outreach to involve African leaders at G8 summits has become customary since 2000. As newly democratic African partners increasingly identified with the core G8 principles of open democracy, individual liberty, and social advance, their relationship with G8 members has developed into a multistakeholder approach appropriate to combating the new generation of disease. The G8 has also worked with a growing number of major multilateral organizations to govern Africans' health.

Competing Assessments

Assessments of the G8's health performance both overall and in regard to Africa have given rise to a vigorous debate among several competing schools of thought (Kirton and Mannell 2007).

In regard to health in Africa, the first school suggests that the G8 has done much harm (Labonté et al. 2004; Lewis 2005; Schrecker et al. 2007). It has not just been unsuccessful in governing health in and for Africa, but has contributed to further disease and death there. Economic growth has continued to trump all other issues at the G8, leading to continual setbacks in Africa. Any commitments to improve health in the region are overridden by economic interests and perhaps an implicit racist attitude on the part of the G8.

The second school sees limited advance (Aginam 2005, 2007). It argues that the G8 may have helped spur a few global health advances for Africa. But it claims that, on the whole, the G8 has had no major impact on the continent.

The third school sees steady improvement due to the high level of specialized capabilities that the G8 members bring (Price-Smith 2002). It claims that G8

African health governance has steadily improved, as its technical and economic capacity puts it in a better position than most other governors.

The fourth school emphasizes the remaining gaps, including in delivering the decisions it has made (Kirton et al. 2007; Kirton and Kokotsis 2007; Kirton and Guebert 2009b). It argues that the G8 has not fully comprehended what needs to be done. The G8 should thus focus on how it can generate better outcomes in Africa.

The fifth school suggests that the Group of 20 (G20) is superior to the G8, due to the G20's broader, more diverse membership (Chand et al. 2010; Bradford 2007; Evans 2004). The G20 would thus be more effective than the G8 at governing Africa's health. The G20's broader membership covers a larger percentage of the globe. It includes as equal members more countries, particularly the non-G8 members, including South Africa, that struggle from the global health challenges that the G8 has addressed inadequately.

A sixth school suggests a partnership between the G8 and G20 (Kirton and Guebert 2009b). It claims this would enhance global health governance in Africa and elsewhere.

The Argument

This chapter argues that the G8 had, until 2011, a solid, generally strengthening performance in governing African's health. Since 1979, it addressed this area increasingly and more effectively, acknowledging the link between health and development in Africa in ever more ways. From its first deliberation on global health for development in 1979, the G8 moved through a more direct and specific focus on Africa, starting in 1985, to a concrete commitment to improve the health of South Africans in 1991.[2] In 2001, it began to include African leaders regularly as invited participants at its summit. G8 health governance for Africa became an increasingly integral part of the agenda through to 2010. The G8 addressed and advanced a growing number and range of health issues, including those that involved the transborder movement brought by globalization, such as the migration of health workers and the escalating spread of disease. It encouraged the exchange of information, cooperation, and coordination of regulation between sovereign states and among national, regional, and international institutions. However, it showed limited innovation in its conception of sovereignty, despite its foundational anti-Westphalian institutional mission of intervening in the internal affairs of sovereign states to advance the principles of open democracy, individual liberty, and social advance.

This pattern was evident in the decade beginning in 2000, especially in the summits in 2002, 2005, 2006, 2008, and 2010, where health governance in Africa became a critical component of the agenda and overall achievements. Several key

2 Throughout this chapter there are references to the documents issued by the leaders at their annual summits. These documents can be found on the G8 Information Centre website at http://www.g8.utoronto.ca/summit.

summits highlighted both how health in Africa benefited from the G8's work and the governance gaps that remained. However, from 2011 to 2013 health largely disappeared from G8 governance, beyond the nutrition and accountability domains (Kirton and Kulik 2012; Guebert 2012).

The G8's growth as an effective African health governor and the gaps that have remained in meeting the real need can largely be explained by those causes assembled in the concert equality model of G8 governance (Kirton 1989, 1993). The first and most powerful cause has been the increasingly equal vulnerability of each G8 member to a new generation of infectious diseases, starting with HIV/AIDS, arising in Africa and spreading at an unprecedented speed and scope as globalization intensified. Only after the tide turned on HIV/AIDS in 2010 did G8 governance of Africans' health drastically decline.

Second, the old organizations of the United Nations system, led by the World Health Organization (WHO), failed to control these infectious diseases, led by HIV/AIDS, that afflicted Africa and G8 members. After 2010, due to the G8's push, the UN itself seemed on track to advance this and the other two health Millennium Development Goals (MDGs) – those on maternal, newborn, and child health.

Third, with their globally predominant and internally equalizing capabilities, G8 members collectively had the resources, recognition of their responsibility, and burden-sharing formula to provide the needed large-scale response, especially through official development assistance (ODA). After 2010 a rapidly growing Africa appeared able to bear more of the burden itself.

Fourth, G8 members were able and willing to contribute, given their expanding politically commonality with a democratizing Africa. The latter allowed for greater access and confidence that their investments would be effectively deployed. After 2010, G8 attention was diverted to the dramatic democratic revolution in North Africa and the Middle East.

Fifth, the rising political control, capital, continuity, professional competence, and personal conviction of G8 leaders, led by the faith-based commitment of America's George W. Bush, Britain's Tony Blair, and Canada's Stephen Harper, furthered the G8 push. Also important was civil society support and pressure, which became especially active after the early 2000s through to 2010.

Sixth, the constricted, controlled participation at the summit, with the five leaders of major African countries regularly attending since 2001 saw them increasingly act as equals with G8 leaders. Together they pushed a broad range of African development priorities, including health, in a common cause within an interpersonal G8-Africa club, with a new group of African personal representatives in support.

An Overview of G8 African Health Performance

The G8's solid and strengthening performance in advancing Africans' health and the 2010–13 drop is seen in the G8's record across six dimensions of governance (see Appendix 9-A).

Domestic Political Management

On the first dimension, domestic political management, G8 African health performance has been mixed. Leaders have increasingly received attention and approval from their domestic constituents and civil society advocates for the G8's attention to and achievements here. In 2005, Tony Blair received virtually unanimous approval from his domestic media by the end of his 2005 Gleneagles Summit for its action on African development and health (Kirton 2005). However, nongovernmental organizations (NGOs) tend to be critical of the G8, claiming that it does not do enough to help the poorest and most vulnerable, who have been exploited for economic gains. Campaigns highlighted what still needed to be done.

The Muskoka Initiative on Maternal, Newborn, and Child Health, the centrepiece achievement of the 2010 summit, secured strong public support thanks to its large focus and impact on Africa. There was only limited criticism from NGOs, mass media, and mass public opinion.

Deliberation

The second dimension, deliberation, refers to the G8's choice to discuss specific issues and help set the global agenda as a result (see Appendix 9-B). The summit began to address Africans' health indirectly in 1979, just five years after the leaders began meeting. It alluded to the suffering of people in the Horn of Africa due to famine by emphasizing the need to assist developing countries in overcoming malnutrition. In 1985, the summit directly recognized the specific struggles of African peoples due to famine and committed to work with developing countries to fight disease. In 1991, the G8 offered humanitarian assistance to countries in Africa that were still suffering from famine and its related diseases (see Appendix 9-B).

Yet attention to Africa's health remained intermittent and minimal until the post-Cold War 1996 summit in Lyon, France. There the leaders focused on infectious diseases, especially the impact of HIV/AIDS in Africa. At the 1997 Denver Summit, Africa received its own section in the communiqué. Focused on development, it acknowledged the link between development and health. The 1998 Birmingham Summit gave substantial attention, too.

At the dawn of the twenty-first century, at the 2000 Okinawa Summit, African health received significant attention, as the G8 committed to fight infectious diseases, particularly HIV/AIDS, tuberculosis, and malaria. The 2001 Genoa Summit created the Global Fund to do so. It also acknowledged the food insecurity of sub-Saharan Africa and supported related international relief efforts. Its

"Genoa Plan for Africa" emphasized the need to encourage human development by investing in health, tackling HIV/AIDS, tuberculosis, and malaria, and improving education.

At the 2002 Kananaskis Summit, the G8 introduced its G8 Africa Action Plan, which contained a specific section on improving health and confronting HIV/AIDS. Here the G8 committed to improve health systems, promote the availability of medicines, and support health research. At Gleneagles in 2005, the G8 again paid particular attention to Africa, with a focus on debt relief, aid, trade, and HIV/AIDS. Its communiqué acknowledged a lack of progress in meeting the MDGs.

At the 2007 Heiligendamm Summit, attention to African health reached an all-time high (see Appendix 9-B). It appeared first in the chair's summary where G8 leaders acknowledged the importance of their partnership with African leaders and the heads of the African Union (AU) and New Partnership for African Development (NEPAD), with a particular emphasis on improving health systems and fighting HIV/AIDS, tuberculosis, and malaria. The bulk of the G8's attention came in a separately issued document entitled "Growth and Responsibility in Africa" with a specific section on combating infectious diseases.

African health appeared in a significant, but less substantial, way at the 2010 Muskoka Summit. Here leaders mounted their initiative on maternal, newborn, and child health (MNCH) and reaffirmed their commitment to meeting the MDGs. References to Africa were made in relation to these two goals, as progress globally depended on progress in Africa.

From 2011 to 2013, however, attention to health virtually disappeared. In 2011 there was a reference to the partnership between the G8 and Africa in ensuring accountability on health and food security. In 2013, leaders referred to the good progress made in supporting maternal and child health, particularly in Africa. The new thrust was on food and nutrition, without any link to health.

Direction Setting

On the third dimension, direction setting through affirming principles and norms, African health became a priority principle for the G8 only in 2002, when G8 leaders issued a chair's statement containing only the subjects that the leaders actually discussed (see Appendix 9-A). At the 2005 Gleneagles Summit, health in Africa was given a prominent place. The G8's twenty-first century priority principles centred on the need for more funding, research, international cooperation, and accessible, affordable medicines for Africa in the fight against HIV/AIDS, polio, malaria, tuberculosis, and severe acute respiratory syndrome (SARS), as well as on healthcare reform within the G8. While there was a hint that health for the poor would trump trade, until the 2004 Sea Island Summit after the 2003 SARS outbreak, there was no recognition of health as a security issue or health as a human right (Labonté et al. 2004, 226).

St. Petersburg in 2006 stood out for its affirmation of the centrality of democratic values such as openness, transparency, information exchange, monitoring, surveillance, reporting, ethics, and civil society participation as vital causes of health promotion in the new era of fast-moving, globalized, infectious disease. The chair's summary issued at the 2007 Heiligendamm Summit highlighted the need to achieve the MDGs in Africa. In 2008 the G8 acknowledged the role that better health would play in promoting development in Africa. Health thus became a cause of development in a health-first approach, even if this approach did not expand to a whole-of-government or whole-of-society health for development vision. African health received priority placement in G8 documents for the last time in 2009, when reference was made to supporting financing instruments for health in Africa (see Appendix 9-A).

Decision Making

On the fourth dimension, decision making, G8 leaders made 254 health commitments overall. Most, including general commitments on infectious diseases, implicitly addressed health in Africa, with 58 explicitly dealing with Africa. In addition, the G8 made 33 commitments in other issue areas that contained references to both health and Africa.

The first explicit commitment on health in Africa came at the dawn of the post-Cold War era, at the 1991 London Summit (see Appendix 9-A). Similar commitments came in 1997 and 2001. At the 2002 Kananaskis Summit, every health commitment was made with Africa in mind.

In 2003 the Evian Health Action Plan stated that the leaders "welcome" and "support" initiatives pertaining to HIV/AIDS (G8 2003a). It also made a strong commitment on policy change or resources in providing developing countries with access to essential medicines, vaccine development, and fighting polio. It mobilized $500 million for polio eradication, representing the first financial commitment on health since the establishment of the Global Fund. In 2007, leaders made 12 health commitments on Africa, including those to combat infectious disease, increase access to affordable medicines, and establish sustainable health systems.

From 2011 to 2013 the G8 made no commitments in health or non-health issue areas that referred to Africa and health.

Delivery

The fifth dimension is the members' delivery of summit decisions before the next summit. Here, the G8's compliance with health-related commitments in general (including Africa-related ones) has been high (see Appendix 9-C). Between 1983 and 2012 the G8 complied well with the 56 health commitments that have been assessed by the G8 Research Group, of the total 254 the G8 has made. The average compliance score was +0.51, which is roughly three quarters of the way up the scientific scale. (Compliance is measured on a scale of −1 for failure to comply, 0 for a work in progress, and +1 for full compliance.) Compliance rose steadily in the later years. It was higher when health commitments were given priority placement in the communiqué's opening chapeau or in the chair's summary and came with precise timelines and specific targets (Kirton and Kokotsis 2007; Kirton et al. 2007; Kirton et al. 2009). Of the 10 specific African health commitments assessed, however, the G8's average compliance score was a low +0.20 (see Appendix 9-A).

In 2002 the G8 leaders complied modestly with their African health-related commitments, with a score of +0.5, above the summit average of +0.35 (see Appendices A and D). They pledged to increase the overall effectiveness of the Global Fund and its operations. Within the framework of both the G8 Africa Action Plan and NEPAD, the G8 committed to increase Africa's access to the Global Fund as well as African participation in it. While no new funds were committed, this fostered a new approach to global health, with Africa at its core.

At Sea Island in 2004 compliance with health commitments affecting Africa rose. Although the number of commitments decreased slightly from 2003, leaders committed to eradicating polio by 2005 and to take the necessary steps toward the development of an HIV vaccine through the establishment of the Global HIV Vaccine Enterprise. The enterprise would upgrade research laboratories in Africa, train African scientists, and ensure measures for equitable vaccine access. The G8 delivered a compliance score of +0.56 on this commitment (see Appendix 9-C). In regards to their commitment to financing the gap for polio eradication, the leaders complied at a level of +0.44, falling short by about $50 million in funding.

In 2005, G8 leaders agreed to boost investment and take action to combat HIV/AIDS, malaria, tuberculosis, and other deadly diseases through 18 health-related African commitments. They committed to mobilize $50 billion in aid to Africa, a new deal on trade, the cancellation of debt, and to provide universal access to AIDS treatment by 2010. In addition, the leaders committed to replenish the Global Fund and to support the Polio Eradication Initiative. However, compliance was modest, as the commitment on the Global Fund replenishment scored +0.33 and polio eradication +0.11 (see Appendix 9-C).

In 2007, G8 members' health compliance averaged a high +0.72 (see Appendix 9-C). Individual G8 members brought their own particular values regarding health in Africa, which partially accounted for the high compliance. France often placed the issue of HIV/AIDS at the forefront of its summit objectives; the G8's acknowledgement of the resources needed to meet its goal of universal access and the commitments to a Global Fund replenishment conference thus secured France's support. As a historically strong supporter of the Global Fund, Canada's objective was for the G8 to acknowledge the extent of the HIV/AIDS epidemic as well as renew pledges to the Global Fund; Canada achieved both these goals.

In 2010 compliance with health commitments slipped. The three assessed commitments received an average compliance of only –0.08 (see Appendix 9-C). In them the G8 had promised increased funding for MNCH initiatives, progress on reaching universal access to treatment for HIV/AIDS, and the control and elimination of neglected tropical diseases.

In 2011, the G8 secured a low health compliance of –0.11 with a health commitment to improve MNCH through the Muskoka Initiative. However, it received full compliance on a commitment to protect public health and consumer safety by exchanging information on rogue internet pharmacy sites.

Development of Global Governance

On the sixth dimension, the development of global governance, the G8 had a solid if sporadic performance on Africans' health, by building relevant institutions both inside and outside the G8 (see Appendix 9-A). Within the G8 there was one meeting of health ministers, hosted by Russia in 2006. In addition, the Global Health Security Initiative, containing all G8 members except Russia but with Mexico, began work in 2001. Yet several official-level health bodies were created, starting in 1987 on HIV/AIDS. At Kananaskis in 2002, the Africa Action Plan endorsed "supporting relevant public-private partnerships for the immunization of children and the elimination of micro-nutrient deficiencies in Africa" (G8 2002). Since 2002 no institutions have been created that relate directly to both Africa and health. However, the G8 has consistently engaged with ministerial and official-level bodies both inside and outside of the G8. The most common engagement has been with the G8 health ministers and the UN, WHO, the Global Fund, and the multilateral development banks.

The G8 also actively developed global governance related to African's health outside the G8. It did so above all in response to the prevalence of HIV/AIDS.

Critical Cases in G8 African Health Governance

This strengthening of G8 governance for Africans' health through to 2010 can be further charted by examining more closely the individual summits where the greatest advances were made.

1975–99

At Tokyo in 1979, health first appeared on the G8 agenda and in such a way that Africa was the key concern. The leaders noted the developing countries' struggle to overcome hunger and malnutrition, the latter constituting a direct reference to health. At Venice in 1980, leaders reiterated their concern for the "hundreds of millions of people of developing countries" suffering from chronic malnutrition (G7 1980).[3]

3 Russia only became a full member in 1998; before that the leaders of Canada, France, Germany, Japan, Italy, the United States, the United Kingdom, and the European Union met as the Group of Seven (G7).

Leaders first focused on health in Africa in 1985, when famines were ravaging the continent. At Venice in 1987 they first recognized that the new disease of AIDS was one of the biggest problems in the world. In the "Chairman's Statement on AIDS", Italian Prime Minister Amintore Fanfani noted that international cooperation was necessary to prevent the further spread of AIDS (G7 1987). WHO was identified as "best forum for drawing together international efforts on a worldwide level to combat AIDS" and all countries were encouraged "to cooperate with the WHO and support its special program of AIDS-related activities" (G7 1987). Summit leaders also decided to create their own International Ethics Committee on AIDS, which first met in 1989.

At London in 1991, leaders reiterated their support to fight famine in Africa. They also committed to working with South Africa to improve the health of its citizens. This was the first time the G7/8 promised to assist a specific African country on health.

At Lyon in 1996, the G8's attention to health and Africa grew. Health was identified under its own heading for the first time and the leaders launched the New Global Partnership for Development. They noted that "infectious diseases such as HIV/AIDS, malaria, cholera, ebola, and antibiotic resistant strains of tuberculosis and pneumonia pose an unacceptable threat to people of all nations, disproportionately affecting the populations of the poorest nations" (G7 1996). They endorsed the creation and implementation of mechanisms to aid in the prevention, detection, surveillance, and response to the emergence/re-emergence of infectious diseases. They stressed that they would continue to extend assistance programs, in particular for the benefit of the countries hardest hit by HIV/AIDS and other infectious diseases. They thus started the long and lasting process of linking health and development. They also encouraged cooperation on joint projects, particularly in Africa, as well as Southeast Asia, Latin America, and the Caribbean, through the transfer of expertise on surveillance, prevention, research, diagnosis, and treatment of diseases.

At Denver in 1997, the Group of Seven (G7) focused on working with Africa, particularly sub-Saharan Africa, for development. Leaders promised to ensure African citizens had adequate health care. At Birmingham in 1998, leaders emphasized making globalization work for Africa. The leaders committed to "drastically" reduce child and maternal mortality (G8 1998).

2000 Okinawa

At Okinawa in 2000, G8 leaders recognized that infectious diseases, particularly HIV/AIDS, tuberculosis, and malaria, were major killers and obstacles to escaping poverty (Bayne 2005). The World Bank had declared AIDS to be a development crisis. Shortly before the Okinawa Summit, the UN held its annual international AIDS conference in Durban, South Africa. Its resounding message was that there was a dire need for increased spending on HIV/AIDS in order to provide the most basic care and prevention in sub-Saharan Africa.

Thus, the G8 made infectious disease a major issue. For the first time, an African outreach event was held in the lead-up to the summit. The leaders of Japan, France, Canada, the United Kingdom, and Italy met with leaders from South Africa, Nigeria, Algeria, and Thailand, as well as representatives of the World Bank, WHO, UN Development Programme, and the business community. Health and development were the major themes discussed (Japan, Ministry of Foreign Affairs 2000).

At Okinawa, G8 leaders made the boldest, most ambitious heath commitments to date, including to reduce the number of HIV/AIDS infected people by 25 per cent by 2010, reduce tuberculosis deaths and prevalence by 50 per cent by 2010, and reduce the burden of disease associated with malaria by 50 per cent by 2010. They discussed creating a fund to combat AIDS, malaria, and tuberculosis (G8 2005a). Japan and the United States supported its establishment but most European members were not ready to commit.

2001 Genoa

At Genoa in 2001, the G8 fully endorsed the creation of the Global Fund to Fight AIDS, Tuberculosis, and Malaria. G8 leaders mobilized $1.3 billion for the fund. Non-member countries, foundations, academic institutions, and the private sector were encouraged to contribute to establish the Global Fund as a public-private partnership.

Leaders from South Africa, Nigeria, Algeria, and Senegal participated in the G8 summit itself. The G8 worked with NEPAD to establish the Genoa Plan for Action in Africa. The leader of each G8 member appointed an African personal representative to recommend specific actions that should be taken to, inter alia, improve the health and welfare of Africans.

2002 Kananaskis

At Kananaskis in 2002, the G8 launched the Africa Action Plan to solidify the G8's partnership with Africa. The plan set a strategy to address a wide range of African health challenges. It included improving health standards, debt relief contingent on African countries using the freed-up resources to improve their health systems; continuing the fight against HIV/AIDS, tuberculosis, and malaria, as well as rarer diseases such as river blindness; strengthening health systems and making them sustainable; recruiting and training health professionals; eliminating micronutrient deficiencies; and working to provide access to affordable medicines.

Leaders from South Africa, Nigeria, Senegal, and Algeria again participated, now for a longer time. They were joined by UN secretary general Kofi Annan. Efforts were made to listen to what the African leaders wanted the G8 to do, as opposed to the G8 simply dictating what would be done. This approach was reflected in the final commitments (Kirton and Guebert 2009b).

2003 Evian and 2004 Sea Island

In 2003 and 2004 the Iraq war, the SARS crisis, and a focus on the Middle East diverted the leaders' attention from Africans' health. However, health more broadly remained on the agenda and African participation in the summits expanded. In 2003, the now familiar four leaders of Algeria, Nigeria, South Africa, and Senegal were joined by the Egyptian president and the king of Morocco as chair of the Group of 77, a coalition of developing countries. In 2004, US president George Bush invited the leaders of South Africa, Nigeria, Algeria, Senegal, Ghana, and Uganda to Sea Island.

G8 leaders made several commitments that implicitly addressed Africa. They included reaffirming support for the Global Fund, strengthening healthcare systems, making access to medicines and vaccine more affordable, improving research on diseases mostly affecting developing countries and eradicating polio.

2005 Gleneagles

At Gleneagles in 2005 African health was addressed as robustly and explicitly as it had been at Kananaskis. G8 leaders discussed the major infectious killer diseases in Africa, and the importance of providing free basic health care for all. The number of attending Africans leaders increased as South Africa, Nigeria, Algeria, Senegal, and now Ethiopia, Ghana, and Tanzania came.

G8 leaders ambitiously agreed to secure universal access to treatment for HIV/AIDS sufferers by 2010, an advance on their commitment in 2000 to reduce the prevalence by 25 per cent by 2010. They acknowledged how far behind they were in achieving the MDGs, particularly in Africa. They committed to support African strategies to improve health and create an environment in Africa where health workers and other capable citizens would want to stay. They added commitments to reduce mortality, improve health systems, train health workers, develop a vaccine centre in Africa, and improve the ability African agricultural and food producers to meet health and safety standards. They raised more money for global health than ever before.

The leaders also addressed accountability, taking stock of where they were in reaching their past African health commitments. They included country-specific information on how they would achieve their future commitments in an annex to their statement on Africa.

2006 St. Petersburg

At St. Petersburg in 2006, the first summit hosted by Russia, health as a whole was a priority theme for the first time. In its preparations, Russia had begun with a wide-ranging and ambitious program for the control of infectious diseases, including HIV/AIDS, tuberculosis, malaria, polio, emerging diseases, and avian influenza. The program embraced G8 measures to strengthen global information and analysis monitoring networks for infectious diseases, the prevention and mitigation of epidemiological consequences of natural disasters (such as the shocks of the hurricanes that had ravaged a vulnerable United States in late summer 2005, as well as the Asian tsunami and Pakistani earthquake), and scientific exchanges to study infectious disease agents.

The summit had the smallest African delegation since 2000. Only the leaders of South Africa and the Congo, which was president of the AU, attended. Also present were the heads of the UN and the World Bank, as well as the WHO, represented at the summit for the first time.

The leaders committed to work with Africa to prevent the spread of infectious disease, address inadequate heath systems, stop the outflow of qualified healthcare workers, and improve nutrition. An annex identified the funding and projects that each country would provide, including bilateral and multilateral aid to Africa for health initiatives.

2007 Heiligendamm

At Heiligendamm in 2007, African development was one of two priority themes. Health was a key component. Leaders sought to deal with "urgent problems in Africa relating to economic development, poverty reduction, and the fight against HIV/AIDS", and to expand their relationship with Africa through a partnership for reform (German Presidency of the G8 2006). The G8 sought continuity with its past policies on Africa. Leaders committed to strengthen healthcare systems in Africa, to combat infectious diseases and to work more closely with African governments, international organizations, and the private sector for a more effective approach.

African outreach was much more robust. Leaders from South Africa, Nigeria, Senegal, Algeria, Egypt, Ghana, Ethiopia, and the AU came. Heads of the UN, the World Bank, and the Organisation for Economic Co-operation and Development (OECD) also participated.

2008 Hokkaido-Toyako

At Hokkaido-Toyako in 2008, the Japanese host used its fourth Tokyo International Conference on African Development as a starting point for the G8's discussions on African health. Leaders focused on children's access to basic healthcare services, the shortage of healthcare workers, the importance of clean water and sanitation, and neglected tropical diseases.

Leaders from South Africa, Nigeria, Senegal, Algeria, Ethiopia, Ghana, Tanzania, and the AU attended. The heads of the UN and the World Bank participated. Health was not as prominent on the agenda as had been originally intended, due to rapidly rising food prices in the months leading up to the summit. As a result of this food shock, much of the leaders' attention was diverted to food security.

2009 L'Aquila

At L'Aquila in 2009, G8 leaders reaffirmed their pledge to step up efforts to achieve the MDGs, particularly on child and maternal health in Africa, where progress had fallen the furthest behind. They noted the importance of Africans' role in finding solutions to African health problems and highlighted the African Leaders Malaria Alliance as success in this regard. They committed to strengthening their partnership with Africa. With the current global economic crisis in mind, they supported innovative financing mechanisms for health.

On accountability the G8 health experts group released a 165-page report at the summit, noting past actions that the G8 had taken and what still needed to be done. The report fell short of specifically noting which G8 countries had kept which G8 health commitments their leaders had made.

Leaders from South Africa, Nigeria, Senegal, Algeria, Egypt, Angola, Ethiopia, Libya, and the AU attended. The heads of the UN, World Bank, and the OECD participated, as did the heads of the Food and Agriculture Organization, the World Food Programme, and the International Fund for Agricultural Development.

2010 Muskoka

At Muskoka in 2010, the G8's overall agenda was less ambitious than it had been in the past. Amid the ongoing global economic crisis, leaders were competing and cooperating with the G20 summit that was taking place nearby immediately following the G8 one (Kirton 2013). However, with the G20 now governing economic issues, more time was left for the G8 to focus on African health.

Leaders from South Africa, Nigeria, Senegal, Algeria, Egypt, Ethiopia, and Malawi attended. However, no international organizations were present, for the first time since 1999. African outreach thus remained a much more robust part of the G8 than the G20.

The Muskoka Initiative on Maternal, Newborn, and Child Health was the major achievement. The leaders, along with several outsiders, promised $7.3 billion for the initiative between 2010 and 2015. They also agreed to train medical professionals, to strengthen health innovation networks in Africa, and to do more to reach the MDGs, particularly in Africa where progress was still far behind. Leaders welcomed Africa's increased involvement in the development process and promised to continue to work with Africa for a more prosperous future.

In the lead-up to the summit, G8 leaders had met with African leaders and leaders from the Americas for the first time. This was important as many of the commitments made were targeted at countries such as Malawi, Sudan, and Tanzania, among other African states. The Muskoka Initiative included strengthening monitoring, reporting, and evaluation; building on cost-effective, evidence-based interventions; supporting country-led national health policies and plans that were locally important; and improving accountability. The accountability component was emphasized by the production of the *Muskoka Accountability Report*, which took stock of the G8's recent commitments on development, assessed its performance, and identified lessons for future reporting.

2011 Deauville, 2012 Camp David, and 2013 Lough Erne

Attention to health declined dramatically at Deauville in 2011. It virtually disappeared at Camp David in 2012 and Lough Erne in 2013, even as Africa was featured in the new, related G8 priority of agriculture, food, and nutrition.

Causes of G8 African Health Performance

This strengthening G8 performance on African health especially since 2000 and the plunge from 2011 to 2013 were driven by the six causes identified in the concert equality model of G8 governance, added by a growing push from civil society from 2000 to 2010.

Shock-Activated Vulnerability

The first cause is shock-activated vulnerability, a specific or series of sudden, surprising events or external forces in the same or similar issue area that shocks G8 members into realizing their vulnerabilities and responding through the G8 to protect themselves. At a second level it includes chronic, cumulative harms that reach a catalytic tipping point. Such shocks can also create a societal and state awareness of common, comprehensible harms to humanity that activate the sense of oneness that virtually all humans share (Linklater 2007).

The first health-related shock was the distant Ethiopian famine that dominated media coverage in G8 members in 1984–85. The second, more chronic shock was the rise in AIDS cases and public anxiety, which directly afflicted G8 members with disease and death at home (Kirton and Mannell 2007). The 1987 summit thus introduced AIDS and infectious disease into the leaders' documents. The chair's statement highlighted the vulnerability felt by the leaders by speaking of the severity of the disease and addressing the general panic by calling for increases in public education and asking the medical community for further studies for prevention and treatment. In 1987, HIV/AIDS was perceived as an issue requiring immediate G7 attention, being the only infectious disease the leaders discussed prior to Denver in 1997. The shock of this initial vulnerability, rapidly spreading equally among all G7 members, brought AIDS onto the agenda. HIV/AIDS was mentioned only once more at the summits before 1996. But during the 1990s the physical assault of HIV/AIDS on all G7 members grew. The number of new cases per year peaked for the United States in 1993, France in 1994, Italy and Canada in 1995, and Germany in 1996 (Kirton and Mannell 2007, 127). With a majority of G7 members so severely afflicted by 1996, HIV/AIDS returned to the summit agenda in a major way and left only after 2010.

In 1996 the G7 summit added the equally mysterious outbreak disease of Ebola from Africa, as well as the merely chronic and exotic ones (in G7 countries) of malaria, tuberculosis, cholera, and pneumonia. This broadening was consistent with the new fact and fear that intensifying demographic globalization was bringing the old diseases still prevalent in poorer countries into a long secure G7. At the same time, where fact and familiarity were high, fear was low, and the continuous chronic burden came with no catalytic tipping point, the G7/8 left the diseases alone. Deadly chronic diseases such as cancer and heart disease, which accounted for significant deaths in G7 members, received almost no attention at the summits.

The disease burden of developing countries had profound impacts on their economic capacity and therefore ability to improve their situation. According to WHO, "analysis of data from thirty-one African countries during the period 1980 to 1995 showed that the annual loss of economic growth due to malaria has been as high as 1.3% per year" (Brundtland 2000). For G8 members – the primary providers of ODA – this presented an economic as well as a healthcare burden.

The post-1996 period was defined by a more external focus, one that addressed a fully international health agenda with the introduction of diseases primarily affecting the developing world. This was epitomized by Ebola, which affected people in Africa. This period saw a drastic improvement in the summits' performance, beginning with the introduction of global health at Lyon. Lyon had four health commitments overall, when previously only a single health commitment at a summit had been made. However, health performance did not consistently improve from one summit to the next. Only a few summits stood out during this time of high health performance. And there were few shocks or chronic tipping points to drive the performance surge on MNCH in 2010.

The absence of shocks helps explain the decline and disappearance of African health from the G8 agenda from 2011 to 2013. From 2011 to 2013, vulnerability to the core HIV/AIDS disease had dwindled among G8 members, and no new intrusive health shocks from distant Africa, similar to SARS from Asia, had arisen to take its place. Indeed, the dominant health shocks came from nearby neighbours, such as the swine influenza that instantly affected the United States and Canada from Mexico (Kirton and Guebert 2010). Moreover, within Africa itself, on the HIV/AIDS pandemic, the tide had turned (Mayaki and Sidibé 2013). More generally, the global financial crisis of 2008–12 reduced the mobility-enhancing globalization and openness that had increased G8 members' exposure to Africa on many fronts, while aging populations within the G8 demanded the diversion of health dollars to rising needs at home.

Multilateral Organizational Failure

The second cause of the G8's growing health governance until 2011 is the poor performance of the old organizations of the UN system, led by the WHO, in response to this proliferation of shock-activated vulnerability from the new diseases from Africa (Cooper 1989; Howard 1989; Zacher 1999; Kirton 2009; Renganathan 2013; Blouin et al. 2013).

The years from 1987 to 2009 saw a growing failure of WHO, in coping with rapidly rising new diseases led by HIV/AIDS and the older, pervasive health challenges such as maternal and child health. Responsibility thus shifted to the broader UN system and the World Bank, culminating in the creation of the three health-related MDGs (4, 5, and 6) at the UN's Millennium Summit in 2000.

With infection rates of HIV/AIDS exceeding 40 million worldwide and threatening a new pandemic across Eurasia, by 2000 it became clear that no international institution was doing enough (Kirton and Mannell 2007). WHO in particular had received widespread criticism both from within the organization and from the larger international community. Those within the UN system also recognized that its own internal failures in handling the crisis contributed in part to its severity: "we have to admit that the way global targets were set is not conducive to success simply because the HIV pandemic was acknowledged but not internalized" (Vandemoortele 2003). In an overt display of its lack of confidence in WHO's handling of the AIDS crisis as early as 1993, the UN had taken the Global Programme for AIDS, which was WHO's largest program, out of the WHO's sole control (Godlee 1994, 7). It created UNAIDS instead. Yet the UN itself then had also failed (Lewis 2005, 155). Thus HIV/AIDS became part of the MDGs in 2000.

Despite a review conference in 2005, the UN was unable to convince members to move adequately to meet the health MDGs, leading to the G8 picking up the cause. At Gleneagles in 2005, G8 leaders addressed the lack of progress on the MDGs. They paid particular attention to boosting investment in health and education in Africa and taking action against HIV/AIDS, tuberculosis, and malaria.

The Muskoka Initiative in 2010 arose when the failure to meet or make progress on the two relevant UN MDGs was becoming urgent. The Muskoka Summit took place at the two-thirds mark for meeting the internationally agreed-upon goals by their due date in 2015. Partly in an effort to make progress on MDGs 4 and 5, the G8 leaders agreed to adopt the initiative. They worked in close cooperation with the UN, through to its MDG summit in September 2010 and the Commission on Information and Accountability for Women's and Children's Health created there. With the success of the UN summit in mobilizing an announced $40 billion for MNCH, the G8 then turned its attention to challenges other than African health.

Moreover, new informal, plurilateral institutions arose to govern global health, and ones in which Africa through South Africa was a full, equal member from the start. The G20 summit's indirect health agenda took off, with a focus on the MDGs and the addition of NCDs through its Seoul Development Consensus and its implementing bodies launched at the Seoul Summit in November 2010. The BRICS summit of Brazil, Russia, India, China, and South Africa, born in 2009 and adding South Africa at its Delhi Summit in March 2012, addressed a vibrant health agenda, with new ministerial and official bodies to back it up (Kulik 2013).

Predominant Equalizing Capabilities

The third cause of growing G8 health governance until 2011 is the globally predominant and internally equalizing capability of the members of the group. In sharp contrast to the limited autonomous capacity of the old multilateral organizations' bureaucracies, especially in African countries themselves, the G8 countries increasingly possessed in their own societies and states the globally dominant share of the overall and specialized capabilities required to combat Africa's diseases (see Appendix 9-E). These were shared among G8 members in a way that enabled and required all to contribute, through collective action, in a materially meaningful way.

There is a correlation between high G8 health performance and an increase in the global predominance and internal equality of the G8 members' specialized capabilities (as demonstrated by each country's annual healthcare budget, the number of health facilities, and similar indicators). The G8's global predominance is highlighted by a comparison of G8 healthcare spending and the healthcare capacity of the developing world. After 2010, however, with Africa's overall growth rising and the strengthening of its health systems in several ways, the G8's capabilities could be – and were – shifted elsewhere.

Shifts in relative capability also caused the G8 to lose its traditional global predominance, even if its internal equalization remained. The American-turned-global financial crisis of 2008 and the Eurocrisis erupting in 2010 reduced the G8's collective capabilities relative to the more resilient, rapidly recovering, and previously faster growing emerging economies assembled as equals in the G20 and the BRICS. And Africa itself was rapidly becoming a richer continent, fuelling a view that Africa's health problems could be increasingly left to African governments, regional organizations, and other African actors themselves (Kaberuka 2013). This was especially the case as the financial-economic crisis, and the emphasis on austerity that the G8 and G20 adopted in June 2010, reduced budgets for ODA and broader external financial support in G8 members. This made the G8, as British Prime Minister David Cameron (2013) put in designing his Lough Erne Summit in June 2013, unwilling to succeed by having G8 leaders "whip out a chequebook at the 11th hour" to donate to a particular, high-profile, good global cause. The Muskoka MNCH model was thus explicitly repudiated by December 2010.

Common Principles of Open Democratic Health

The fourth cause is the G8's common principles of open democracy, individual liberty, and social advance and the growing attachment of consequential African countries to these principles as well. These core values increasingly brought G8 members ideologically closer to their new rapidly democratizing African and most outreach partners, which were now embracing democratic development, especially as the twenty-first century began. Together they made it easy for the G8 to move beyond national sovereignty frames into the openness and transparency needed to protect human security both at home and in the African source of the central diseases. These common values also fuelled the functionally appropriate, multistakeholder approaches most appropriate to combat the new generation of disease. Thus the movement bred by globalization and the resulting cadence of openness leading to an awareness of oneness increasing trumped the traditional premium on national sovereignty and security that divided G8 countries and Africa into a separated "us" and "them".

After 2010 the G8's democratic commonality with sub-Saharan Africa was also diminished relatively in a global context. While Africa's democratization remained largely intact, despite setbacks in Mali and elsewhere, G8 attention was diverted to the new democratic revolution erupting in North Africa and the Middle East with the advent of the Arab spring in the spring of 2011 and then the Deauville Partnership that the G8 launched in response. Further afield, the political opening in Myanmar provided another diversionary pull.

Political Cohesion

The fifth cause is domestic political cohesion – the G8 leaders' political control, capital, continuity, competence, conviction, and civil society pressure. From 2001 to 2005, the period when the G8's performance took off, high political control at home by the popularly elected G8 leaders allowed the same seven individuals to come to an unprecedented five summits in a row. This consistency encouraged a sustained, iterative, and expanding treatment of African health over half a decade, as continuity generated experience, self-confidence, a sense of responsibility and accountability, and a determination to get the job done (Bayne 1999).

In 1998 the newly elected Tony Blair as G8 host brought the Rollback Malaria Partnership to the summit. But Birmingham did little to further G8 health governance as a whole. In general, the peaks in G8 African health performance came during the secure years between elections or at the end of a leader's final term. In 2000 the particularly significant peak in health performance came as US president Bill Clinton attended his last summit and the unelected Japanese Prime Minister Yoshiro Mori hosted his first. Clinton's desire for a legacy and an all-encompassing effort domestically and internationally to push forward the agenda items on which he had previously been holding off for the sake of popular support drove summit progress, even if the actual birth of the Global Fund had to wait until Genoa the next year. The 2002 Kananaskis Summit's high deliberation and decision making coincided with the leadership of Jean Chrétien, attending the summit for the tenth time and hosting it for the second. The 2004 Sea Island Summit's focused deliberation and decreased decision making came as host George Bush was entering a very tight electoral race for his second term later that same year and needed to be seen as conservative as well as effective in his commitments.

In 2005, with a committed Tony Blair hosting his second summit, after eight years of summit experience and having just received his third majority mandate at home, many gains on African health were made. From the United States, a re-elected George Bush helped as well (Helleiner and Cameron 2006). In 2006, while there were several new leaders, domestic publics across the G8 picked infectious disease as the second most popular issue they wanted the summit to address, with those in the United States and Canada putting it in first place, and those in Russia, France, and Britain in second spot (Global Markets Institute 2006).

The role of civil society in pushing the G8 to address African health had been increasing since 1998 and especially since the early 2000s (Hajnal 1999, 2002). Since the beginning of the HIV pandemic in the early 1980s, civil society had encouraged G8 governments to commit more resources to address HIV/AIDS and other infectious diseases. It consistently represented the needs of marginalized groups and extended prevention services to hard-to-reach communities. Through grassroots advocacy campaigns, civil society organizations eventually led to an international commitment to fight HIV/AIDS. The first substantial instance of the impact of civil society was through Jubilee 2000 at the Birmingham Summit and then, NGOs more broadly in the formation of the Global Fund at both the 2000 and 2001 summits.

In 2005, there was intense involvement of civil society in the lead-up to the Gleneagles Summit (Baruchel and Dasilva 2005). The most prominent coalition was the Global Call to Action Against Poverty (GCAP), which was a world-wide alliance of existing coalitions, civil society organizations, NGOs, trade unions, faith-based groups, individuals, and other campaigners. Among GCAP's largest members were Action Aid, Amnesty International, CIVICUS, Oxfam, Red Cross, UNICEF, World Vision, and World Wildlife Fund. Its objectives were to eliminate poverty and achieve the MDGs. In the final communiqué, the G8 leaders at Gleneagles agreed to one of the demands of civil society, affirming that the G8 would double aid for Africa by 2010.

During the discussions leading up to the 2010 Muskoka Summit, civil society was present in full force behind the scenes (Steiner 2012a, 2012b). A coalition of NGOs dedicated to the health and welfare of children – led by World Vision, Save the Children, and Plan Canada – met with Canadian G8 officials as early as the summer of 2008 to discuss Canada's agenda for the summit. After discussions and deliberations, Harper announced that the Muskoka Initiative would be the main issue for the summit. On June 26, 2010, Canada and the other G8 members plus organizations such as the Bill and Melinda Gates Foundation and the UN Foundation pledged a total of $5 billion toward maternal, newborn, and child health. This achievement surprised many observers as the Harper government had not indicated global health in general or MNCH in particular as a main priority in earlier years. Civil society organizations were thus important in making MNCH the centrepiece in 2010. They were the primary reason for Harper's financial commitment to the cause.

After Muskoka, the G8 leaders changed and civil society organizations focused on new issues, notably nutrition, food, and agriculture. Concurrently, G8 attention to Africans' health dropped. To be sure, US president Barack Obama and Germany's Angela Merkel remained with Stephen Harper at the summit table, with Obama and Harper having been re-elected comfortably. But they were joined by four newly or recently elected leaders: the UK's David Cameron (replacing Gordon Brown, the G8's most passionate campaigner against poverty), France's François Hollande in 2012 (who defeated Nicolas Sarkozy, the only G8 leader ever to have served as health minister), Italy's Mario Monti in 2012 and Enrico Letta in 2013, and Japan's Naoto Kan in 2011, Yoshihiko Noda, and Shinzo Abe in 2013. And throughout most of austerity-affected G8 members, public support for development and Africa slipped; in the United States it dipped to very low levels indeed.

The Constricted, Controlled Participation of the G8 Leaders' Club

The sixth cause is the constricted, controlled membership and participation in the G8 summit club. This allowed the same G8 leaders to meet face to face, annually, and, increasingly as equals, with the same four core African partners in the still constricted G8 club. It allowed them also reach out to other stakeholders at the ministerial and official levels below (Hajnal 1999).

Most directly, as both a cause and consequence of G8 leaders' concern with African health, the annual presence from 2001 to 2009 of the same four leaders of Africa's major democratic powers at the summit fuelled the take-off of G8 African health governance in the twenty-first century, particularly in its concentration on those diseases that were devastating Africa most. The same four leaders were joined since 2003 by other regulars, such as Ghana.

The assured participation of Africa's big four ended after the Muskoka Summit. Another trend began at the 2009 L'Aquila Summit, when a large number of leaders assembled to discuss food security on the last day. Starting in 2011 came an ad hoc, à la carte collection of African leaders, often from smaller countries, invited to discuss the particular non-health issues chosen by the G8 leaders.

The G8's constricted, controlled participation had altered, as invitations were now issued according to the priority of the moment rather than to the weighty regulars who had repeatedly come from Africa to discuss a broad agenda since 2001.

Conclusion

The G8 had a solid and generally strengthening performance in governing health for Africa beginning in 1979, increasing through to 1999, peaking from 2000 to 2010, and retreating back to its initial focus on malnutrition in 2011–13. Overall, G8 performance on health generally rapidly rose through to 2010. In the several instances in which G8 action on specific issues was more prominent, the most common target was Africa. The initial surges were seen on famine-related illnesses dating back to 1979. During the late 1980s the G8 became increasingly concerned about the impact of HIV/AIDS, especially due to its infectious nature. In the early 2000s the G8 made significant progress in identifying the linkages between development and health, particularly through its Africa Action Plan in 2002 and at the Gleneagles Summit in 2005. In 2010 the Muskoka Initiative on Maternal, Newborn, and Child Health again showed the G8's successful push for Africans' health.

Globalization has led to many challenges in governing global health, whether in terms of the spread of infectious disease, data sharing during pandemics, or food insecurity. In response, the G8 increasingly looked away from the Westphalian concept of sovereignty toward a global sovereignty where the world as a whole has a stake in Africa's health.

G8 governance for Africans' health, however, remains incomplete. G8 attention has dropped since 2011. Several regions in Africa still lag significantly in their health outcomes behind the rest of the developing world, particularly evident when measuring progress on the internationally agreed MDGs. While countries in Europe and Central Asia are on track either to meet or make significant progress on MDGs 4 and 5 on child and maternal health, sub-Saharan Africa has been less successful in reducing under-five and maternal mortality and malnutrition. The Muskoka Initiative, adopted by the G8 in 2010, was an attempt to accelerate progress in meeting targets that the other major multilateral institutions had left behind. It will take the same kind of commitment and focus that the G8 showed in Muskoka for the G8 to provide effective leadership for Africans' health as a whole, as the 2015 due date for the delivery of the MDGs arrives.

References

Aginam, Obijifor (2005). *Global Health Governance: International Law and Public Health in a Divided World.* Toronto: University of Toronto Press.

Aginam, Obijifor (2007). "Diplomatic Rhetoric or Rhetorical Diplomacy: The G8 and Global Health Governance". In *Governing Global Health: Challenge, Response, Innovation*, Andrew F. Cooper and John J. Kirton, eds. Aldershot: Ashgate, pp. 147–55.

Baruchel, Hanae and Steve Dasilva (2005). "Global Civil Society Action at the 2005 G8 Gleneagles Summit". G8 Research Group, Toronto. http://www.g8.utoronto.ca/evaluations/csed/csed2005.pdf (December 2013).

Bayne, Nicholas (1999). "Continuity and Leadership in an Age of Globalisation". In *The G8's Role in the New Millennium*, Michael R. Hodges, John J. Kirton, and Joseph P. Daniels, eds. Aldershot: Ashgate, pp. 21–44.

Bayne, Nicholas (2005). *Staying Together: The G8 Summit Confronts the 21st Century*. Aldershot: Ashgate.

Besada, Hany (2009). "Coming to Terms with Southern Africa's HIV/AIDS Epidemic". In *Innovation in Global Health Governance: Critical Cases*, Andrew F. Cooper and John J. Kirton, eds. Farnham: Ashgate, pp. 155–78.

Blouin, Chantal, Mark Pearcey, and Valerie Percival (2013). "Instruments for Global Health Diplomacy in the UN System Beyond the WHO". In *Global Health Diplomacy: Concepts, Issues, Actors, Instruments, Fora, and Cases*, Ilona Kickbusch, Graham Lister, Michaela Told, et al., eds. New York: Springer, pp. 199–212.

Bradford, Colin I. (2007). "Reaching the Millennium Development Goals". In *Governing Global Health: Challenge, Response, Innovation*, Andrew F. Cooper and John J. Kirton, eds. Aldershot: Ashgate, pp. 79–86.

Brundtland, Gro Harlem (2000). "Address at the Opening Dinner of the Massive Effort Advocacy Meeting". Winterthur, October 3. http://www.who.int/director-general/speeches/2000/english/20001003_massive_effort.html (December 2013).

Cameron, David (2013). "Prime Minister's Letter to G8 Leaders". London, January 2. http://www.g8.utoronto.ca/summit/2013lougherne/130102-cameron.html (December 2013).

Chand, Sudeep, J. Stephen Morrison, Peter Piot, et al. (2010, June 23). "From G8 to G20, Is Health Next in Line?" *Lancet*. Published online. http://c657621.r21.cf2.rackcdn.com/commissioners/lancetg8g20.pdf (January 2014).

Cooper, Andrew F. (2013). "The G8/G20 and Global Health Governance". In *Global Health Diplomacy: Concepts, Issues, Actors, Instruments, Fora, and Cases*, Ilona Kickbusch, Graham Lister, Michaela Told, et al., eds. New York: Springer, pp. 243–52.

Cooper, Andrew F., John J. Kirton, Franklyn Lisk, et al., eds. (2013). *Africa's Health Challenges: Sovereignty, Mobility of People, and Healthcare Governance*. Farnham: Ashgate.

Cooper, Richard N. (1989). "International Cooperation in Public Health as a Prologue to Macroeconomic Cooperation". In *Can Nations Agree? Issues in International Economic Cooperation*, Richard Cooper, Barry Eichengreen, Gerald Holtham, et al., eds. Washington DC: Brookings Institution, pp. 178–254.

Evans, Tim (2004). "The G20 and Global Public Health". Paper prepared for the conference on The G20 at Leaders' Level? organized by the International Development Research Centre, February 29, Ottawa. http://www.l20.org/publications/25_63_g20_ottawa_evans.pdf (January 2014).

G7 (1980). "Declaration". Venice, June 23. http://www.g8.utoronto.ca/summit/1980venice/communique (December 2013).

G7 (1987). "Chairman's Statement on AIDS". Venice, June 10. http://www.g8.utoronto.ca/summit/1987venice/aids.html (December 2013).

G7 (1996). "Chairman's Statement [Political Declaration]: Toward Greater Security and Stability in a More Cooperative World". June 29, Lyon. http://www.g8.utoronto.ca/summit/1996lyon/chair.html (December 2013).

G8 (1998). "Communiqué". Birmingham, May 15. http://www.g8.utoronto.ca/summit/1998birmingham/finalcom.htm (December 2013).

G8 (2002). "G8 Africa Action Plan". Kananaskis, June 27. http://www.g8.utoronto.ca/summit/2002kananaskis/africaplan.html (December 2013).

G8 (2003). "Health: A G8 Action Plan". Evian, June 2. http://www.g8.utoronto.ca/summit/2003evian/health_en.html (December 2013).

G8 (2005). "Africa". Gleneagles, July 8. http://www.g8.utoronto.ca/summit/2005gleneagles/africa.html (December 2013).

German Presidency of the G8 (2006). "Focuses of the G8 Presidency". October 18. http://www.g8.utoronto.ca/summit/2007heiligendamm/2007focus.html (December 2013).

Global Markets Institute (2006). "G8 Summit in St. Petersburg". Goldman Sachs, New York.

Godlee, Fiona (1994). "WHO in Retreat: Is It Losing Its Influence?" *British Medical Journal* 309(6967): 1491–5.

Guebert, Jenilee (2012). "Global Health at the G8: Integration, In Decline or Simply Stalled?" Global Health Governance (Blog). June 11. http://blogs.shu.edu/ghg/2012/06/11/global-health-at-the-g8-integration-in-decline-or-simply-stalled-jenilee-m-guebert/ (December 2013).

Hajnal, Peter I. (1999). *The G7/G8 System: Evolution, Role, and Documentation.* Aldershot: Ashgate.

Hajnal, Peter I., ed. (2002). *Civil Society in the Information Age*. Aldershot: Ashgate.

Helleiner, Eric and Geoffrey Cameron (2006). "Another World Order? The Bush Administration and HIPC Debt Cancellation". *New Political Economy* 11(1): 125–40. doi: 10.1080/13563460500494958.

Howard, Lee (1989). "The Evolution of Bilateral and Multilateral Cooperation for Health in Developing Countries". In *International Cooperation for Health: Problems, Prospects, and Priorities*, Michael R. Reich and Eiji Marui, eds. Dover MA: Auburn House.

Japan. Ministry of Foreign Affairs (2000). "Summit Meeting in Tokyo among President Olusegun Obasanjo of the Federal Republic of Nigeria, President Thabo Mbeki of the Republic of South Africa, President Abdelaziz Bouteflica of the Democratic People's Republic of Algeria, Prime Minister Chuan Leekpai of the Kingdom of Thailand and G8 Leaders". Tokyo, July 20. http://www.g8.utoronto.ca/summit/2000okinawa/devs.htm (December 2013).

Kaberuka, Donald (2013). "Africa Can Give the World the Economic Pulse It Needs". In *The Russia G20 Summit: St Petersburg 2013*, John J. Kirton and Madeline Koch, eds. London: Newsdesk, pp. 124–6. http://www.g8.utoronto.ca/newsdesk/stpetersburg.

Kirton, John J. (1989). "Contemporary Concert Diplomacy: The Seven-Power Summit and the Management of International Order". Paper presented at the annual convention of the International Studies Association, March 29–1 April, London. http://www.g8.utoronto.ca/scholar/kirton198901 (July 2010).

Kirton, John J. (1993). "The Seven Power Summits as a New Security Institution". In *Building a New Global Order: Emerging Trends in International Security*, David Dewitt, David Haglund, and John J. Kirton, eds. Toronto: Oxford University Press, pp. 335–57.

Kirton, John J. (2005). "Gleneagles G8 Boosts Blair at Home". Toronto, August 1. http://www.g8.utoronto.ca/evaluations/2005gleneagles/coverage.html (December 2013).

Kirton, John J., ed. (2009). *Global Health*. Farnham: Ashgate.

Kirton, John J. (2013) G20 Governance for a Globalized World. Farnham: Ashgate.

Kirton, John J. and Jenilee Guebert (2009). "Canada's G8 Global Health Diplomacy: Lessons for 2010". *Canadian Foreign Policy* 15(3): 85–105.

Kirton, John J. and Jenilee Guebert (2010). "North American Health Governance: Shocks, Summitry, and Societal Support". *Revista Norteamericana* 5(1): 221–44. http://www.scielo.org.mx/scielo.php?script=sci_arttext&pid=S1870-35502010000100008 (July 2012).

Kirton, John J. and Ella Kokotsis (2007). "Keeping Faith with Africa's Health: Catalysing G8 Compliance". In *Governing Global Health: Challenge, Response, Innovation*, Andrew F. Cooper, John J. Kirton, and Ted Schrecker, eds. Aldershot: Ashgate, pp. 157–80.

Kirton, John J. and Julia Kulik (2012). "A Summit of Significant Success: G20 Los Cabos Leaders Deliver the Desired Double Dividend". June 19. http://www.g20.utoronto.ca/analysis/120619-kirton-success.html (December 2013).

Kirton, John J. and Jenevieve Mannell (2007). "The G8 and Global Health Governance". In *Governing Global Health: Challenge, Response, Innovation*, Andrew F. Cooper, John J. Kirton, and Ted Schrecker, eds. Aldershot: Ashgate, pp. 115–46.

Kirton, John J., Nikolai Roudev, and Laura Sunderland (2007). "Making G8 Leaders Deliver: An Analysis of Compliance and Health Commitments, 1996–2006". *Bulletin of the World Health Organization* 85(3): 192–9.

Kirton, John J., Nikolai Roudev, Laura Sunderland, et al. (2009). "Explaining Compliance with G8 Leaders' Health Commitments, 1996–2006". In *Innovation in Global Health Governance: Critical Cases*, Andrew F. Cooper and John J. Kirton, eds. Farnham: Ashgate, pp. 257–84.

Kirton, John J. and Junichi Takase, eds. (2002). *New Directions in Global Political Governance: The G8 and International Order in the Twenty-First Century*. Aldershot: Ashgate.

Kulik, Julia (2013). "Reducing the Economic Burden of Non-communicable Diseases in the BRICS: Lessons from Brazil". January 25, BRICS Research Group, Toronto. http://www.brics.utoronto.ca/biblio/Kulik-NCDs-Brazil.html (December 2013).

Labonté, Ronald, Ted Schrecker, David Sanders, et al. (2004). *Fatal Indifference: The G8, Africa, and Global Health*. Ottawa: International Development Research Centre.

Lewis, Stephen (2005). *Race Against Time: Searching for Hope in AIDS-Ravaged Africa*. Toronto: House of Anansi.

Linklater, Andrew (2007). *Critical Theory and World Politics: Citizenship, Sovereignty, and Humanity*. Abdingdon: Routledge.

Mayaki, Ibrahim Assane and Michel Sidibé (2013). "Advancing the Africa-G8 Partnership: Towards an AIDS-Free Generation". In *The UK Summit: The G8 at Lough Erne 2013*, John J. Kirton and Madeline Koch, eds. London: Newsdesk, pp. 188–9. http://www.g8.utoronto.ca/newsdesk/stpetersburg.

Price-Smith, Andrew (2002). *The Health of Nations: Infectious Disease, Environmental Change, and Their Effects on National Security and Development*. Cambridge MA: MIT Press.

Renganathan, Elik (2013). "The World Health Organization as a Key Venue for Global Health Diplomacy". In *Global Health Diplomacy: Concepts, Issues, Actors, Instruments, Fora, and Cases*, Ilona Kickbusch, Graham Lister, Michaela Told, et al., eds. New York: Springer, pp. 173–87.

Schrecker, Ted, Ronald Labonté, and David Sanders (2007). "Breaking Faith with Africa: The G8 and Population Health". In *Governing Global Health: Challenge, Response, Innovation*, Andrew F. Cooper and John J. Kirton, eds. Aldershot: Ashgate, pp. 181–205.

Steiner, Sherrie (2012a). "Faith-Based Accountability Mechanism Typology". SAGE Open 2(2). doi: 10.1177/2158244012450705.

Steiner, Sherrie (2012b). "Religious Soft Power as Accountability Mechanism for Power in World Politics". *SAGE Open* 1(3). doi: 10.1177/2158244011428085.

Vandemoortele, Jan (2003). "The MDGs and Pro-Poor Policies: Can External Partners Make a Difference?", December, United Nations Development Programme, New York. http://depot.gdnet.org/gdnshare/pdf2/gdn_library/annual_conferences/fifth_annual_conference/vandemoortele_paper.pdf.

World Health Organization (2010). "World Health Statistics 2010". Geneva. http://www.who.int/entity/whosis/whostat/EN_WHS10_Full.pdf (January 2014).

World Health Organization (2013a). "World Health Statistics 2013". Geneva. http://www.who.int/gho/publications/world_health_statistics/EN_WHS2013_Full.pdf (January 2014).

World Health Organization (2013b). "World Malaria Report 2013". Geneva. http://www.who.int/malaria/publications/world_malaria_report_2013/report/en/index.html (December 2013).

Zacher, Mark W. (1999). "Global Epidemiological Surveillance: International Cooperation to Monitor Infectious Diseases". In *Global Public Goods: International Cooperation in the 21st Century*, Inge Kaul, Isabelle Grunberg, and Marc A. Stern, eds. New York: Oxford University Press for the United Nations Development Programme, pp. 266–83.

Appendix 9-A African Health Performance Chart, 1975–2013

	Deliberation	Direction Setting	Decision Making	Delivery	Development of Global Governance		Participation	
Summit	*# Words*	*# Paragraphs*	*Commitments*	*Compliance*	*In*	*Out*	*African*	*Other*
1975	0	0	0	N/A	0	0	0	0
1976	0	0	0	N/A	0	0	0	0
1977	0	0	0	N/A	0	0	0	0
1978	0	0	0	N/A	0	0	0	0
1979	0	0	0	N/A	0	0	0	0
1980	0	0	0	N/A	0	0	0	0
1981	0	0	0	N/A	0	0	0	0
1982	0	0	0	N/A	0	0	0	1
1983	0	0	0	N/A	0	0	0	0
1984	0	0	0	N/A	0	0	0	0
1985	17	0	(1)	N/M	0	0	0	0
1986	0	0	0	N/A	0	0	0	1
1987	0	0	0	N/A	0	0	0	1
1988	0	0	0	N/A	0	0	0	0
1989	0	0	0	N/A	0	0	5	10
1990	0	0	0	N/A	0	0	0	0
1991	98	0	1 (1)	N/M	0	1	0	1
1992	34	0	0	N/A	0	0	0	0
1993	0	0	0	N/A	0	0	0	1
1994	0	0	0	N/A	0	0	0	0
1995	0	0	0	N/A	0	0	0	0
1996	84	1	0	N/A	0	0	0	5
1997	86	0	1	0.0 (1)	0	0	0	1
1998	140	0	0	N/A	0	1	0	0
1999	0	0	0	N/A	0	0	0	0
2000	115	0	0	N/A	0	0	3	5
2001	350	0	1	N/M	0	4	5	7
2002	672	1	18 (11)	0.5 (1)	0	1	4	2
2003	586	2	(1)	N/M	2	4	4	13
2004	178	2	(1)	N/M	0	0	6	8
2005	1,718	2	11 (2)	0.22 (2)	3	8	3	9
2006	1,749	1	6	N/M	2	18	2	9
2007	2,556	3	12	0.63 (2)	6	30	2	10
2008	663	1	5 (12)	0.04 (3)	0	6	7	12
2009	1,009	2	2 (4)	0.56 (1)	1	16	8	19
2010	633	0	1	N/M	5	5	6	4
2011	44	0	0	N/A	1	2	8	2
2012	153	0	0	N/A	0	0	6	0
2013	73	0	0	N/A	0	0	6	1
Average	280.97	0.38	1.48 (0.85)	0.20	0.51	2.46	1.92	3.13

Notes:

Deliberation: the number of words in the paragraphs containing references to Africa and health and their cognate terms in each G8 summit's official document.

Direction Setting: the number of paragraphs in the G8 summit's chair's summary, chapeau, or preamble that contain references to Africa and health and their cognate terms.

Decision Making: the number of G8 commitments in the health issue area that refer to Africa and its cognate terms. Numbers in parentheses indicate commitments in other issue

areas that also refer to health and Africa or their cognate terms.
Delivery: compliance scores are measured on a scale from –1 to +1, with –1 indicating no compliance, 0 indicated work in progress, and +1 indicating full compliance. A commitment is fully complied with if a G8 member succeeds in achieving the specific goal set out in the commitment.
Development of Global Governance: the number of new African health-related G8 institutions created at internal and external levels at or by the summit, or during the hosting year, with at least one meeting take place during the hosting year.
Participation: African – the number of leaders from African countries invited to participate in official summit sessions, including representatives from the African Union; other – the number of leaders from non-member countries invited to participate in summit sessions, including representatives from international organizations.
N/A: not available; N/M: not measured.

Appendix 9-B G8 Conclusions on Health and Africa, 1975–2013

Year	# of Words	% of Total Words	# of Paragraphs	% of Total Paragraphs	# of Documents	% of Total Documents	# of Dedicated Documents
1975	0	0	0	0	0	0	0
1976	0	0	0	0	0	0	0
1977	0	0	0	0	0	0	0
1978	0	0	0	0	0	0	0
1979	0	0	0	0	0	0	0
1980	0	0	0	0	0	0	0
1981	0	0	0	0	0	0	0
1982	0	0	0	0	0	0	0
1983	0	0	0	0	0	0	0
1984	0	0	0	0	0	0	0
1985	17	.54	1	2.4	1	50	0
1986	0	0	0	0	0	0	0
1987	0	0	0	0	0	0	0
1988	0	0	0	0	0	0	0
1989	0	0	0	0	0	0	0
1990	0	0	0	0	0	0	0
1991	98	1.2	2	3.6	2	40	0
1992	34	.45	1	.60	1	25	0
1993	0	0	0	0	0	0	0
1994	0	0	0	0	0	0	0
1995	0	0	0	0	0	0	0
1996	84	.55	1	.48	1	20	0
1997	86	.66	1	.71	1	20	0
1998	140	2.3	1	1.7	1	25	0
1999	0	0	0	0	0	0	0
2000	115	.85	2	1.4	1	20	0
2001	350	5.6	6	8.2	2	29	0
2002	672	5.8	22	14	2	29	0
2003	586	3.5	8	4.8	3	20	0
2004	178	.57	3	.80	2	10	0
2005	1,718	8.7	30	13	4	27	0
2006	1,749	5.7	21	9.3	4	31	0
2007	2,556	8.9	19	7.1	3	38	0

Appendix 9-B continued

Year	# of Words	% of Total Words	# of Paragraphs	% of Total Paragraphs	# of Documents	% of Total Documents	# of Dedicated Documents
2008	663	4.1	4	2.5	2	20	0
2009	1,009	3.3	7	2.3	4	40	0
2010	633	8.8	5	9.4	2	100	0
2011	44	.30	1	.54	1	33	0
2012	153	4.2	1	2.5	1	50	0
2013	73	.54	1	.42	1	25	0
Average	280.9	1.7	3.5	2.2	1	16.7	0

Notes:
Data are drawn from all official English-language documents released by the G8 leaders as a group. Charts are excluded.
# of Words: the number of African health-related subjects for that year, excluding document titles and references. Words are calculated by paragraph because the paragraph is the unit of analysis.
% of Total Words: the total number of words in that year's documents.
# of Paragraphs: the number of paragraphs containing references to African health for that year. Each bullet point is recorded as a separate paragraph.
% of Total Paragraphs: the total number of paragraphs in all documents for that year.
# of Documents: the number of documents containing African health-related subjects, excluding dedicated documents.
% of Total Documents: the total number of documents for that year.
# of Dedicated Documents: the number of documents that contain a health-related subject in the title for that year.

Appendix 9-C G8 Health Compliance, 1983–2012

	Health	Canada	France	Germany	Italy	Japan	Russia	United Kingdom	United States	European Union	Average
1	1983	1			1				1		1.00
2	1997	1	1					1	1		1.00
3	1997	–1	–1	1	–1	0		1	1		0.00
4	1998	1	1	0	–1	0	–1	1	1	1	0.33
5	1998	1	1	–1	–1	–1	–1	1	1	1	0.11
6	1999	1	1	–1	1	1	0	1	1		0.63
7	1999	0	0	0	0	0	0	0	0		0.00
8	2000	1	1	1	1	1		1	1	1	1.00
9	2000	1		0	0	1	0		0	1	0.43
10	2000	1	1	1	1	1		1	1	1	1.00
11	2000	1	1	1	1	1		1	1	1	1.00
12	2000	1	1	1	0	1	–1	1	1	1	0.67
13	2001	1	1	1	1	0	1	1	0		0.75
14	2001	1	1	1	1	1	1	1	1	1	1.00
15	2002	0	0	0	0	0	0	0	0		0.00
16	2002	1	1						1		1.00
17	2002	0		0		0		0	0	0	0.00
18	2002	1	1	1	1	1	–1	–1	1		0.50
19	2002	1	0	0	0	1	0	1	0		0.38
20	2002	1	1	1	1	1	1	1	1	1	1.00
21	2002	1	0	0	1	0	0	0	0		0.25
22	2002	1	0	0	–1	0	0	1	1	1	0.33
23	2003	1	1	1	1	1		1	1		1.00
24	2003	1	1	1	1	1	1	1	1	1	1.00
25	2003	1	1	0	1	1	1	1	1	1	0.89
26	2003	1	1	1	1	1	1	1	1	1	1.00
27	2003	1	1	0	1	1	0	1	1	1	0.78
28	2003	1	0	0	0	0		0	0	0	0.13
29	2004	1	1	1	1	–1	–1	1	1	1	0.56
30	2004	1	–1	1	–1	0	1	1	1	1	0.44
31	2005	–1				1	1		0		0.25
32	2005	0	1	0		1		–1	0	1	0.29
33	2005	1	1	1	1	1	1	1	1	1	1.00
34	2005	0	0	0	–1	1	1	0	1	1	0.33

Appendix 9-C continued

	Health	Canada	France	Germany	Italy	Japan	Russia	United Kingdom	United States	European Union	Average
35	2005	1	–1	1	–1	–1	–1	1	1	1	0.11
36	2005	1	0	0	0	1	1	1	1	1	0.67
37	2006	1	1	–1	1	–1	1	1	1		0.50
38	2006	1	1	0	0	1	1	0	1	0	0.56
39	2006	1	0	0	0	0	0	0	1	0	0.22
40	2006	1	0	1	–1	0	1	1	1	0	0.44
41	2006	0	0	0	0	0	0	1	0		0.13
42	2007	1	1	1	0	1	0	1	1	0	0.67
43	2007	1	1	1	1	1	1	1	1	1	1.00
44	2007	1	1	0	–1	0	–1	1	1	1	0.33
45	2007	1	1	0	0	1		1	1	0	0.63
46	2007	1	1	1	1	1	1	1	1	1	1.00
47	2007	1	1	1	0	0	1	1	1	0	0.67
48	2008	1	1	1	1	0	0	1	1	–1	0.56
49	2008	0	–1	–1	–1	0	–1	1	1	–1	–0.33
50	2009	1	1	0	–1	1	0	1	1	1	0.56
51	2009	1	0	0	0	1	0	1	0	–1	0.22
52	2010	1	–1	1	–1	–1	–1	–1	–1	–1	–0.56
53	2010	1	0	0	–1	1	0	–1	1	1	0.22
54	2010	1	0	1	–1	–1	0	1	1	–1	0.11
55	2011	1	–1	1	–1	–1	1	–1	–1	1	–0.11
56	2012	1	1	1	1	1	1	1	1	1	1.00
	Average	0.80	0.50	0.42	0.14	0.42	0.23	0.65	0.71	0.56	0.51

Note: The list of G8 commitments on health is available from the G8 Information Centre website at http://www.g8.utoronto.ca/evaluations/#commitments.

Appendix 9-D G8 Performance, 1975–2013

Year	Grade	Domestic Political Management		Deliberation			Direction Setting	Decision Making	Delivery	Development of Global Governance		Participation		
		# communiqué compliments	Spread	# days	# statements	# words	# references to core values	# commitments	Compliance	# ministerials created	# official groups created	# members	# participants	# international organizations
1975	A-	2	29%	3	1	1,129	5	14	0.57	0	1	6	0	0
1976	D	0	0%	2	1	1,624	0	7	0.09	0	0	7	0	0
1977	B-	1	13%	2	6	2,669	0	29	0.08	0	1	8	0	0
1978	A	1	13%	2	2	2,999	0	35	0.36	0	0	8	0	0
1979	B+	0	0%	2	2	2,102	0	34	0.82	1	2	8	0	0
1980	C+	0	0%	2	5	3,996	3	55	0.08	0	1	8	0	0
1981	C	1	13%	2	3	3,165	0	40	0.27	1	0	8	0	0
1982	C	0	0%	3	2	1,796	0	23	0.84	0	3	9	0	0
1983	B	0	0%	3	2	2,156	7	38	-0.11	0	0	8	0	0
1984	C-	1	13%	3	5	3,261	0	31	0.49	1	0	8	0	0
1985	E	4	50%	3	2	3,127	1	24	0.01	0	2	8	0	0
1986	B+	3	25%	3	4	3,582	1	39	0.58	1	1	9	0	0
1987	D	2	13%	3	7	5,064	0	53	0.93	0	2	9	0	0
1988	C-	3	25%	3	3	4,872	0	27	-0.48	0	0	8	0	0
1989	B+	3	38%	3	11	7,125	1	61	0.08	0	1	8	0	0
1990	D	3	38%	3	3	7,601	10	78	-0.14	0	3	8	0	0
1991	B-	1	13%	3	3	8,099	8	53	0	0	0	9	1	0
1992	D	1	13%	3	4	7,528	5	41	0.64	1	1	8	0	0
1993	C+	0	0%	3	2	3,398	2	29	0.75	0	2	8	1	0
1994	C	1	13%	3	2	4,123	5	53	1.00	1	0	8	1	0
1995	B+	3	25%	3	3	7,250	0	78	1.00	2	2	8	1	0
1996	B	1	13%	3	5	15,289	6	128	0.41	0	3	8	1	4

Appendix 9-D continued

		Domestic Political Management		Deliberation			Direction Setting	Decision Making	Delivery	Development of Global Governance		Participation		
Year	Grade	# communiqué compliments	Spread	# days	# statements	# words	# references to core values	# commitments	Compliance	# ministerials created	# official groups created	# members	# participants	# international organizations
1997	C-	16	88%	3	4	12,994	6	145	0.13	1	3	9	1	0
1998	B+	0	0%	3	4	6,092	5	73	0.32	0	0	9	0	0
1999	B+	4	22%	3	4	10,019	4	46	0.38	1	5	9	0	0
2000	B	1	11%	3	5	13,596	6	105	0.81	0	4	9	4	3
2001	B	1	11%	3	7	6,214	3	58	0.55	1	2	9	0	0
2002	B+	0	0%	2	18	11,959	10	187	0.35	1	8	10	0	0
2003	C	0	0%	3	14	16,889	17	206	0.66	0	5	10	12	5
2004	C+	0	0%	3	16	38,517	11	245	0.54	0	15	10	12	0
2005	A-	8	67%	3	16	22,286	29	212	0.65	0	5	9	11	6
2006		6	44%	3	15	30,695	256	317	0.47	0	4	10	5	9
2007		12	100%	3	8	25,857	86	329	0.51	0	4	9	9	9
2008	B+	8	78%	3	6	16,842	33	296	0.48	1	4	9	15	6
2009	B	13	67%	3	10	31,167	62	254	0.53	2	9	10	28	10
2010	C	10	89%	2	2	7,161	32	44	0.46	0	1	10	9	0
2011	B+	14	67%	2	5	19,071	172	196	0.54	1	0	10	7	4
2012	B+	7	67%	2	2	3,640	42	81	0.60	0	1	10	4	1
2013		7	44%	2	4	13,494	71	214	N/A	0	0	10	6	1
Total	N/A	138	N/A	106	218	388,448	899	3978	16.26	16	95	339	128	58
Average		3.54	28%	2.72	5.59	9,960	23.05	102.00	0.43	0.41	2.44	8.69	3.28	1.49

Notes:
Grade: Grades up to and including 2005 are given by Nicholas Bayne; from 2006 on are given by John Kirton and the G8 Research Group using a different framework and method.
Domestic Political Management: communiqué compliments are explicit references to G8 members in the official documents; spread is percentage of the full 20 members that received compliments contained in the official documents.
Deliberation: the duration of the summit in days; the number of statements issued by the summit; and the total number of words contained in the statements.
Direction setting: the number of references in the summit documents to the G8's core values of democracy, social advance, and individual liberty.
Decision making: the number of commitments contained in the summit documents as defined and identified by the G8 Research Group.
Delivery: compliance scores on selected commitments assessed by Ella Kokotsis (1990–95) and the G8 Research Group (1996–2012)
Development of Global Governance: the number of new institutions created at the ministerial and official levels at or by the summit, or during the hosting, year, at least in the form of having one meeting take place.
Participation: the number of G8 members in attendance; the number of invited leaders in attendance; the number of international organizations represented at the summit. Russia started as a participant in 1991 and became a full member in 1998.
N/A=not available.

Appendix 9-E African and Global Health Capability

	Life Expectancy at Birth (years)									Healthy Life Expectancy at Birth (years)			Neonatal Mortality Rate (per 1,000 live births)
	Male			Female			Both Sexes			Male	Female	Both	
	1990	2000	2011	1990	2000	2011	1990	2000	2011	2007	2007	2007	2011
Africa	48	49	55	51	52	58	50	50	56	45	46	45	34
Global	62	64	68	67	68	72	64	66	70	58	61	59	22

	Cholera	Leprosy	Malaria	Measles	Meningitis
	2011	2011	2011	2011	2012
Africa	110,915	17,953	20,168,253	194,364	28,281
Global	589,854	224,334	23,826,496	354,820	NA

	Physicians (number)	Physicians (per 10,000 population)	Nurses and Midwives (number)	Nurses and Midwives (per 10,000 population)	Dentists (number)	Dentist (per 10,000 population)	Pharmacists (number)	Pharmacists (per 10,000 population)
	2000–09	2005–12	2000–09	2005–12	2000–09	2005–12	2000–09	2005–12
Africa	174,510	2.5	802,076	9.1	25,798	0.4	56,212	0.6
Global	8,747,790	13.9	17,548	29	2,008,518	2.6	2,525,705	0.3

	Total Expenditure on Health as % of GDP		General Government Expenditure on Health as % of Total Spent on Health		Private Expenditure on Health as a % of Total Spent on Health		General Government Expenditure on Health as % of Total Government Expenditure		External Resources for Health as % Total Spent on Health	
	2000	2010	2000	2010	2000	2010	2000	2010	2000	2010
Africa	5.5	6.2	44.0	47.2	56.0	52.8	8.1	9.6	6.6	12.0
Global	8.2	9.2	56.4	58.9	43.6	41.4	13.5	15.1	0.4	1.2

Source: World Health Organization (2010c, 2013g).

PART IV
Connecting Health and Climate Change in Global Governance

Chapter 10

The Impact of Climate Change on Health Governance and Sovereignty in Africa

Nelson Sewankambo, James K. Tumwine and Hany Besada

In recent years, the scientific community has reached a consensus: human activity is largely contributing to the atmospheric build-up of greenhouse gases, increasing global temperatures to unprecedented levels, and causing changes in the hydrologic cycle (Parry et al. 2007; Rosenzweig et al. 2008). These factors will affect access to natural resources, particularly water, arable land, and vegetation as well as vulnerable ecosystems. Regions with relatively low adaptive capacity due to poverty and inequality, inadequate governance structures, high levels of corruption, lack of infrastructure, competing health concerns, and poor service delivery will be most severely affected. According to the Intergovernmental Panel on Climate Change (IPCC), Africa is expected to feel the brunt of the planet's fury and face the most serious and immediate impacts as a result of climate change. In 1992, the United Nations Framework Convention on Climate Change (UNFCCC) recognized that the adverse effects of climate change will be felt in states least responsible for the cause of those effects and also least able to adapt to this global assault.

Climate change is a major developmental challenge for present and future generations, particularly the impoverished populations in low- and middle-income countries that are the most vulnerable to adverse impacts including health threats. According to the International Monetary Fund (2013b), 36 of the 50 most impoverished countries in the world are located there. This has important policy implications for health governance and sovereignty in Africa. The susceptibility to climate change is especially acute given that the extent of spatial patterns of impacts is particularly unpredictable. Policy planning is difficult because of changing climate projections and unreliable data. This situation is aggravated by the interaction of multiple environmental and human stresses, occurring at various levels accompanied in many countries by poor governance and lack of transparency and accountability.

African governments have been applauded by multilateral institutions and western governments in recent years for undertaking much-needed economic reforms, addressing issues of peace and security, strengthening good governance and accountability, and advancing political pluralism. Indeed, Africa is shining with small but important victories in communities and regions from north to south and east to west. From 2004 to 2012, the continent experienced record annual economic growth of more than 5.2 per cent (International Monetary Fund 2013a, 3). This rate of growth declined by approximately 50 per cent in 2009 due to the global financial crisis, bounced back to 5.6 per cent in 2010, but by 2012 declined to 4.9 per cent. In the same period, the numbers of new HIV infections in Africa stabilized while AIDS-related deaths declined in some African states (UNAIDS 2013b). It is all the more important to address climate change if Africa's recent accomplishments are to be safeguarded.

Governance

Governance means different things to different people. Most would take it as a set of processes including decision making, implementation, and, possibly, evaluation of which things get done or not done (United Nations Economic and Social Commission for Asia and the Pacific [UN ESCAP] 2013). The process can be complex depending on the issues. In climate change and health, the main actors might include government, cultural or religious communities and their leaders, financial institutions, the media, universities, trades unions, political parties, bloggers, donors, development partners, civil society actors, and others such as lobbyists and activists, as witnessed at the annual conferences of the parties (COPs) to the UNFCCC.[1]

In the words of the UN Economic and Social Commission for Asia and the Pacific (2013), good governance has several components: "It is participatory, consensus oriented, accountable, transparent, responsive, effective and efficient, equitable and inclusive and follows the rule of law. It assures that corruption is minimized, the views of minorities are taken into account and that the voices of the most vulnerable in society are heard in decision-making. It is also responsive to the present and future needs of society". It would be instructive to determine to what extent climate change and its impacts on health in sub-Saharan Africa are amenable to this concept. While there have been experiences with participatory decision making in the health sector, such experiences with climate change and health are limited (Tumwine 1989).

In climate change and health governance, the issues are akin to those of primary health care where involvement of communities in making decisions that affect their health seems to have tangible benefits. In the state of Kerala in India, half-hearted attempts to introduce reforms to address fiscal crises affecting local government functions, erosion of public health functions, and a perceived decrease in the quality of public health services met with little success. Policy makers realized that uncoordinated social sector spending was further complicated

1 The 2011 United Nations Climate Change Conference concluded a legally binding deal comprising all countries, to be formulated by 2015 and take effect by 2020. A management framework for the Green Climate Fund was adopted; the fund is to distribute $100 billion per year to assist poorer countries to adapt to climate changes.

by the reduced maintenance of public health facilities and decreased funding of drugs with increasing levels of salaries and benefits. The situation called for more participatory decision making in health, more accountability, and strengthened finances. Governance in health and climate change as an issue at the community level, in particular, should involve working with local communities to identify the critical issues and design ways of adaptation using indigenous knowledge and best practices.

Several nongovernment organizations (NGOs), such as World Vision and Tearfund, have initiated work on climate change. Yet very few programs have addressed climate change and health at the community level. This is unfortunate because, while the emergency public health impacts of climate change, such as epidemics, may need top-down national or state action, community-based action is often critical (Ebi and Semenza 2008). Top-down interventions that deal with poorly informed communities and an "un-engaged" public often meet with little success as they fail to take into account issues that directly affect critical decisions that must be made (Semenza et al. 1996). In this regard, Tearfund and World Vision unveiled the Climate Change and Environmental Degradation Risk and Adaptation Assessment (CEDRA) in 2009. As an environmental tool for agencies in low-income countries, it has encouraged community-based action (Wiggins 2009). CEDRA assists NGOs and donor agencies to understand not only environmental degradation but also the science of climate change in combating the adverse effects of climate change at the community level.

According to its author, Sarah Wiggins (2009, 3), the tool "helps agencies working in developing countries to access and understand the science of climate change and environmental degradation and to compare this with local community experience of environmental change ... Using CEDRA, agencies can prioritise which environmental hazards may pose a risk to their existing projects and project locations, enabling them to make decisions to adapt some projects, stop doing some projects or start new ones".

When assessing participatory governance, several authors have looked at a number of scenarios, such as nonparticipation, tokenism, and citizen power (de Schutter and Riemer 2009; see also Matovu 2011; Murray et al. 2010). Tokenism involves passing on information and at times consultation. Citizens' power involves a situation of "partnership, delegated power and citizen decision making and control" (de Schutter and Riemer 2009, 6). In previous work in Zimbabwe, true community involvement in primary healthcare programs was often characterized by tokenism rather than true decision making, delegated power, or citizen's control. True community involvement involves activism, use of participatory techniques such as CEDRA, participatory learning and action, and other approaches.[2] Current health programs in sub-Saharan Africa have largely used tokenism to push for

2 Participation learning and action uses approaches and methodologies that stress the need for the full participation of people in the processes of learning about their needs and opportunities, and steps needed to address them.

interventions such as higher coverage rates of vaccination, polio eradication, and prevention of mother to child transmission of HIV and for disease control such as malaria and tuberculosis programs. Even where there has been true decentralization of budgets and decision making, as in Uganda and Zambia, early gains from decentralization are beginning to get eroded with the push for a return to centralization. Future work in climate change and health must draw lessons from these experiences; otherwise the danger of reinventing the wheel is real and will lead to similar unsatisfactory results.

Transparency, accountability, openness, inclusiveness, and participation are defining characteristics of good governance processes that enable the implementation of wise, evidence-based policies that are effective and coherent across levels and sectors. As Diarmid Campbell-Lendrum and Manjula Lusti-Narasimhan (2009) have written, for all of its complexities, the basic challenge of climate change policy is the apparent conflict between the drive to maximize short-term individual or national gains (increasing per capita gross domestic product [GDP] through use of cheap fossil fuel energy) and the need for long-term protection of shared benefits (reducing climate change and minimizing global damage to natural and human systems.

To underpin decision making, African states need to identify the defining values of their societies, including social justice, sustainable development, equality, human dignity, equity, and human rights.

The vision for future health on the continent should be based on an African perspective. It should be ambitious, with a consensus on what is required for both the environment and human well-being to achieve sustainable development. This will require concerted action and change along at least five pathways: good governance, progressive green (low-carbon) health service, a green economy, creativity and innovation, and knowledge and education. The governance pathway will have to involve, recognize, and empower people as citizens whose rights are respected while concurrently strengthening both a national and continental identity. There is a need for creating an Africa-wide shared normative framework that includes relevant climate-related policies, salutatory instruments, and statutes for the enforcement of law and order based on shared desired objectives for environment and human well-being. Climate change policies must be brought into the mainstream governance of individual countries and ensure relevance to the local context, underpinned by the recognition that what is good for tackling climate change is similarly good for health. Policies needed for adaptation and mitigation against climate change will affect health by acting on many social determinants of health and health inequities.

The UNFCCC

At its establishment in 1994, the UNFCCC had two objectives: to reduce greenhouse gas emissions and to provide funding from members of the Organisation for

Economic Co-operation and Development (OECD) to developing countries that required financial support to adapt to climate change. Mitigation and adaptation were identified by the UNFCCC as the two main strategies for limiting climate change's negative effects. In general, low- and middle-income countries in Africa, and elsewhere, have focused on adaptation so as to limit the predicted damage caused by climate change. Ever since the UNFCCC was established, many governments have submitted their national adaptation programs of action (NAPAs) to the Global Environment Facility (GEF) for funding.[3]

This funding comes from OECD members that have pledged to provide financial support – over and above existing aid flows – to developing countries that require assistance to adapt to the impact of climate change. NAPAs represent identified national priorities and proposed strategies for adaptation. Individual country governments develop their strategies through an approach that involves the people at the grassroots, civil society organizations, government leaders, and funders. Of the 50 countries that submitted NAPAs by November 2013, 34 are African (UNFCCC 2013a).[4] From a health governance perspective it might be instructive to understand why some of the eligible countries have not submitted NAPAs.

To what extent do existing UNFCCC governance mechanisms contribute to the process of addressing the impacts of climate change specifically on health governance and sovereignty in Africa? In the context of the UNFCCC's two objectives three fundamental questions emerge: How should health-related issues be addressed better in the successor to the Kyoto Protocol and in the NAPAs of African states? How should raising and managing funds to meet the needs of African countries to address health challenges arising from climate change be addressed better? What other governance considerations need to be made so as to empower African countries as sovereign states to successfully overcome the climate change–health challenges they will likely confront in the future? Although governance issues related to the health impacts of climate change are part of the overall landscape of governance arrangements for adaptation and mitigation, there are peculiarities that need to be added to the overall discussion of climate change.

Social and other health inequities that affect or are affected by climate change in Africa pose significant governance challenges. Maximum efforts must be made to ensure that prevention and management of the health effects of climate change are integrated and mainstreamed into countries' overall health programs. The

---

3 The GEF brings together 183 countries and NGOs, international institutions, multilateral organizations, and the private sector to address global environmental issues affecting the world while supporting national sustainable development initiatives to mitigate and adapt to the adverse effects of climate change.

4 Those countries are Angola, Benin, Burkina Faso, Burundi, Cape Verde, Central African Republic, Chad, Democratic Republic of Congo, Djibouti, Equatorial Guinea, Eritrea, Ethiopia, Gambia, Guinea, Guinea-Bissau, Lesotho, Liberia, Madagascar, Malawi, Mali, Mauritania, Mozambique, Niger, Rwanda, São Tomé and Principe, Senegal, Sierra Leone, Somalia, Sudan, Tanzania, Togo, Uganda, Yemen, and Zambia.

breadth of those health impacts extend beyond the obvious to include the effects on workers' health and productivity, particularly for those employed in outdoor environments that are hot and humid, such as farm and construction workers, miners, and manufacturers. Both the direct and indirect adverse effects of climate change on the populations are receiving increasing attention (Patz et al. 2005; Haines et al. 2006; Costello et al. 2009; *Nature* 2009; Costello et al. 2011; Nilsson et al. 2012).

Health Co-benefits of Adaptation and Mitigation

Inequities may be addressed through contraction and convergence by the fair-shares network that ensures an equal per-head carbon entitlement (Haines et al. 2009). The governance implications for both adaptation and mitigation must be considered in relation to the health impacts of climate change in order to reap the maximum significant positive co-benefits from mitigation policies in terms of better health, improved productivity, lower rates of accidents and morbidity, and improved sense of comfort and social well-being. Major ethical and political concerns become evident (McMichael et al. 2004; Campbell-Lendrum et al. 2007; Friel et al. 2008; Patz et al. 2008). Africa's development has lagged behind all other continents. Since health and well-being are central to development, the current and potential health impacts of a changing climate should drive climate policy in Africa and elsewhere. The full range of benefits from that climate change policy includes both adaptation and mitigation since ancillary health co-benefits can arise. Andy Haines (2009) and others have drawn global attention to the fact that "the public health benefits of mitigation policies have not had sufficient prominence in international negotiations" (see also Wilkinson et al. 2009; Woodcock et al. 2009; Markandya et al. 2009; Friel et al. 2009; Smith et al. 2009). At COP15 in Copenhagen in 2009 there was glaring underrepresentation of any such discussions by government, NGOs, and health professionals. More recent meetings have attempted to bring health more fully into the agenda. At COP16 in Cancun in 2010, health was mentioned briefly by the director general of the WHO in her video statement and health risks were raised in side events organized by the WHO (2010a). For COP17 held in Durban in 2011, WHO was expected to devise a policy proposal but the human health implications of climate change were again relegated to side-event status (WHO 2011b).

Discussions on climate change within the context of development and poverty-reduction strategies more broadly were not adequately discussed at COP15 but were discussed in side events at COP16 and COP17. No progress was made in 2013 at COP19 in Warsaw. Ultimately, any pledges made to Africa should examine how to implement climate change in development assistance, such as in healthcare provision and adaptive strategies to combat a rise of malaria and other diseases. Malaria occupies a prominent place as a disease shaped by climate change on a large scale. Rising temperatures affect the transmission and spread of mosquitoes, their increased density within sprawling urban and rural communities, and the increasing likelihood of infection. Indeed, with rising temperatures, mosquitoes will seek higher elevations, further intensifying the spread and transmission of malaria in areas once immune to the disease. By 2080 malaria will affect between 260 million and 320 million more people as a result of that that migration of mosquitoes (Lindsay and Martens 1998). The prevalence of mosquitoes is further increased with global warming, an over ten-fold increase with every unit increase (0.1 degree Celsius) in temperature (Pascual et al. 2006).

Dengue fever is also very sensitive to climate change. It is prominent in urban areas as a result of inadequate clean water storage. Increased precipitation and global temperatures raise the rate of infection (Menne et al. 2002). Up to 6 billion people will be at risk in contacting the disease as a result of climate change by 2085, compared to 3.5 billion people if there are no major global weather changes (Hales et al. 2002). This prompts the question of how much development assistance is going to Africa to combat the spread of malaria and other diseases and help it adapt to changing weather patterns.

Food insecurity and undernutrition, inadequate and unsafe water, exposure to indoor smoke, infectious disease conditions such as malaria and diarrheal diseases, all of which are among the leading health risks in sub-Saharan African countries, show significant sensitivity to climate change and vice versa. Some health interventions such as the proper management of AIDS and prevention of infant HIV/AIDS are also climate sensitive because access to good nutrition is essential for success.

There is growing evidence to support the link between the impact of climate change and conflict. Climate change–related civil conflicts and violence over scarce resources and migration are not uncommon in Africa. They, too, are important drivers of ill health and premature death (Holdren 2008). Rising temperatures have increased the likelihood of intra and interstate conflicts in Africa. With agriculture accounting for more than 90 per cent of employment and 50 per cent of the continent's GDP, African states are particularly vulnerable to changes in the environment (Burke et al. 2009). Climate models measuring global temperature changes in Africa predict an increase in armed conflicts by up to 54 per cent by 2030, or an additional 393,000 battle deaths (Burke et al. 2009). This has been well illustrated by events in Rwanda, Darfur in Sudan, and the Democratic Republic of Congo (Diamond 2005; Faris 2007; Coghlan et al. 2006; Coghlan et al. 2008).

To cook and provide heat, Africa's poor rely on burning solid household fuels indoor mainly in the form of biomass (wood, charcoal, and agricultural residues). Improving combustion efficiency and cleanliness of energy fuels presents a well-recognized co-benefit to health (Smith 1994). Mainstreaming climate-related programming into central planning for improved health service delivery will, therefore, be a double win. Governance in health should address the actors and all-purposeful mechanisms and measures aimed at steering social systems toward preventing, mitigating, or adapting to the health risks posed by the impacts of climate change. The increasing visibility and influence of nonstate actors in global climate change politics is well illustrated by their numbers, activism, and protests at the annual COP meetings, which are attended by thousands of journalists and thousands of NGO representatives.

Numbers of indigenous nongovernmental actors in individual countries have been increasing. In preparation for COP15 in 2009 in Copenhagen, for example, African states joined together to enhance solidarity on climate change and speak with one voice. In the lead-up to the meeting, the African Union held extensive discussions on the need for a coherent continental position on climate change. It approved the Algiers Declaration in May 2009 on African Common Platform to Copenhagen and put together a Conference of African Heads of State and Government on Climate Change in August 2009. The leaders' conference carried forward several key political messages to COP15. African delegates voiced ideas of sustainable development, anticipating that the goals of poverty reduction, economic development, and environmental protection could be assessed and evaluated comprehensively.

In addition, the African delegates at Copenhagen argued that industrialized states bore the responsibility for current global environmental changes and that developing states were owed compensation for the socioeconomic and environmental losses they were suffering. African mitigation efforts would be voluntary and would require technology transfer, adequate funding, and capacity building. African states wanted serious reforms to the existing financial mechanisms, particularly with regard to accessibility while demanding that industrialized states commit between 0.5 per cent and 1.5 per cent of their GDP for climate change strategies in developing countries. COP15 represented the first serious attempt by the continent to come up with a set agenda spearheaded by a single delegation that was empowered to negotiate on behalf of member states.

This emerging order has implications. Although there are increasing national and regional organizations in Africa, very few have climate change as a major area of focus. The reasons for this need to be understood in order to inform appropriate construction of governance structure beyond the realms of the nation-state and its responsibilities. The emergence of many nonstate actors with their own guiding principles, values, rules, norms, and procedures may lead to fragmentation, non-productive competition for resources, and the sidelining of state machinery and mechanisms (like the climate change units created by African states). Governments might become complacent and adopt a laissez-faire attitude, thereby failing to invest the required resources. Private sector donors are also important in ensuring that adequate sources of funding are available for climate change programs. However, it is unclear what drives many organizations into climate change programming and activities.

Governing climate change-induced disease and ill health will likely bring in a wide range of actors from individuals, through local communities to the national level, and thus governance arrangements below the state at all levels of social organization. It remains uncertain whether continental or regional actors (above the state level) will emerge to collaborate effectively with governments to steer Africa's climate change-related health issues. Such health effects are clearly in the domain of global health. States are necessary for taking adaptation and mitigation measures in order to satisfactorily address at least the most important priority health issues. There is a need for an intersection between global health governance and health governance by individual states. Effective adaptation requires local action and taking local circumstances into consideration. Measures to reduce greenhouse gases must also address and improve global health.

Health should be part of a new development model that focuses on improving human well-being, in line with sustainable development. Health and climate change present a complexity that requires contextualizing the debate and coherently framing the issues that are relevant to policymakers, researchers, and communities.

Promoting Awareness and Capacity Building

Adaptation is highly local and local institutions play a major role in ensuring success (Agrawal 2008). Similarly there are many aspects of mitigation such as avoiding deforestation that can only succeed with the participation of local institutions. Africa should build a strong base for local relevance, sustainability, and local applicability of practical interventions and strategies, through government stewardship and leadership by strengthening the roles of local institutions and harnessing indigenous knowledge. The literature on the importance and role of local institutions in adaptation to climate change generally has not adequately emphasized the place of such institutions in addressing the effects of climate change on health governance (Nyong et al. 2007). Likewise the role of indigenous knowledge in addressing similar issues has not been studied in detail and thus its potential remains unknown (Nyong et al. 2007; Orlove et al. 2010).

Regarding the promotion of awareness and action on the impact of climate change in a global health context, Michael St. Louis and Jeremy Hess (2008) have proposed four strategies for "pursuing both action and a collaborative learning exercise to deepen understanding and synergy between the community involved in traditional global health programs and the community involved in global climate change science and policy". This approach should be adapted in sub-Saharan countries for communities involved in traditional health programs and those in climate change science and policy at state or regional or continental levels. The adapted approach involves the following strategies:

> Maintain and promote mutual awareness of climate change with national, regional, continental, and global health communities, and serve as role models individually and institutionally for associated best practices applicable locally.

> Incorporate technical approaches and strategies in current national, regional, and continent-wide health programs that will facilitate mitigation and adaptation to climate change.
>
> Align state health policies and priorities with larger principles and frameworks that support sustainable national development in general, and mitigation of, and adaptation to climate change specifically and harness regional or continental synergies whenever feasible.
>
> Help strengthen the evidence base and accessible information about workable and affordable interventions that affect the impact of climate change on poor and vulnerable populations, and cause productive responses to those effects (St. Louis and Hess 2008).

Effective health communication is critical if Africa is to reduce the harmful effects of climate change. However, it is challenging in this slowly emerging field because so many knowledge gaps exist. Climate change requires thoughtful communication, given that the current discourse features scientific complexity, considerable uncertainty, ample misinformation, and many vested interests – with the resulting potential to frighten, confuse, and alienate people (Frumkin et al. 2008). Moreover, those who would communicate about climate change have little evidence to guide them. Nonetheless, this should not lead to paralysis and inaction. Lessons can be drawn from the global efforts to control tobacco use (Nilsson et al. 2009). It took 50 years from the identification of the scientific evidence on the association between tobacco use and harmful health effects and premature death to the entry into force the WHO Framework Convention on Tobacco Control (FCTC).[5]

Africa must participate actively and ensure that binding climate change international policy is in place and implemented to improve human well-being and prevent ill health. It should also take lessons from the HIV/AIDS epidemic. In the early 1980s when the AIDS epidemic emerged in Africa, the global community in general and Africa in particular knew nothing about the disease. The world may be better off today with climate change because many of the likely health effects are an exacerbation of pre-existing conditions for which much is known. This should not, however, result in complacency as entirely new challenges may emerge. Although AIDS has galvanized greater attention and efforts in Africa and globally, the continent still suffers from the ravages of the epidemic. In 2012, sub-Saharan Africa was home to 70 per cent (25 million) of the world's population of people living with HIV and 75 per cent (1.2 million) of AIDS deaths (amfAR 2013;

5 The first treaty adopted under the auspices of WHO, FCTC came into force in 2005 and aims to protect individuals from the harmful effects of tobacco consumption and exposure. It provides a framework of national, regional, and international tobacco control measures. With 168 countries signatories and 177 as parties to the treaty, it is has close to universal appeal and support (see the FCTC website at http://www.who.int/fctc/en).

UNAIDS 2011). The disease has stretched health systems to the limit and led to a reversal of many health gains.

Strengthening Health Systems in the Context of Climate Change

The struggle against the HIV/AIDS epidemic has existed for more than a quarter of a century. Africa, given its population relative to the rest of the world, has experienced the greatest impact, with more than its share of the problem. It affects all segments of society. The epidemic has been a defining challenge for African health systems. The health effects of climate change will likely compound that challenge many times. There are important experiences that can serve as lessons for the climate change–health nexus on governance and sovereignty in Africa. Moreover, AIDS is also undermining human and social capital in Africa: the traditional coping strategies of households are overwhelmed, making the population more vulnerable to the effects of climate change (Commission for Africa 2005, 2010). Efforts to address HIV and climate change have reached the top of the international political agenda and generated two vigorous global social movements that have each called for a common and shared responsibility between developing and developed countries. In the late 1980s and as part of WHO's Global Program on AIDS, AIDS began to be framed as a social and human rights issue (Wehrwein 1998). The nature and origins of the global warming that will likely affect the poor people of Africa the most, who have caused it the least, support a strong argument for climate change and its effects to be considered a social and human rights issue.

Engagement with communities, entrepreneurs, philanthropists, political leaders, and prominent personalities has been critical in enhancing and strengthening the struggle against HIV/AIDS. Climate change and health governance should do the same. Mitigation and adaptation have equivalents in HIV prevention and HIV treatment, care, and support respectively. Food security in receiving increasing attention in Africa's war against AIDS because it is a significant contributor to ensuring adequacy of HIV prevention, treatment, care, and support programs.

Major considerations at the heart of the AIDS efforts in Africa include community mobilization and education, social justice and equity considerations. They also include seeking benefit for the poor and marginalized, enhancing service delivery coupled with technology transfer and capacity building, raising concern for sustainable development, engaging in advocacy and activism, developing a multisectoral approach, implementing innovations, discovering new knowledge supported by a massive research machinery, aggressively mobilizing funds (from the public and private sectors), and heightening the focus on transparency and accountability. In the long run AIDS has received a much greater share of official development assistance (MacKellar 2005). Initiatives such as the Global Fund to Fight AIDS, Tuberculosis, and Malaria and the US President's Emergency Plan for AIDS Relief (PEPFAR) have provided hope to millions of HIV-positive patients across Africa and have altered the administration of health care on the continent.[6] Critics, however, have expressed concern over the dangers of disease-specific programming with particular emphasis on AIDS. They suggest that such an approach weakens the general health system for provision of comprehensive primary health care. Programming to address climate change-related health effects should therefore not become stand-alone silos that, in addition to weakening the health system, might lead to increased transaction costs for countries and system inefficiencies.

AIDS poses a significant threat to state sovereignty. Many African governments have feared that openness would lead to the stigmatization of individual countries and a collapse in international trade. Therefore, there have been different approaches to combat the AIDS epidemic.

At the one extreme, South Africa's leadership chose to deny the existence of both the epidemic and scientifically proven approaches to AIDS prevention, treatment, and care, with the devastating results that the country has one of the highest HIV population rates in Africa. An estimated 270,190 people died of AIDS in the country in 2011 (UNAIDS 2012e). In the same year, the rate of HIV prevalence in the general population is 17.3 per cent. In total, an estimated 5.6 million South Africans were living with HIV in 2011, more than any other country in the world (UNAIDS 2012e). Although South Africa has a long history of political activism, it took a long time before AIDS activism kicked in and built up momentum to have any impact.

On the other hand, Uganda's leadership openly accepted the severity of the epidemic in the early 1980s. This prompted the implementation of aggressive national programs that have resulted in a decline in the overall HIV prevalence, although this alleged achievement has not been without controversy (Parkhurst 2002). For African countries, strengthening health systems may provide a significant part of the response to an appropriate adaptation to climate change.

Africa's advances have come against the backdrop of a lack of political will to deal with the inequities in access to preventive interventions such as condoms

---

6 The Global Fund was launched in 2002 to redirect resources toward fighting HIV/AIDS, malaria, and tuberculosis. It has provided 20 per cent of all international funding to combat HIV/AIDS. By November 2012, it had provided approximately 4.2 million people with antiretroviral treatment (ART) across the globe (see Global Fund to Fight AIDS 2012a). PEPFAR, established by US President George Bush in 2003, has been described as the largest ever global initiative dedicated to tackling a single disease. From 2003 to 2008, it provided $15 billion ($10 billion in new money) to fund desperately needed drugs (U.S. President's Emergency Plan for AIDS Relief 2008). As of September 2012, the United States had supported ART for more than 5.1 million people worldwide and is the largest donor to the Global Fund, having provided more than $7 billion (U.S. President's Emergency Plan for AIDS Relief 2013). As a result of these two programs, nearly 7 million of the estimated 8 million individuals in low- and middle-income countries receive treatment (U.S. President's Emergency Plan for AIDS Relief 2013). They have both had a tremendous impact on increasing access to AIDS treatment on the African continent.

and information and to HIV treatment and care. The same scenario might play out with respect to the health effects of climate change if Africans do not show strong leadership in getting the global community to act responsibly.

AIDS and climate change resources can be used wisely to support the health system and through the formation of an alliance between the two major challenges of present and future generations. A key link is human resources – the health workers who have not yet begun to lobby and lead a people's movement against climate change. The United Kingdom's Climate and Health Council is one such organization of mainly health workers that advocates for the prominence of health arguments in climate change policies. It is to be emulated in Africa.

The global health workforce crisis has received heightened global attention, with Africa having the most severe shortage of health workers (Joint Learning Initiative 2004; WHO 2006; WHO 2008c). There are major efforts in the health sector to find creative ways to improve the numbers, distribution (between urban and rural settings), and performance of health workers at all levels. As part of this process, there is an opportunity for the health sector to show leadership, creativity, and innovation at local, national, regional, and continental levels by transforming from being silent observers to actively confronting the climate change challenge.

Physicians have demonstrated their ability to tackle pressing challenges affecting humanity such as nuclear war (Lown et al. 1981). They were actively involved against tobacco use (Sullivan 1990; American College of Chest Physicians 1995). Since Africa is the continent most at risk for the negative impacts of climate change, the health workers on the continent can lead a crusade for continental justice to produce fundamental change in the manner health issues are addressed in the context of climate change. Physicians should also more broadly participate in lobbying and advocacy for activities that are outside health but where successes have great health co-benefits in Africa. These include speaking for enhanced food security and a sub-Saharan Green Revolution, improving access to renewable energy, and ensuring sustainable development in Africa.

Research Governance

Research regarding the contribution of climate change to the global burden of disease has contributed to the understanding of the importance of this issue (WHO 1990; McMichael et al. 2003; McMichael et al. 2004). It has further emphasized the links between climate change and different aspects of health (Parry et al. 2007). The report published by the UCL-Lancet Commission on Managing the Health Effects of Climate Change further suggests that the highest regional burden of climate change is likely to be borne by sub-Saharan Africa, with 34 per cent of the global disability-adjusted life years attributable to climate change located there (Costello et al. 2009). Since sub-Saharan Africa has just over 12 per cent of the world's population, this reflects a three-fold population-based risk for adverse effects of climate change among Africans compared with the global population.

There is scanty scientific evidence about the intersection of climate change and population health in Africa, both because of the lack of understanding of the progress and nature of climate change and the widespread lack of community-based health data. The generation of African-based scientific information on the health impacts, the health co-benefits, and harms derived from adaptation and mitigations measures against global warming may influence governance and motivate action among African states. Evidence-based policies are needed in order to minimize harms while maximizing positive co-benefits from adaptation and mitigation policies for improved productivity, better health, and social well-being.

The IPCC's Fourth Assessment Report acknowledges the lack of certainty about the health effects of climate change (Parry et al. 2007). The absence of adequate scientific evidence hinders planning and the efficient use of available resources. However, this lack of data should not lead to a lack of action. WHO (2009e) has recommended expanded research into health and climate change. Africa is a fertile ground for conducting independent scientific analyses of the potential health impacts of addressing climate change. Research should focus on many different aspects, including building time-series data sets linked to meteorological data and health outcomes, behaviour changes, disease surveillance; identifying and quantifying the benefits and harms to public health arising from adaptation and mitigation policies; determining the appropriate mix of adaptation and mitigation of greatest benefit in different African environments; developing and refining a variety of methodological approaches to researching different scientific questions relevant to Africa; and formulating, evaluating and determining the economic costs of adaptive and mitigation strategies.

Infectious diseases tend to be considered first when contemplating the effects of climate change on health (Shope 1991). There are, however, other effects that may well be equally, if not more, important, such as the physiological effects of heat extremes (Kjellstrom 2009). There is also a serious governance challenge issue for Africa in terms of future policy aimed at supporting research institutions and universities to develop and be able to generate the required scientific information. Africa lacks the research capacity to take advantage of and use the existing global climate models and also to link health and climate change phenomena. This inadequacy underscores the need for more research in Africa and by African scientists in partnership with advanced climate research centres (mainly based in the north), and for the creation of African health and climate research groups (Pierce et al. 2009; Byass 2009a, 2009b).

Despite increasing media coverage on the theme of African peoples' potential vulnerability to actual and predicted changes in climate at the global level, detailed scientific evidence remains scanty. In developing countries, the impact may be more serious than that in developed countries, yet the data are sparse in general. Much existing work has looked at the effects of climate change on specific diseases, without connecting to overall changes in population health. Good governance will facilitate the strengthening of research infrastructure in African countries and thus accelerate development, and increase support for cross-disciplinary research and the maintenance of prospective longitudinal population demographic surveillance sites, many of which are under the umbrella of the INDEPTH Network in various African countries (Evans and AbouZahr 2008). In Ethiopia erratic seasonal patterns of rainfall have been linked to disease epidemics, which produced to a 2.5-fold increase in local overall population mortality over a two-year period (Emmelin et al. 2008). Brodie Morgan Ramin and Anthony McMichael (2009), acknowledging the paucity of evidence-based results, present five hypothetical case results illustrating what they believe to be the major issues.

Africans should identify research gaps and develop an African research agenda with research priorities for the continent but with provisions for individual states to address individual peculiarities and contexts. Africa here can learn from other efforts at the global level (Parry et al. 2007; Neira 2009). A much stronger network of researchers in the southern hemisphere would be invaluable to Africa.

Funding

Funding is needed as a governance strategy for reducing harm from the effects of climate change and for managing ill health associated with climate change shocks. Health services research and capacity building are generally underfunded in Africa. They can barely afford to absorb added health challenges without increased resources. Africa's thriving private sector can make an important contribution to providing healthcare services across the continent, particularly in fragile states. The health community should lose no chance to advocate for increased funding that will be used across government departments working directly on climate change adaptation and mitigation measures with the potential for co-benefits to health. In the face of new challenges, developing countries often face a development dilemma of how to finance new problems, leading inevitably diverting funds from existing development priorities such as education and health or taking loans from international financial institutions. It is a moral imperative for developed countries to come up with funds to help Africa and other vulnerable countries address the impacts of climate change since the developing countries have had a negligible role in its creation.

The Least Developed Countries Fund, administered by the GEF and funded by OECD members, provides support to African governments and others to adapt to the impact of climate change after the submission of their NAPAs. Mobilizing increased funding comes with new challenges and costs that must be managed appropriately. African countries must increase their absorptive capacity, transparency, and accountability so as to gain trust from the many new organizations playing a role in global health and also to benefit from existing funders in global health such as the Bill and Melinda Gates Foundation, Wellcome Trust, the Rockefeller Foundation, PEPFAR, and the Global Fund. There is fear that the attention and resources of funders and development partners might be diverted from existing health challenges to the more distant impacts of climate change. Recipient countries need to show greater transparency and accountability as part of their governance mechanisms in order to build greater confidence among the funders who provide the resources to support adaptation and mitigation activities.

The lack of adequate funding should not lead to political paralysis and inaction by individual governments. Those governments should instead show leadership and stewardship for what can be done with the resources available in the public and private sectors and within communities. Existing indigenous knowledge, which local communities have used so far in adapting to climate change, should be emphasized. This knowledge can be harnessed and enriched with relatively limited resources based on locally appropriate scientific knowledge.

Family Planning and Population Growth

The demographic trends in sub-Saharan Africa reveal a continent with the most rapidly increasing population in the world (United Nations Population Fund [UNFPA] 2012). High rates of population growth have not been factored adequately into policy discussions of climate mitigation and even much less so in those of adaptation to climate change. Reproductive health services deserve special consideration in a governance discussion that relates to health impacts of climate change in Africa. Diarmid Campbell-Lendrum and Manjula Lusti-Narasimhan (2009) have argued that "climate change and population, taken individually, are among the most contentious issues in public policy; bringing the two issues together is a recipe for controversy". Leo Bryant and his colleagues (2009) have recently shown that the NAPAs of most of the least developed countries, many of which are in Africa, cited population pressure as a detrimental factor, compromising their ability for adaptation and therefore a local priority for action.

There is need to close the gap between recognition of the need and implementation of effective programs on the ground. Universal access to reproductive health and rights is an essential element for achievement of the Millennium Development Goals (MDGs). Caution is required to avoid pitfalls experienced during the dehumanizing population control programs that were implemented in some developing countries in the 1960s and '70s (Kasun 1999). Concurrently there is recognition of the urgent need to address the human rights of individuals who wish to control their fertility for their own well-being and that of their families. Approximately 222 million women in developing countries, including in Africa, have an unmet need for family planning services (UNFPA 2012). Access to a range of safe and effective services that satisfy people's needs is a human right and a key determinant of reproductive health outcomes (RamaRao et al. 2003).

Some have suggested that voluntary, rights-based family planning programs in the developing world should be integrated into adaptation efforts, thus making climate change a priority shared by health and environment ministries (Bryant et al. 2009; Campbell-Lendrum and Lusti-Narasimhan 2009). Family planning should be presented primarily as addressing the rights of individuals to improve their well-being but also as having important climate change co-benefits. The co-benefits of slower population growth include less pressure on and degradation of natural resources, less human vulnerability to climate change-induced natural disasters, and less demand for resources such as agricultural land, food, and fresh water otherwise lessened by climate change.

Ethiopia is as an example of best practices regarding the integration and mainstreaming of family planning services in climate change adaptation. Family planning services are included in the country's agricultural sector of the NAPA (Ethiopia Ministry of Water Resources and National Meteorological Agency 2007; Bryant et al. 2009). The Watershed Management project in the Wichi province of Metu Woreda demonstrated that such integration within a project framework aimed at sustainable development is possible (Deribe 2007; Bryant et al. 2009).

Conclusion

A changing global environment has significant impacts on both the incidence and spread of diseases across the continent. The effects of climate instability are expected to fall disproportionately on Africa's poor and will risk reversing the gains of the past decade in alleviating poverty, raising life expectancy, and controlling the spread of infectious diseases. Across the continent, extreme weather conditions exacerbate inequalities in access to health care, putting millions of Africans at risk. With limited adaptive capacity in Africa, industrialized countries must make good on their promises for increased but sustainable financial support, technical assistance, and capacity building to Africa.

Climate change has adversely affected human health in Africa in a variety of ways. It will continue to do so unless innovative mitigation and adaptive steps are taken concurrently by the international community, African governments, and civil society groups across the continent. In terms of governance, better assessments of climate change politics are needed. In a globalized environment, the control and management of health services are no longer the domain of national governments. Increasingly, transnational arenas of health and climate change governance have allowed for the inclusion and importance of nonstate actors. They have also led to the configuration of key sites of private, hybrid, and public authority and management of climate issues. With increased emphasis on multiple-actor and multilevel perspectives in global governance, civil society groups play an important role in health governance as it relates to climate change in Africa. Local initiatives, indigenous technologies, and programs led by state and nonstate actors and supported by the international community would go a long way in addressing the effects of climate change on the continent's fragile health sector. These efforts need to be part of Africa's socioeconomic development strategies. It is impractical to address them in isolation.

References

Agrawal, Arun (2008). “The Role of Local Institutions in Adaptation to Climate Change and Conflict in Africa”. Paper prepared for the Social Dimensions of Climate Change, Social Development Department, World Bank, 5–6 March, Washington DC. http://www.icarus.info/wp-content/uploads/2009/11/agrawal-adaptation-institutions-livelihoods.pdf (October 2013).

American College of Chest Physicians (1995). “Smoking and Health: Physician Responsibility”. *Chest* 108(4): 1118–21. doi: 10.1378/chest.108.4.1118.

amfAR (2013). “Statistics: Worldwide”. New York. http://www.amfar.org/about-hiv-and-aids/facts-and-stats/statistics- -worldwide/ (November 2013).

Bryant, Leo, Louise Carver, Colin D. Butler, et al. (2009). “Climate Change and Family Planning: Least-Developed Countries Define the Agenda”. *World Health Bulletin* 87(11): 852–7. http://www.who.int/bulletin/volumes/87/11/08-062562.pdf

Burke, Marshall B., Edward Miguel, Shanker Satyanath, et al. (2009, 23 November). “Warming Increases the Risk of Civil War in Africa”. *Proceedings of the National Academy of Sciences*. doi: 10.1073/pnas.0907998106.

Byass, Peter (2009a, 11 November). “Climate Change and Population Health in Africa: Where Are the Scientists?” *Global Health Action*. doi: 10.3402/gha.v2i0.2065.

Byass, Peter (2009b). “The Unequal World of Health Data”. *PLoS Medicine* 6(11). doi: 10.1371/journal.pmed.1000155.

Campbell-Lendrum, Diarmid, Carlos Corvalán, and Maria Neira (2007). “Global Climate Change: Implications for International Public Health Policy”. *World Health Bulletin* 85(3): 161–244. http://www.who.int/bulletin/volumes/85/3/06-039503/en/ (October 2013).

Campbell-Lendrum, Diarmid and Manjula Lusti-Narasimhan (2009). “Taking the Heat Out of the Population and Climate Debate”. *World Health Bulletin* 87(11): 807. http://www.who.int/bulletin/volumes/87/11/09-072652/en/ (October 2013).

Coghlan, Benjamin, Richard J. Brennan, Pascal Ngoy, et al. (2006). “Morality in the Democratic Republic of Congo: A Nationwide Survey”. *Lancet* 367(9504): 44–51.

Coghlan, Benjamin, Pascal Ngoy, Flavien Mulumba, et al. (2008). “Mortality in the Democratic Republic of Congo: An Ongoing Crisis”. International Rescue Committee, New York. http://www.rescue.org/sites/default/files/migrated/resources/2007/2006-7_congomortalitysurvey.pdf (October 2013).

Commission for Africa (2005). “Our Common Interest”. Report of the Commission for Africa, London. http://www.commissionforafrica.info/2005-report (October 2012).

Commission for Africa (2010). “Still Our Common Interest”. London. http://www.commissionforafrica.info/wp-content/uploads/2010/09/cfa-report-2010-full-version.pdf (October 2013).

Costello, Anthony, Mustafa Abbas, Adriana Allen, et al. (2009). "Managing the Health Effects of Climate Change: Lancet and University College London Institute for Global Health Commission". *Lancet* 373(9676): 1693–733. http://www.ucl.ac.uk/global-health/project-pages/lancet1/ucl-lancet-climate-change.pdf (October 2013).

Costello, Anthony, Mark Maslin, Hugh Montgomery, et al. (2011). "Global Health and Climate Change: Moving from Denial and Catastrophic Fatalism to Positive Action". *Philosophical Transactions of the Royal Society* 369(1942): 1866–82. http://rsta.royalsocietypublishing.org/content/369/1942/1866.full (October 2013).

de Schutter, Jacqueline and Manuel Riemer (2009). "Participatory Decision-Making Models in the Context of Environmental Justice: Are They Working?" Paper prepared for "Earth System Governance: People, Places and the Planet", 2009 Amsterdam Conference on the Human Dimensions of Global Environmental Change, December 2–4, Amsterdam. http://www.earthsystemgovernance.org/ac2009/papers/AC2009-0151.pdf (October 2013).

Deribe, Shewaye (2007). "Wichi Integrated Wetland-Watershed Management Project". Presentation prepared for the International Conference on Population, Health, and Environment: Integrated Development for East Africa, 14–16 November, Addis Ababa. http://www.ehproject.org/PDF/phe/deribe-wichi.pdf (October 2012).

Diamond, Jared (2005). *Collapse: How Societies Choose to Fail or Succeed.* revised edn. New York: Penguin.

Ebi, Kristie L. and Jan C. Semenza (2008). "Community-Based Adaptation to the Health Impacts of Climate Change". *American Journal of Preventive Medicine* 35(5): 501–7.

Emmelin, Anders, Mesganaw Fantahun, Yemane Berhane, et al. (2008, December 16). "Vulnerability to Episodes of Extreme Weather: Butajira, Ethiopia, 1998–1999". *Global Health Action* 2. http://www.globalhealthaction.net/index.php/gha/article/view/1829/2088 (October 2013).

Ethiopia. Ministry of Water Resources and Ethiopia. National Meteorological Agency (2007). "Climate Change Adaptation Programme of Action (NAPA) of Ethiopia". Addis Ababa. http://unfccc.int/resource/docs/napa/eth01.pdf (October 2012).

Evans, Tim and Carla AbouZahr (2008, 14 November). "INDEPTH @ 10: Celebrate the past and illuminate the future". *Global Health Action* 1. http://www.globalhealthaction.net/index.php/gha/article/view/1899/2003 (October 2013).

Faris, Stephen (2007). "The Real Roots of Darfur". *Atlantic Monthly*, pp. 67–9. (October 2013).

Friel, Sharon, Alan D. Dangour, Tara Garnett, et al. (2009). "Public Health Benefits of Strategies to Reduce Greenhouse-Gas Emissions: Food and Agriculture". *Lancet* 374(9706): 2016–25.

Friel, Sharon, Michael Marmot, Anthony J. McMichael, et al. (2008). "Global Health Equity and Climate Stabilisation: A Common Agenda". *Lancet* 372(9650): 1677–83.

Frumkin, Howard, Anthony J. McMichael, and Jeremy J. Hess (2008). "Climate Change and the Health of the Public". *American Journal of Preventive Medicine* 35(5): 401–2.

Global Fund to Fight AIDS, Tuberculosis, and Malaria (2012). "Global Fund Support Extends Antiretroviral Treatment to 4.2 Million People". Geneva, November 29. http://www.theglobalfund.org/en/mediacenter/newsreleases/2012-11-29_Global_Fund_support_extends_antiretroviral_treatment_to_4,2_million_people/ (October 2012).

Haines, Andy, Sari Kovats, Diarmid Campbell-Lendrum, et al. (2006). "Climate Change and Human Health: Impacts, Vulnerability, and Mitigation". *Lancet* 367(9528): 2101–9. http://dx.doi.org/10.1001/jama.291.1.99.

Haines, Andy, Paul Wilkinson, Cathryn Tonne, et al. (2009). "Aligning Climate Change and Public Health Policies". *Lancet* 374(9707): 2035–8.

Hales, Simon, Neil de Wet, John Maindonald, et al. (2002). "Potential Effect of Population and Climate Changes on Global Distribution of Dengue Fever: An Empirical Model". *Lancet* 2002(360): 9336. 830–34.

Holdren, John P. (2008). "Science and Technology for Sustainable Well-Being". *Science*, pp. 424–34. http://www.sciencemag.org/content/319/5862/424.full (October 2013).

International Monetary Fund (2013a). "Regional Economic Outlook: Sub-Saharan Africa Keeping the Pace". October, Washington DC. https://www.imf.org/external/pubs/ft/reo/2013/afr/eng/sreo1013.pdf (January 2014).

International Monetary Fund (2013b). "World Economic Outlook Database". Washington DC, October. http://www.imf.org/external/pubs/ft/weo/2013/01/weodata/index.aspx (October 2013).

Joint Learning Initiative (2004). "Human Resources for Health: Overcoming the Crisis". Harvard University, Cambridge MA. http://www.who.int/hrh/documents/JLi_hrh_report.pdf (October 2012).

Kasun, Jacqueline (1999). *The War Against Population: The Economics and Ideology of World Population Control*. 2nd edn. San Francisco: Ignatius Press.

Kjellstrom, Tord (2009, March 6). "Climate Change, Direct Heat Exposure, Health, and Well-Being in Low and Middle Income Countries". *Global Health Action* 2. http://www.globalhealthaction.net/index.php/gha/article/view/1958/2183 (October 2013).

Lindsay, Steve and Pim Martens (1998). "Malaria in the African Highlands: Past, Present, and Future". *World Health Bulletin* 76(1): 33–45. http://whqlibdoc.who.int/bulletin/1998/Vol76-No1/bulletin_1998_76(1)_33-45.pdf (October 2013).

Lown, Bernard, James Muller, Eric Chivian, et al. (1981). "The Nuclear-Arms Race and the Physician". *New England Journal of Medicine* 304(12): 726–9.

MacKellar, Landis (2005). "Priorities in Global Health Assistance for Health, Aids, and Population (HAP)". OECD Development Centre Working Papers No. 244, Organisation for Economic Co-operation and Development, Paris. http://www.oecd-ilibrary.org/content/workingpaper/725643456002 (November 2013).

Markandya, Anil, Ben G. Armstrong, Simon Hales, et al. (2009). "Public Health Benefits of Strategies to Reduce Greenhouse-Gas Emissions: Low-Carbon Electricity Generation". *Lancet* 374(9706): 2006–15.

Matovu, George (2011). "New Participatory Instruments in Local Governance: Cases from Rwanda, South Africa, and Uganda". Paper presented at the Commonwealth Local Government Research Colloquium, March 13–15, Cardiff. http://www.lgma.org.au/downloads/File/Matovu%20-%20New%20Participatory%20Instruments1-1%20-%20African%20Case%20Studies.pdf (October 2013).

McMichael, Anthony J., Diarmid Campbell-Lendrum, Carlos Corvalán, et al., eds. (2003). *Climate Change and Human Health: Risks and Responses*. Geneva: World Health Organization. http://whqlibdoc.who.int/publications/2003/924156248X_eng.pdf (October 2013).

McMichael, Anthony J., Diarmid Campbell-Lendrum, Sari Kovats, et al. (2004). "Global Climate Change". In *Comparative Quantification of Health Risks: Global and Regional Burden of Disease Attributable to Selected Major Risk Factors*, Majid Ezzati, Alan D. Lopez, Anthony Rodgers, et al., eds. Vol. 1. Geneva: World Health Organization, pp. 1543–650.

Menne, Bettina, Nino Kunzli, and Roberto Bertollini (2002). "The Health Impacts of Climate Change and Variability in Developing Countries". *International Journal of Global Environmental Issues* 2(3/4): 181–205. doi: 10.1504/IJGENVI.2002.002399.

Murray, Jessica, Busani Tshabangu, and Natasha Erlank (2010). "Enhancing Participatory Governance and Fostering Active Citizenship: An Overview of Local and International Best Practices". *Politikon: South African Journal of Political Studies* 37(1): 45–66.

Nature (2009, July 2). "Time for Early Action". 460(12). Editorial. doi: 10.1038/460012a.

Neira, Maria (2009). "Foreword". *Global Health Action* 2. http://www.globalhealthaction.net/index.php/gha/article/view/2109/2545

Nilsson, Maria, Robert Beaglehole, and Rainer Sauerborn (2009). "Climate Policy: Lessons from Tobacco Control". *Lancet* 374(9706): 1955–6.

Nilsson, Maria, Birgitta Evengård, Rainer Sauerborn, et al. (2012). "Connecting the Global Climate Change and Public Health Agendas". *PLoS Med* 9(6): e1001227. doi: 10.1371/journal.pmed.1001227.

Nyong, Anthony, Francis Adesina, and Balgis Osman Elasha (2007). "The Value of Indigenous Knowledge in Climate Change Mitigation and Adaptation Strategies in the African Sahel". *Mitigation and Adaptation Strategies for Global Change* 12(5): 787–97. doi: 10.1007/s11027-007-9099-0. http://dx.doi.org/10.1007/s11027-007-9099-0.

Orlove, Ben, Carla Roncoli, Merit Kabugo, et al. (2010). “Indigenous Climate Knowledge in Southern Uganda: The Multiple Components of a Dynamic Regional System”. *Climatic Change* 100(2): 243–65. doi: 10.1007/s10584-009-9586-2.

Parkhurst, Justin O. (2002). “The Ugandan Success Story? Evidence and Claims of HIV-1 Prevention”. *Lancet* 360(9326): 78–80.

Parry, Martin, Osvaldo Canziani, Jean Palutikof, et al., eds. (2007). *Climate Change 2007: Impacts, Adaptation, and Vulnerability. Contribution of Working Group II to the Fourth Assessment Report of the Intergovernmental Panel on Climate Change*. Cambridge: Cambridge University Press. http://www.ipcc.ch/publications_and_data/publications_ipcc_fourth_assessment_report_wg2_report_impacts_adaptation_and_vulnerability.htm (October 2013).

Pascual, Mercedes, Jorge A. Ahumada, Luis Fernando Chaves, et al. (2006). “Malaria Resurgence in the East African Highlands: Temperature Trends Revisited”. *Proceedings of the National Academy of Sciences* 103(15): 5829–34. doi: 10.1073/pnas.0508929103.

Patz, Jonathan A., Diarmid Campbell-Lendrum, Tracey Holloway, et al. (2005). “Impact of Regional Climate Change on Human Health”. *Nature* 438(7066): 310–17. doi: 10.1038/nature04188.

Patz, Jonathan A., Diarmid Campbell-Lendrum, Holly Gibbs, et al. (2008). “Health Impact Assessment of Global Climate Change: Expanding on Comparative Risk Assessment Approaches for Policy Making”. *Annual Review of Public Health* 29: 27–39. doi: 10.1146/annurev.publhealth.29.020907.090750.

Pierce, David W., Tim P. Barnett, Benjamin D. Santer, et al. (2009). “Selecting Global Climate Models for Regional Climate Change Studies”. *Proceedings of the National Academy of Sciences* 106(21): 8441–6. doi: 10.1073/pnas.0900094106.

RamaRao, Saumaya, Marlina Lacuesta, Marilou Costello, et al. (2003). “The Link Between Quality of Care and Contraceptive Use”. *International Family Planning Perspectives* 29(2). http://www.guttmacher.org/pubs/journals/2907603.html (October 2013).

Ramin, Brodie Morgan and Anthony J. McMichael (2009). “Climate Change and Health in Sub-Saharan Africa: A Case-Based Perspective”. *EcoHealth* 6(1): 52–7. doi: 10.1007/s10393-009-0222-4.

Rosenzweig, Cynthia, David Karoly, Marta Vicarelli, et al. (2008). “Attributing Physical and Biological Impacts to Anthropogenic Climate Change”. *Nature* 453(7193): 353–7. doi: 10.1038/nature06937.

Semenza, Jan C., Carol H. Rubin, Kenneth H. Falter, et al. (1996). “Heat-Related Deaths during the July 1995 Heat Wave in Chicago”. *New England Journal of Medicine* 335(2): 84–90. doi:10.1056/NEJM199607113350203.

Shope, Robert (1991). “Global Climate Change and Infectious Diseases”. *Environmental Health Perspectives* 96: 171–4.

Smith, Kirk R. (1994). “Health, Energy, and Greenhouse-Gas Impacts of Biomass Combustion in Household Stoves”. *Energy for Sustainable*

Development 1(4): 23–9. http://www.whrc.org/policy/pdf/India/Smith_1994.pdf (October 2013).

Smith, Kirk R., Michael Jerrett, H. Ross Anderson, et al. (2009). "Public Health Benefits of Strategies to Reduce Greenhouse-Gas Emissions: Health Implications of Short-Lived Greenhouse Pollutants". *Lancet* 374(9707): 2091–103.

St. Louis, Michael E. and Jeremy J. Hess (2008). "Climate Change: Impacts on and Implications for Global Health". *American Journal of Preventive Medicine* 35(5): 527–38.

Sullivan, Louis (1990). "An Opportunity to Oppose: Physicians' Role in the Campaign against Tobacco". *Journal of the American Medical Association* 1990(264): 12. 1581–2. http://jama.jamanetwork.com/article.aspx?articleid=383349 (October 2013).

Tumwine, James K. (1989). "Community Participation as Myth or Reality: A Personal Experience from Zimbabwe". *Health Policy and Planning* 4(2): 157–61. doi: 10.1093/heapol/4.2.157.

UNAIDS (2011). "UNAIDS World AIDS Day Report 2011: How to Get to Zero Faster". Geneva. http://www.unaids.org/en/media/unaids/contentassets/documents/unaidspublication/2011/jc2216_worldaidsday_report_2011_en.pdf (October 2013).

UNAIDS (2012). "UNAIDS World AIDS Day Report 2012: Results". Geneva. http://www.unaids.org/en/media/unaids/contentassets/documents/epidemiology/2012/gr2012/JC2434_WorldAIDSday_results_en.pdf (October 2013).

UNAIDS (2013). "Global Report: UNAIDS Report on the Global AIDS Epidemic 2013". Geneva. http://www.unaids.org/en/media/unaids/contentassets/documents/epidemiology/2013/gr2013/UNAIDS_Global_Report_2013_en.pdf (January 2014).

United Nations Economic and Social Commission for Asia and the Pacific (2013). "What Is Good Governance?", Bangkok. http://www.unescap.org/pdd/prs/ProjectActivities/Ongoing/gg/governance.asp (October 2013).

United Nations Framework Convention on Climate Change (2013). "NAPAs Received by the Secretariat". Bonn. http://unfccc.int/adaptation/workstreams/national_adaptation_programmes_of_action/items/4585.php (November 2013).

United Nations Population Fund (2012). "By Choice, Not By Chance: Family Planning, Human Rights, and Development". Geneva. http://www.unfpa.org/webdav/site/global/shared/documents/publications/2012/EN-SWP2012_Report.pdf (November 2013).

United States President's Emergency Plan for AIDS Relief (2008). "Making a Difference: Funding". Washington DC. http://www.pepfar.gov/documents/organization/100073.pdf (November 2013).

United States President's Emergency Plan for AIDS Relief (2013). "Latest Results". Washington DC. http://www.pepfar.gov/funding/results/index.htm (November 2013).

Wehrwein, Peter (1998). "Jonathan Mann and Mary Lou Clements-Mann Killed in Airplane Crash". *Lancet* 352(9131): 888.

Wiggins, Sarah (2009). "CEDRA Climate Change and Environmental Degradation Risk and Adaptation Assessment". Tearfund. http://preventionweb.net/go/11964 (October 2013).

Wilkinson, Paul, Kirk R. Smith, Michael Davies, et al. (2009). "Public Health Benefits of Strategies to Reduce Greenhouse-Gas Emissions: Household Energy". *Lancet* 374(9705): 1917–29.

Woodcock, James, Phil Edwards, Cathryn Tonne, et al. (2009). "Public Health Benefits of Strategies to Reduce Greenhouse-Gas Emissions: Urban Land Transport". *Lancet* 374(9705): 1930–43.

World Health Organization (1990). "Potential Health Effects of Climatic Change: Report of a WHO Task Group". WHO/PEP/90/10, Geneva. http://whqlibdoc.who.int/hq/1990/WHO_PEP_90_10.pdf (December 2013).

World Health Organization (2006). "The World Health Report 2006: Working Together for Health". World Health Organization, Geneva. http://www.who.int/whr/2006/en/ (October 2012).

World Health Organization (2008). "The Kampala Declaration and Agenda for Global Action". Geneva. http://www.who.int/entity/workforcealliance/Kampala%20Declaration%20and%20Agenda%20web%20file.%20FINAL.pdf (October 2013).

World Health Organization (2009). "Protecting Health from Climate Change: Global Research Priorities". Geneva. http://www.who.int/globalchange/publications/9789241598187/en/ (October 2013).

World Health Organization (2010). "Health Coverage at the 16th Conference of the Parties to the UN Framework Convention on Climate Change". 29 November–10 December, Cancún, Mexico. http://www.wits.ac.za/files/res843b46a0ac83418f98d98ad8d8f3279c.pdf (October 2013).

World Health Organization (2011). "Improving Coherence of Climate Change, Health, and Development Policy: Update and Policy Proposals for UNFCCC CoP17 in Durban". Geneva. http://www.who.int/globalchange/mediacentre/events/2011/WHO_Health_in_UNFCCC_COP17_.pdf (October 2013).

Chapter 11
Innovation for Integrated Climate–Health Governance for Africa

Franklyn Lisk

There is ample evidence that climate change affects human development, predominantly through the adverse effects of extreme weather and climate events on health (Costello et al. 2009; Intergovernmental Panel on Climate Change [IPCC] 1997; Oxfam 2008; United Nations Environment Programme [UNEP] 2008; World Health Organization [WHO] 1997; 2008a). The link between climate and health is clearly evident in developing regions, particularly in sub-Saharan Africa – the world's poorest region and the region with the largest share of the world's burden of disease. More recently, sub-Saharan Africa has witnessed increasing incidence of droughts, floods, coastal storms, and changes in biodiversity that have increased vulnerability to malnutrition and climate-sensitive diarrheal and infectious diseases (African Development Bank [AfDB], Asian Development Bank, United Kingdom Department for International Development et al. 2003; Gambia 2008).

While extreme weather events are not new in Africa's history, the opinion of experts is that warming of the climate system – global warming – is deepening the region's vulnerability to disaster and health risks (United Kingdom Department for International Development 2004; IPCC 2007b; 2007d; Simms and Reid 2005; Stern 2007; G8 2005c; Huq et al. 2006). Despite evidence of the adverse effects of climate change on health, existing global governance systems have failed to address contemporary global health issues adequately as those changes interact with changes in climate. For example, even though the threat posed to human development by climate change and global infectious diseases such as the HIV/AIDS epidemic are similar and interlinked, the similarities and connections have received minimal recognition in global health governance innovation.

The inadequacy of existing global governance systems to respond effectively is exacerbated by state failures to deal with public health issues that have transnational implications, such as responding to the threat of pandemics. Poor and weak states may be unable to exercise ultimate responsibility to protect and provide for their citizens when faced with a global health crisis. At the same time, states may resent external and local pressures to cooperate with "outsiders" on national health concerns, which they consider as interference and even perceive as a threat to their sovereignty (International Commission on Intervention and State Sovereignty 2001; Garrett 2007; Cooper et al. 2007). Governments have been unwilling to assume accountability to the international community on matters they regard as sensitive, such as those relating to the need to address public health as a human right, including providing access for women to sexual and reproductive health services, or to the need to provide information on locally discovered viruses (Holbrooke and Garrett 2008). This results in a schism between state responsibility and international accountability. Efforts to integrate health and climate change concerns in a common global governance framework could, in effect, result in a tug of war between sovereign responsibilities entrusted to the state, on the one hand, and the external obligations of the state to the international community, on the other.

The jurisdictional tussle over health sovereignty between national interest and foreign influence underlines the importance of identifying innovations that are most promising for designing and promoting a global governance framework that links climate change concerns and human health. Given the duty of the state to assume responsibility for health in its territory, innovations in global health governance for the adaptation to the effects of climate change must allow for national health sovereignty as well as for the role and governance of designated and relevant international institutions. This sovereignty is required in order to respond appropriately and adequately at both the national and global levels to the interlinked challenge of health and climate change in a globalizing and increasingly interdependent world. Sovereignty also implies the redesign of global governance on the basis of an "innovation agenda" that addresses climate change as an element of health sovereignty and at the same time holds promise for effective changes in global health governance that reflect both national priorities and global standards (Šehović 2014; Cooper and Kirton 2009). The harmonization of national interest with international concern in an integrated global governance framework is challenging and could be problematic in some cases.

This chapter explores the nature and problématique of the link between health and climate change, with special reference to sub-Saharan Africa, as a new challenge in global health governance. It argues that the recent emergence and re-emergence of several diseases can be attributed in varying degrees to climate change-induced environmental and ecological factors derived mainly from human interactions with eco-systems and consequent changes in biodiversity and habitat through greenhouse gas emission, deforestation, use of pesticides, overfishing, overgrazing, and so on. It highlights the link between poor governance in responding to the impact of climate change on human well-being and security as well as the failure of global health governance to address major health conditions that exist predominantly in the developing regions. The combination of the two interlinked problems of poor climate change governance and inappropriate health governance could have a devastating impact on livelihoods and human well-being, particularly in resource-poor countries such as those in sub-Saharan Africa. Of all the socioeconomic conditions associated with poverty reduction and the achievement of sustainable development, health ranks among the most important.[1] Given that health and climate change share similarities in terms of impacts on human well-being and development, the interlinking of health and climate change provides possibilities for incorporating the two issues in an integrated manner in a common global governance framework. An integrated global health governance framework that recognizes the link between the determinants of health and the effects of climate change could be useful for addressing climate change–related health challenges and the failures in existing global health governance to deal with them.

This chapter begins with a conceptual framework for understanding and analysing the interaction between climate change and health. It next examines the different pathways that connect climate change to health status and identifies elements in the adaptation to climate change that could complement and support appropriate innovations in global health governance. This examination is followed by a review of current global and regional efforts to mitigate and adapt to the impacts of climate change on health, with particular reference to the situation of sub-Saharan Africa, where climate change has its greatest effect on countries that have the least resources to respond. The analysis is undertaken through a policy response framework centred on intergovernmental initiatives and efforts made within the dominant framework of the United Nations Framework Convention on Climate Change (UNFCCC) to address the adaptation needs of resource-poor developing countries.[2] From the standpoint of the interest of developing countries and particularly those in sub-Saharan Africa, and following the principles of equity, mutual responsibility, and global social justice, the chapter highlights salient points in the negotiations leading to and conclusions of the much hyped 15th session of the Conference of the Parties (COP) to the UNFCCC in Copenhagen in December 2009 (COP15), which was supposed to agree on a new pact to replace the Kyoto Protocol after its expiry in 2012, and successive sessions – COP16 in Cancun in 2010, COP17 in Durban in 2011, and COP18 in Doha in 2012 (UNFCCC 2009, 2010, 2011, 2012).[3] In conclusion, the chapter assesses how fuller recognition of the climate change–health connection within the UNFCCC framework could contribute to the innovations in global health governance

1 Several of the Millennium Development Goals (MDGs) relate to health and environmental factors (see WHO 2005b).

2 The UNFCCC, which came into existence in 1992, is the principal international instrument of the United Nations to address the effects of climate change, on the basis of international cooperation while recognizing the principle of sovereignty of states. Signatories to the convention constitute a Conference of Parties (COP), which is the supreme decision-making body for the implementation and monitoring of the convention.

3 COP19 in Warsaw in November 2013 closed with a deal on loss and damage mechanisms designed to help developing countries cope with the impacts of climate change, and also agreed that countries should submit "emission plans" by the first quarter of 2015 that will come into force as of 2020.

required for facilitating the adaptation of developing countries to climate change, while still acknowledging individual state sovereignty.

The Climate Change–Health Link: A Conceptual Framework

Conceptually, health and climate change is viewed as "long wave" events of global importance, with wide intergenerational socioeconomic consequences and humanitarian implications (World Bank 2010b; Richards 2003; Smith 2006; Roberts 2001). The interactions between these two global concerns are based on important identifiable pathways that connect the two and are characterized by regional variations in the impacts of climate change and differences in the health status of the population. In resource-poor settings such as sub-Saharan Africa, long-term changes in temperature and rainfall will affect health through pathways such as infectious disease, food insecurity, population displacement and migration, and competition for scarce resources such as water and land. The combined impacts of the adverse effects of climate change, on the one hand, and the relatively poor health status of the majority of the population, on the other, increase vulnerability to poverty and undermine gains in well-being, with potentially serious consequences for effective health governance and the capacity of sovereign states to protect and provide health care for their citizens. The impacts of the interactions of health and climate change will vary with physical conditions and socioeconomic factors. Such a complex and interlinked situation requires a comprehensive and integrated system of global health governance for dealing with the challenges of adaptation to climate change. The complexity of the climate change–health link has, until recently, been further compounded by the relative neglect of this aspect in international negotiations on climate change.

While there is broad consensus that climate change exacerbates existing health challenges in developing countries, insufficient attention has been paid in the context of the UNFCCC to the direct and immediate impact of climate change on human development that includes health (Najam et al. 2003; Agrawala 2005). Part of the reason for this, perhaps, is limited data and evidence of direct and indirect health impacts of climate change, which could have constrained work in this area by the IPCC.[4] Analysis at the international level of the impact of climate change on society has been carried out mainly in the context of global environmental and energy issues with an emphasis on medium- to long-term effects (Simms et al. 2004).[5] Although one of the guiding principles of the UNFCCC (1992) relates to the "specific needs and special circumstances" of developing countries and their

4 The IPCC is a UN-appointed body, made up of technical experts, established in 1988 to obtain and assess climate information for the United Nations, particularly for the UNFCCC.

5 This can be discerned, for example, from the general orientation of various IPCC assessment reports on global warming.

vulnerability to "the adverse effects of climate change", global climate change negotiations have focused more on limiting greenhouse gas emissions associated with human activity and less on the direct and immediate effects on human development in poor countries that have contributed least to global warming. This reflects an attempt to deal with the cause of the problem, and is driven mainly by the stated "ultimate objective" of the UNFCCC.[6] What is needed is a broader policy response framework that focuses on two important conceptual issues of relevance to the situation of resource-poor developing countries regarding the temporal and spatial interaction of climate and health: vulnerability and adaptation.

Given that the potential health effects of climate change are immense, the management of health issues attributable to climate variations implies a need to emphasize human vulnerability to both current and future impacts. The concept of vulnerability in this context represents a combination of two concerns: first, exposure to the impacts of climate change and, second, the ability to cope with the consequences of climate change due to economic, social, and institutional factors. Given the different pathways that connect climate change and health, and the range of socioeconomic factors that determine the interactions of the two dimensions of vulnerability, there is a strong case for putting climate change on the international development agenda as a health issue, as distinct from its environmental impacts and energy implications. Also important are the impacts of contemporary changes in climate on human development, rather than as distinct from medium- and long-term projections of the damage that climate change will cause.

Adaptation in the context of managing the health effects of climate change refers to the response by governmental, global intergovernmental, and multilateral institutions to changes in climate and the impacts of those changes. Adaptation is crucial for reducing vulnerability by building on and strengthening existing coping mechanisms, as reflected in country profiles presented in the Africa Adaptation Programme (2010). The issue of adaptation received hardly any attention during the first decade of international negotiations, when the UNFCCC focused on financial and institutional mechanism for mitigation. With the impacts of climate change becoming more visible in developing countries, particularly through the vulnerability of individuals and communities to climate-induced health risks, and the realization that coping with these impacts was a necessity, more attention has been given to adaptation policy in international negotiations since 2001 (IPCC 2001a, Summary for Policymakers; Oxfam 2008; UNFCCC 2013b, 2007; Huq 2005). The governance response to the need for adaptation in the context

6 The ultimate objective of the UNFCCC (1992, article 2) is to achieve "stabilization of greenhouse gas concentrations in the atmosphere at a level that would prevent dangerous anthropogenic interference with the climate system", on the basis of an international agreement among the parties concerned on climate change. The most high-profile agreement reached within the framework of the UNFCCC is the Kyoto Protocol, which was adopted in 1997 and set binding targets for reduction in greenhouse gas emissions that entered into force in 2005.

of the UNFCCC therefore seeks to assist those states most vulnerable to the risks associated with changes in climate yet least capable of preparing for and managing impacts.

The need for an integrated system of global health governance that does not conflict with the precept of health sovereignty, but also meets the global challenge of governing climate change adaptation for reducing health risks, can be approached from two perspectives. The first is the institutional system of international organizations, multilateral institutions, and the state in terms of their governance structures and mechanisms, taking into account the impact of these structures on power relationships and decision-making authority. The second is the nature of policy at both the international and domestic levels required for the transformation or expansion of the system of global health governance to accommodate linkages between climate change and health. In both cases, the state is the dominant actor, although other important nonstate actors might be involved. The primacy of governmental authority is reflected in longstanding governance arrangements. Within intergovernmental entities in the multilateral system, member states or their representatives offer direction and guidelines for the decisions collectively taken by those institutions in their name. Similarly, member states negotiate and ratify treaties on global health and climate change issues as well as take action to implement them at national and regional levels. Therefore, the sovereign state will play a major role in any initiative to redesign global health governance for addressing the adaptation to climate change.

The Pathways of Climate Change–Health Interaction

Most of the humanitarian disasters globally between 1900 and 2000 were climate-related. Virtually all, particularly in the developing world, entailed health risks and emergencies (McMichael et al. 2003; Mitchell and Tanner 2006; Faris 2007; Jarman 2007; Stern 2007; World Food Programme 2009). New patterns of disease have been driven by temperature and rainfall variation over time (WHO 2008a). The effects of climate change on health are generally manifested in immediate threats and medium- to long-term risks stemming from drought and sea-level rise that could affect livelihoods and human well-being through different pathways: worsening poverty and inequality; the spread of infectious diseases; food insecurity; the displacement of populations and forced migration; and increased competition for scarce resources, such as food, water, and land. In the case of sub-Saharan Africa, the contemporary situation offers a fuller understanding of the current (and future) impacts of climate change and health and the main pathways through which they interact.

Poverty and Inequality

Climate change is already affecting the lives of people worldwide, but the impact is likely to be most severe and felt soonest by the world's poorest people. More than 90 per cent of mortality and morbidity related to disasters associated with climate change has occurred in regions where some of the poorest people live (World Meteorological Organization 2007, 2013; McMichael et al. 2003, ch. 9). The poor may be more vulnerable to climate change simply because of where they live – for example, in exposed areas such as flood plains and slums on unstable hill slopes that are at most risk to natural disasters such as floods and coastal hurricanes. They have less access to resources to withstand the damage to property, infrastructure, and livelihoods that climate change brings. The Commission on the Social Determinants of Health and an earlier path-breaking report on health and economic development both noted that social inequalities among societies constitute a major cause of poor health and are responsible for millions of needless and untimely deaths in the poorest countries (Commission on Macroeconomics and Health 2001; Commission on Social Determinants of Health 2008). The inequity of climate change – with rich countries causing most of the problem and poor countries currently suffering most of the consequences – is inextricably linked to health inequity, and threatens to derail progress in achieving the health targets set in the Millennium Development Goals (MDGs) (WHO 2005b). The 2007/8 Human Development Report of the United Nations Development Programme ([UNDP]), which focused on climate change, pointed out that "climate shocks" such as droughts, floods and storms – predicted to become more frequent as the planet warms – already drive poverty, with the world's poor facing the most immediate and severe costs of climate change and the threat of "unprecedented reversals" in poverty reduction and health.

There is a vicious circle. Inequalities between rich and poor increase vulnerability to the impacts of climate change and its effects on health exacerbate inequalities between poor and rich. Those impacts accentuate the existing health challenges faced by the poorest countries, such as those in sub-Saharan Africa, where populations depend on climate-sensitive sectors (such as rain-fed agriculture and coastal fishing) for their nutritional requirements and livelihoods, and have limited resources and institutional capacities to cope.[7] From a global governance perspective, the "poverty pathway" connecting climate change and health raises issues of equity and justice. The need for climate justice is grounded in the understanding that it is the world's poorest who are most vulnerable to the impact of climate change on their well-being, yet they are least responsible for its cause. As the poorest continent, Africa is at the frontline and is a barometer for how poorly the world is performing to avoid negative consequences. The report of the Commission on Africa (2005) stressed that climate change-induced threats to agricultural productivity and food security, health, water, and energy security will undermine the continent's ability to develop. Using the AIDS epidemic as an illustration, the report makes the important point that the reduction of poverty and

7 Climate change and global warming are already leading to oceanic acidification and increased surface water temperatures, which affect fish stocks and threaten the livelihoods of small-scale fishing communities along the west coast of South Africa (Mannak 2009).

socioeconomic inequalities is crucial to the management of the health effects of climate change.

Pattern and Burden of Disease

Changes in temperature and extreme weather events due to climate change can cause downstream effects on the environment that will affect health directly and indirectly and aggravate the burden of disease. Temperature rise has been associated with the spread of malaria epidemics, as a result of the presence of mosquitoes at higher altitudes once free of the disease. The number of people worldwide at risk of contracting the deadly dengue fever is projected to double in the next 50 years as a consequence of climate change (Costello et al. 2009). With rapid urbanization in developing countries, global warming is likely to increase the spread and transmission rates of vector-borne and infectious diseases, especially in sprawling, densely populated local communities in developing regions. The epidemiological outcome of climate change on the pattern and burden of disease can be profound, especially in poor developing countries where existing vulnerabilities to poor health are high and available resources for maintaining the health of the population are already overstretched.

The spread of HIV/AIDS in sub-Saharan Africa, which has reached pandemic proportions, is a case in point. HIV/AIDS and climate change are two important long-wave global concerns on the international development agenda. They share similarities in terms of their medium- and long-run impacts on human development and its sustainability, and they interact to intensify these impacts. The severity of the impact of climate change on HIV/AIDS is influenced by the location and timing of the interaction between the two (UNEP and UNAIDS 2008). The interaction therefore has an uneven spatial distribution globally, regionally, and locally. Populations with high HIV prevalence rates will likely be more vulnerable to a worsening or prolongation of the epidemic due to climate change. This situation places the people of the southern African sub-region – the area worst affected by HIV/AIDS on the continent – at the greatest risk to the interaction of climate change and HIV/AIDS. In the past decade, countries such as Angola, Benin, Ethiopia, Kenya, Malawi, Mozambique, Zambia, and Zimbabwe that have been affected by one or more of the environmental hazards linked to the impact of climate change – droughts, water shortages, floods, coastal storms, and hurricanes – have had to deal with the spread of vector-borne and other infectious diseases.

Food Insecurity

One of the most important pathways through which climate change threatens human health in poor countries and communities is its effect on food insecurity and malnutrition. Chronic and acute malnutrition is a major cause of infant mortality in sub-Saharan Africa and South Asia, where the majority of the world's poor people live and rely on local ecosystems as the dominant source of staple food.

Droughts are disastrous for food production in sub-Saharan Africa because many countries in the region depend on rain-fed agriculture, and have limited capacity and resources to cope when the rains do not come.

Temperature, sea-level rise, and rainfall variation due to climate change are known to damage agricultural production and increase vulnerability to food insecurity, particularly where production is undertaken by smallholder and subsistence farmers, traditional pastoralists, and artisanal fishers. In 2002, about 15 million people in southern Africa were affected by food insecurity brought about mainly by change in rainfall levels and patterns. Many communities in the sub-region are today struggling to cope with rainfall variability: in the half century between 1950 and 2000, summer rainfall over Southern Africa declined by 20 per cent (Institute for Development Studies and Tearfund 2006). In Malawi, famine in 2001, 2005, and 2006 has been attributed to the effects climate change – drought and flood – that damaged crops and disrupted farming. Climate change-linked food insecurity has been compounded by the current global food crisis, highlighted by the rise in food prices since 2008, which has extended the problem to urban-based food-insecure populations. Lack of ability to meet food needs either through production of purchase could result in under-nutrition, which would impair health.

From a health governance perspective, a case can be made for greater equity in global food distribution to combat the adverse effects of climate change on food security in poor developing countries. An estimated one quarter to one third of people living in the rich countries is over-nourished, in contrast to the situation in sub-Saharan Africa where the majority of the population is likely to be under-nourished. Thus a more equitable distribution of global food production and consumption would go a long way toward defusing the global food crisis and would also improve the health for both the starving in poor countries and the over-fed and obese populations in the rich countries.

Displacement of Populations and Forced Migration

Climate change and its adverse effects on human settlement and livelihood can trigger population migration, as people move from arid or flooded environments in search of more hospitable and secure locations. The manifestations of climate change have precipitated temporary and sometimes permanent movements of people throughout sub-Saharan Africa, with repercussions for their health and well-being (Myers 1997; Reuveny 2008; Stern 2007). The movement of population in large numbers could increase the risk of health problems and vulnerability to the transmission of infectious diseases. The risk of contracting HIV has been observed to be higher among migrants and refugees: for example, the need to provide sex in exchange for money, shelter, or protection exposes female migrants to coercive and unsafe sex with multiple partners, as does the engagement of male foreign migrant workers in transactional sex (Samuels and Spraos 2008; Spiegel et al. 2007; UNEP and UNAIDS 2008).

In addition to the adverse health effects on displaced and mobile populations, climate change–related disasters could reduce existing human capital stock through mortality and emigration. This could affect the effectiveness of the delivery of health and basic services when and where most needed such as during emergencies. The confluence of increased risk of poor health and reduced human capital due to climate change is likely to worsen poverty in resource-poor countries and disadvantaged communities.

Competition for Scarce Resources

Population growth and large-scale population movement will interface with climate change in ways that intensify pressure and competition for scarce resources such as food, water, and land. Changes in temperature and rainfall is already causing shortages in the supply of fresh water in many parts of the world, leading to increasing competition for this most important basic human resource (Bates et al. 2008). Increased competition for diminishing water and food resources will be catastrophic for the poorest, who are most vulnerable. It could entail enormous financial costs for countries already very poor.

Responding to the impact of climate change on livelihood and infrastructure could lead to the diversion of public funds toward disaster relief and management, away from productive activities and the provision of basic social services needed to improve living standards. Public expenditure on climate change-related humanitarian crises and disaster management and reconstruction will likely have a huge opportunity cost in terms of alternative investments in vital development programs and basic social services. State sovereignty in terms of the responsibility to protect and provide health care and other basic services for citizens is eroded by the fiscal implication of responding to the effects of climate change through the allocation of scarce funds to deal with an expanding range of deadly infectious diseases and other human needs accentuated by disasters and emergencies.

Governance Response Framework for Climate Change–Health Interactions

There is a consensus at the international and national levels about the threat to human health posed by climate change, especially for people living in poverty and lacking access to essential health care, and about the need to reduce vulnerability to the adverse health consequences of climate change. Management of the health effects of climate change will require an integrated global governance framework that connects climate change responses and health outcomes. This would involve interaction between sovereign states and global and regional intergovernmental institutions. A governance response framework that integrates climate change and health would require international cooperation on a range of policies needed to tackle climate change as a current global concern with significant development and financial implications, and on the adoption of a "global public goods" approach as the basis for action (Cooper and Kirton 2009; UK Department for International

Development 2006; Sohn et al. 2005). Both the IPCC and the UNFCCC consider global warming to be a global crisis affecting all countries. It is therefore in the interest of both rich and poor countries to act collectively to promote the rapid diffusion of low carbon and clean energy technologies globally.

The UCL Lancet Commission on Managing the Health Effects of Climate Change argued that that an integrated health governance response framework aimed at reducing the adverse health effects of climate change would require action on at least three fronts (Costello et al. 2009). First, policies must be adopted within the UNFCCC mechanism to reduce carbon dioxide emissions and thereby slow down global warming. Second, policy should be directed at events linking climate change to health risks, such as waterborne and poverty-linked infectious diseases. Third, appropriate public health systems and institutional arrangements should be put in place at the national level to deal with adverse health outcomes.

Action in the UNFCCC

The international community met at COP15 in Copenhagen in December 2009 to negotiate the successor to the Kyoto Protocol. Experience from the implementation of Kyoto suggested that it would not be easy to negotiate an international agenda to control global warming and provide assistance for adaptation to climate change to the satisfaction of everyone concerned. But there were reasons to believe that progress could be achieved in Copenhagen. A unilateral approach to adaptation assistance had been established at the COP12 in Nairobi in November 2006. It was largely endorsed by the COP13 in Bali in December 2007, which brought together countries that are parties to the UNFCCC. At Bali both developed and developing countries agreed to negotiate a new treaty on climate change – the successor to the Kyoto Protocol – by the end of 2009. The Bush administration, which had repudiated the Kyoto Protocol that had been signed by the Clinton administration, agreed in Bali to the principle of emission limits and showed an interest in supporting new multilateral programs to finance clean energy technology and protect the environment, including forest conservation. The Obama administration was now strongly committed to clean energy and green growth. There was a precedent in the US that gave rise to optimism. Twenty years earlier, Ronald Reagan's United States provided global leadership in the negotiations of the Montreal Protocol on Substances That Deplete the Ozone Layer.[8] At the same time, the EU proposed new emission regulations that were ahead of the US. China and India acknowledged the need for emission limits that they regarded as consistent with their rapid industrialization and growth strategies.

Copenhagen was an opportunity for both developed and developing countries to address the negative impacts of climate change by committing themselves to a

8 The Montreal Protocol was ratified by the US Senate and ultimately by nearly 200 countries and territories, and has proved largely successful in limiting and phasing out ozone-depleting chemicals.

low-carbon future and support for adaptation including integrating vulnerability reduction into wider development policies such as health. Moving poor countries on to low-carbon development requires large-scale financial and technical assistance, as well as incentives to replace fossil fuel systems with clean energy technology such as solar and wind power. Financing adaptation to climate change – which is now an integral part of the UNFCCC – is costly for most African countries, and could even threaten past development gains in some areas. The rich developed countries are expected to help the poorer developing countries in meeting this cost, which seems fair from an equity and social justice standpoint: the less developed and poor countries that have contributed the least to global warming are most affected by the impacts of climate change. Copenhagen was expected to result in the establishment of an adaptation fund that would be financed by the successor to the Clean Development Mechanism (CDM) that was established within the framework of the Kyoto Protocol.[9] In this context, there would now be now a basis for integrating development challenges, including health problems, in the governance response framework of the UNFCCC.

However, Copenhagen was inconclusive in terms of reaching a consensus among the parties on an agenda for action. The Copenhagen Accord that emerged from the negotiations was a last-minute political compromise brokered by the US, China, India, Brazil, and South Africa, but had little legitimacy. There were no binding agreements on limiting emissions, or timeframes for reaching targets. Long-term commitments on the transfer of resources from developed to developing countries for adaptation to climate change were tentative. Copenhagen also failed to reach agreement on setting a deadline for signing a new global climate treaty. It was a missed opportunity for immediate action to shine the spotlight on human development issues regarding health and poverty reduction, and to extend the provision of financial and technical assistance for adaptation to include the impacts of climate change on health and wider development objectives.

Africa went to Copenhagen with a common position – the first time that Africa fielded a single team empowered to negotiate at the global level on behalf of all members of the African Union (AU). At the heart of the common position was an insistence that rich countries should agree at Copenhagen to aggressive and binding emission cuts in line with UNFCCC recommendations, and that Africa expected adequate, additional, and predictable funding for adaptation, as well as support for mitigation including technology transfer and technical assistance to boost national capacity to exploit clean energy opportunities. Africa, on the basis of its united stand, was apparently taken seriously at Copenhagen. The AU was cautiously receptive to the accord, which it considered an important first step toward a meaningful global agreement with favourable global governance implications.

9 The CDM allows rich countries with emission-reduction commitments to invest in developing countries projects for emission reduction that cost less than home-country projects – so-called carbon credits and offsetting of carbon footprints.

COP16 at Cancun in December 2010 emphasized a shared vision for long-term cooperative action to meet the environmental and development challenges of climate change and achieve the ultimate objective of the UNFCCC. In terms of governance innovation, the Cancun Adaptation Framework called for enhanced action and international cooperation, with a view to integrating climate change adaptation into relevant economic, social, and environmental policies as appropriate. This provides some leeway for integrating climate change and health in a common and integrated response framework. Another outcome of Cancun of some relevance to democratic governance was the decision to establish the Green Climate Fund as a financial mechanism for funding adaptation and mitigation efforts: it was agreed that the fund will be governed by a board of 24 members, comprising an equal number of members from developing and developed country parties; provision was made to ensure broad-based representation from among the developing countries themselves, including from small island states and least developed countries (LDCs).

The Durban Platform for Enhanced Action, which emerged from COP17 at Durban in December 2011, included a consensus to achieve a universal legal agreement on climate change as soon as possible and no later than 2015. The main aim of the UNFCCC was again to stop global warming by limiting global carbon emissions and, for the first time, it agreed on a "road map" to which all parties – including the US, China, India, and the EU – are committed. There was also commitment on some form of legally binding treaty for a second commitment period to extend the Kyoto Protocol until 2020, when a new agreement would come into force. In terms of governance innovation to integrate climate change and health, very little came out of Durban beyond the endorsement of a work program concerning vulnerability and adaptation to climate change, which implied addressing health and other climate-linked development challenges of resource-poor countries. Durban also decided to create the Least Developed Countries Fund to support the implementation of the special work program of the LDCs. This could also apply to health risks from exposure to climate-induced disasters.

For sub-Saharan Africa, the provision of financial and technical assistance for adaptation to climate change should go beyond the introduction of low and clean energy sources to include assistance for addressing the damaging link between devastation of natural resources that provide food and medicines for the poor in developing countries, on the one hand, and, on the other, the depletion of which leads to food insecurity and disease. This underlines the need for deforestation policies to be part of the next climate change agreement, and why action on this issue should be shaped and led by the countries from regions such as sub-Saharan Africa and Latin America where forests are important to livelihoods and human well-being.

Institutional Challenges of an Integrated Climate–Health Governance Response

Institutional arrangements for an effective and equitable governance response to the health consequences of climate change remain a major challenge for many developing countries, especially those in sub-Saharan Africa. The difficulty of coordinating environmental and health concerns in a common operational framework is compounded by the usual vertical segmentation of sectoral responsibilities at different levels of government. Responding to the health effects of climate change requires the coordination of the responsibilities of the environmental and health sectors, not only at national level but also as they relate to the relationship of individual states with regional and global institutions. The sectoral segmentation implicit in the respective global mandates of UN and multilateral institutions – notably the World Health Organization dealing with health matters and the UN Environment Programme with environmental concerns – makes it difficult for international agencies to work with and support government agencies and ministries outside their mandate. At the same time turf wars make inter-agency collaboration hard to put into practice. Two cases are presented below to illustrate innovative efforts to overcome institutional challenges to an integrated climate–health governance response: the case of WHO, which has acted to address climate change as a health issue, and the initiative taken by the African Development Bank (AfDB), a regional development finance institution, to integrate climate change into wider development objectives including health.

World Health Organization

In a report entitled "Climate Change and Health" presented to its executive board in November 2009, WHO (2008a) stated: "There is a strong, global, scientific consensus that warming of the climate system is a fact and is affecting human health". Based on growing evidence of the link between the two issues, the World Health Assembly had adopted a resolution in May 2008 requesting the WHO director general to hold consultations on the preparation of a "workplan for scaling up WHO's technical support to Member States for assessing and addressing the implications of climate change for health and health systems" (WHO 2008a). Although the workplan was intended to serve as a common framework for action by all countries, it recognizes differences in climate, levels of socioeconomic development, culture, health systems, and health status between regions and countries. Accordingly, the consultative process for implementing actions contained in the WHO workplan had been organized on a regional basis. The problem of climate change and health interactions was likely to be most severe in the less developed countries that do not have the capacity and resources to cope with the health risks associated with the impacts of climate change. The workplan was therefore designed to support health systems in low- and middle-income countries and small island states, where vulnerability to the impacts of climate change is further compounded by lack of ability to introduce climate change adaptation and mitigation strategies and policies.

As part of its implementation of its workplan globally, WHO launched a global campaign to raise awareness of the effects of climate change on health and to ensure that health was fully considered in the negotiations leading to and at the Copenhagen conference. WHO believed that increased awareness was important both for prompting actions to reduce greenhouse gas emissions and for supporting strategies central to climate change adaptation programs. As part of its preparation for Copenhagen, WHO worked in partnership with other UN organizations at the global level, and with sectors other than health such as energy, agriculture, and transport at national and regional levels, in order to ensure that health protection and health promotion objectives were incorporated into climate change adaptation and mitigation policies at all levels in an integrated global governance response framework.

In the sub-Saharan Africa region, the WHO workplan focused on the provision of guidance and technical assistance for enhancing capacity to assess health vulnerability and risks due to climate change and for implementing strategies and action programs to protect human health as part of adaptation to climate change. This focus is consistent with the overall aim to incorporate climate change considerations into the pursuit of health and related development objectives at all levels. The global coverage of the WHO workplan facilitated the sharing of knowledge and exchange of information on good practices for integrating climate and health in a common operational framework, as well promoting partnerships between developed and developing countries and between health agency and other global institutions.

The African Development Bank

The AfDB recognizes that its region is particularly vulnerable to the impacts of climate change, as evidenced by the bank's provision of financial assistance to repair damaged infrastructure and transport networks due to floods and other natural disasters in a number of countries in the region. As a development finance institution, the AfDB sees the impact of climate change in the region more as a short- to medium-term adaptation challenge to manage the damage caused by climate change to infrastructure as well as to support publicly provided services so as to mitigate the impact on economic performance, rather than as a challenge pertaining to long-term limits on greenhouse gas emissions. The AfDB is therefore committed to helping its regional members adjust to the new challenge of the impact of climate change on their economies and economic performance by promoting an integrated climate risk management approach that incorporates climate-change considerations into economic development objectives, which could include health and other social objectives. The AfDB uses this approach to assess potential synergies with relevant policies pertaining to health, environment, and gender. With long-term sustainability in mind, the AfDB's Clean Energy Investment Framework relates climate change issues to its urban development and natural resources strategies and also serves as one of its mechanisms for mainstreaming environmental and health concerns into its operations (AfDB 2008; AfDB et al. 2003).

Conclusion: Integrated Innovations in Global Health Governance

Climate change adaptation requires improved coordination and accountability in global governance. Existing deficiencies in climate change negotiation at the global level, which manifest themselves in fragmentation, institutional turf wars, and vested interests, need to be addressed through integrated governance innovations. In terms of such innovations in global health governance, there is a need to work on all fronts to increase the momentum for international action. This involves working through the developed countries (G8 led by the US and the EU), with the emerging and leading developing economies (G20), and with individual countries, toward a common global agenda and action plan. It also raises many challenges for political leaders at the global level, national policy makers, private businesses, international nongovernmental organizations, and pressure groups at the local community level. A common and binding global deal on an integrated climate change and (public) health framework as well as the recognition of climate change as a health issue are important innovations that underline the importance of the UNFCCC. If there could be agreement in the UNFCCC negotiations along the lines of this broader agenda, and also in uniting the world behind a common position for avoiding climate change-linked environmental catastrophes and humanitarian disasters, and if the global community acts quickly with the right type of global institutional support and improved governance of global institutions – with the richer countries taking responsibility and leading the way – the UNFCCC may well provide pathways for effectively addressing climate change-linked health and related poverty problems.

Several innovations are required for integrating governance of climate change adaptation with global health governance. First, climate change should be recognized as a contemporary challenge that encompasses present global priority development issues such as poverty, food insecurity, and health. Climate change adaptation should be mainstreamed into national and international development agendas, recognizing that climate change poses a huge threat to all aspects of human development including health and the achievement of the MDGs. Second, the emphasis of climate change governance should be on promoting proactive responses as a priority, rather than promoting reactive ones. Efforts should be focused on helping society and local communities in sub-Saharan Africa develop an understanding of the main climate change risks and their impact on livelihoods including health, and should encourage strong participation of the local population in policy and action plans to reduce vulnerability. Third, based on a policy framework that integrates health and climate change, there should be investment in building long-term health–climate change resilience including reinforcing and making use of existing health infrastructures and institutions to undertake climate change adaptation activities. Fourth, given the moral implications of the imbalances between those adversely affected by climate change and those responsible for the problem, there is a need to increase development assistance from rich to poor countries for adaptation to the effects of climate change. The UNFCCC conferences in Doha in December 2012, Warsaw in November 2013, Venezuela in December 2014, and beyond offer such on an adequate and sustainable basis, as well as the opportunity to reduce poverty within a climate change adaptation program.

For this to happen, the UNFCCC should widen its focus by incorporating key components of human development – such as food security, health, and human security – into its negotiations and agreements, rather than focusing only on avoiding the negative consequences of climate change and setting targets for greater use of new energy technologies. Governance innovations for making the management of climate change concerns more development-oriented are needed within the framework of the UNFCCC. Apart from agreeing to fund adaptation to climate change in African countries, the UNFCCC process should encourage governments in the region and their external partners to integrate climate variability and climate risk factors into health and development planning. Such a wider and development-oriented agreement would be the basis for enhancing the capacity of African countries to adapt to climate changes positively in a manner that complements their aspiration to achieve long-term sustainable development.

Finally, and in relation to the achievement of the health targets of MDGs, the opportunities created by the negotiation of a new UNFCCC protocol are amenable to the introduction of governance innovations that could make use of climate change adaptation to reduce poverty. The integration of climate change adaptation governance with global health governance should emphasize the adoption of a pro-poor adaptation strategy, aimed at providing assistance to poorer countries to cushion the impacts of climate change on health and other development issues while at the same time recognizing their sovereignty on national development matters. This calls for a conceptualization of health sovereignty that captures the response to the challenges of climate change in a globalized and increasingly interdependent world, and the introduction of innovative policy instruments to deal with health-related aspects of adaptation to climate change. Change is required in the governance structures of relevant global multilateral institutions to reflect the new conceptualization of global health governance in the evolving global order and a changing world. Conditions exist for realizing this new conceptualization of integrated global health governance that is needed to manage the health effects of climate change. The global financial crisis has stimulated governments of the rich industrialized countries to give more attention to green "new deals" that emphasize reindustrialisation based on low-carbon energy. Negotiations since Copenhagen have remained focused on the shared vision of governments of both developed and developing countries to reduce carbon emissions drastically by setting new global warming targets for up to 2050. There is now more attention within the UNFCCC paid to adapting to and avoiding the negative effects of climate change. With strong economic growth performance, developing countries – including those in sub-Saharan Africa – are better placed to improve the quality and efficiency of their public health systems.

References

Africa Adaptation Programme (2010). "Africa Adaptation Programme: An Insight into AAP and Country Project Profiles". United Nations Development Programme. http://www.undp.org/content/dam/undp/library/Environment%20and%20Energy/Climate%20Change/UNDP_GOJ_HR.pdf (January 2014).

African Development Bank (2008). "Integrating Climate Change Adaptation into AfDB Group Operations". Internal memo, Tunis.

African Development Bank, Asian Development Bank, United Kingdom. Department for International Development, et al. (2003). "Poverty and Climate Change: Reducing the Vulnerability of the Poor through Adaptation". World Bank, Washington DC. http://www.unpei.org/sites/default/files/publications/Poverty-and-Climate-Change.pdf (January 2014).

Agrawala, Shardul, ed. (2005). *Bridge Over Troubled Waters: Linking Climate Change and Development*. Paris: Organisation for Economic Co-operation and Development.

Bates, Bryson, Zbigniew W. Kundzewicz, Shaohong Wu, et al. (2008). "Climate Change and Water: Technical Paper VI". Intergovernmental Panel on Climate Change, Geneva. https://www.ipcc.ch/publications_and_data/publications_and_data_technical_papers.shtml (December 2013).

Commission for Africa (2005). "Our Common Interest". Report of the Commission for Africa, London. http://www.commissionforafrica.info/2005-report (October 2012).

Commission on Macroeconomics and Health (2001). "Macroeconomics and Health: Investing in Health for Economic Development". World Health Organization, Geneva. http://www.cid.harvard.edu/archive/cmh/cmhreport.pdf (October 2012).

Commission on Social Determinants of Health (2008). "Closing the Gap in a Generation: Health Equity through Action on the Social Determinants of Health. Final Report of the Commission on Social Determinants of Health". World Health Organization, Geneva. http://www.who.int/social_determinants/thecommission/finalreport/en/index.html (December 2013).

Cooper, Andrew F. and John J. Kirton, eds. (2009). *Innovation in Global Health Governance: Critical Cases*. Farnham: Ashgate.

Cooper, Andrew F., John J. Kirton, and Ted Schrecker, eds. (2007). *Governing Global Health: Challenge, Response, Innovation*. Aldershot: Ashgate.

Costello, Anthony, Mustafa Abbas, Adriana Allen, et al. (2009). "Managing the Health Effects of Climate Change: Lancet and University College London Institute for Global Health Commission". *Lancet* 373(9676): 1693–733. http://www.ucl.ac.uk/global-health/project-pages/lancet1/ucl-lancet-climate-change.pdf (October 2013).

Faris, Stephen (2007). "The Real Roots of Darfur". *Atlantic Monthly*, pp. 67–9. http://www.theatlantic.com/magazine/archive/2007/04/the-real-roots-of-darfur/305701/ (January 2014).

G8 (2005). "Gleneagles Plan of Action: Climate Change, Clean Energy, and Sustainable Development". Gleneagles, July 8. http://www.g8.utoronto.ca/summit/2005gleneagles/climatechangeplan.html (December 2013).

Gambia (2008). "Climate Change in the Gambia". Department of State for Forestry and the Environment, Banjul.

Garrett, Laurie (2007). "The Challenge of Global Health". *Foreign Affairs* 86(1): 14–38. http://www.foreignaffairs.com/articles/62268/laurie-garrett/the-challenge-of-global-health (January 2014).

Holbrooke, Richard and Laurie Garrett (2008). ""Sovereignty" That Risks Global Health". *Washington Post*, August 10. http://www.washingtonpost.com/wp-dyn/content/article/2008/08/08/AR2008080802919.html (December 2013).

Huq, Saleemul (2005). "Adaptation to Climate Change: A Paper for the International Climate Change Taskforce". Institute for Public Policy Research, London. http://www.ippr.org/ecomm/files/adaptation.pdf (January 2014).

Huq, Saleemul, Hannah Reid, and Laurel A. Murray (2006). "Climate Change and Development Links". International Institute for Environment and Development, London. http://pubs.iied.org/14516IIED.html?k=climate%20change%20and%20development%20links (January 2014).

Institute for Development Studies and Tearfund (2006). "Overcoming the Barriers: Mainstreaming Climate Change Adaptation in Developing Countries". Tearfund Climate Change Briefing Paper 1, Tearfund, London. http://www.tearfund.org/webdocs/website/Campaigning/Policy%20and%20research/Overcoming%20the%20barriers%20briefing%20paper.pdf (December 2013).

Intergovernmental Panel on Climate Change (1997). *The Regional Impacts of Climate Change: An Assessment of Vulnerability*. Geneva: http://www.ipcc.ch/ipccreports/sres/regional/index.php?idp=0 (December 2013).

Intergovernmental Panel on Climate Change (2001). *Climate Change 2001: Impacts, Adaptation, and Vulnerability. Contribution of Working Group II to the Third Assessment Report of the Intergovernmental Panel on Climate Change*. Cambridge: Cambridge University Press. http://www.ipcc.ch/ipccreports/tar/wg2/ (December 2013).

Intergovernmental Panel on Climate Change (2007a). *Climate Change 2007: Mitigation. Contribution of Working Group III to the Fourth Assessment Report of the Intergovernmental Panel on Climate Change*. Cambridge: Cambridge University Press. http://www.ipcc.ch/publications_and_data/publications_

ipcc_fourth_assessment_report_wg3_report_mitigation_of_climate_change.htm (December 2013).
Intergovernmental Panel on Climate Change (2007b). *Climate Change 2007: The Physical Science Basis. Contribution of Working Group I to the Fourth Assessment Report of the Intergovernmental Panel on Climate Change.* Cambridge: Cambridge University Press. http://www.ipcc.ch/publications_and_data/publications_ipcc_fourth_assessment_report_wg1_report_the_physical_science_basis.htm (December 2013).
International Commission on Intervention and State Sovereignty (2001). "The Responsibility to Protect: Report of the International Commission on Intervention and State Sovereignty". December. http://responsibilitytoprotect.org/ICISS%20Report.pdf (December 2013).
Jarman, Melanie (2007). *Climate Change.* London: Pluto Press.
Mannak, Miriam (2009). "Climate Change Threatens Livelihoods Along Africa's Coast". *Inter Press Service*, February 19. http://www.ipsnews.net/2009/02/environment-climate-change-threatens-livelihoods-along-africa39s-coast (December 2013).
McMichael, Anthony J., Diarmid Campbell-Lendrum, Carlos Corvalán, et al., eds. (2003). *Climate Change and Human Health: Risks and Responses.* Geneva: World Health Organization. http://whqlibdoc.who.int/publications/2003/924156248X_eng.pdf (October 2013).
Mitchell, Tom and Thomas Tanner (2006). "Adapting to Climate Change: Challenges and Opportunities for the Development Community". Tearfund, London. http://www.tearfund.org/webdocs/website/Campaigning/policy%20and%20research/Adapting%20to%20climate%20change%20discussion%20paper.pdf (December 2013).
Myers, Norman (1997). "Environmental Refugees". *Population and Environment* 19(2): 167–82.
Najam, Adil, Saleemul Huq, and Youba Sokona (2003). "Climate Negotiations beyond Kyoto: Developing Countries Concerns and Interests". *Climate Policy* 3(3): 221–31. doi: 10.1016/S1469-3062(03)00057-3.
Oxfam (2007). "Adapting to Climate Change: What's Needed in Poor Countries, and Who Should Pay". Oxfam Briefing Paper 104, May 29. http://www.oxfam.org/sites/www.oxfam.org/files/adapting%20to%20climate%20change.pdf (January 2014).
Oxfam (2008). "Double Disaster: How Climate Change and HIV Are Twinning to Devastate Southern Africa's Poor". Oxfam Global Centre of Learning, Pretoria.
Reuveny, Rafael (2008). "Ecomigration and Violent Conflict: Case Studies and Public Policy Implications". *Human Ecology* 36(1): 1–13.
Richards, Michael (2003). "Poverty Reduction, Equity, and Climate Change: Global Governance Synergies or Contradictions?", Overseas Development Institute, London. http://www.odi.org.uk/sites/odi.org.uk/files/odi-assets/publications-opinion-files/2408.pdf (January 2014).

Roberts, J. Timmons (2001). “Global Inequality and Climate Change”. *Society and Natural Resources* 14(6): 501–9. doi: 10.1080/08941920118490.

Samuels, Fiona and Helen Spraos (2008). “HIV and Emergencies: Haiti”. Overseas Development Institute, London. http://www.odi.org.uk/publications/3265-haiti-hiv-aids-emergencies (December 2013).

Šehović, Annamarie Bindenagel (2014). *HIV/AIDS and the South African State*. Farnham: Ashgate.

Simms, Andrew, Julian Oram, and Petra Kjell (2004). *The Price of Power: Poverty, Climate Change, the Coming Energy Crisis, and the Renewable Revolution*. London: New Economics Foundation.

Simms, Andrew and Hannah Reid (2005). “Africa: Up in Smoke? The Second Report from the Working Group on Climate Change and Development”. New Economics Foundation and International Institute for Environment and Development, London. http://pubs.iied.org/9560IIED.html (December 2013).

Smith, D. Mark (2006). *Just One Planet: Poverty, Justice, and Climate Change*. Warwickshire: Intermediate Technology Publications.

Sohn, Jon, Smita Nakhood, and Kevin Baumert (2005). “Mainstreaming Climate Change Considerations at the Multilateral Development Banks”. WRI Issue Brief, World Resources Institute, Washington DC. http://www.wri.org/sites/default/files/pdf/mainstreaming_climate_change.pdf (January 2014).

Spiegel, Paul B., Anne Rygaard Bennedsen, Johanna Claas, et al. (2007). “Prevalence of HIV Infection in Conflict-Affected and Displaced People in Seven Sub-Saharan African Countries: A Systematic Review”. *Lancet* 369(9580): 2187–95.

Stern, Nicholas (2007). *The Economics of Climate Change: The Stern Review*. Cambridge: Cambridge University Press.

United Kingdom. Department for International Development (2004). “Climate Change in Africa”. Key Sheet 10. http://www.eldis.org/vfile/upload/1/document/0708/DOC15876.pdf (December 2013).

United Kingdom. Department for International Development (2006). “Eliminating World Poverty: Making Governance Work for the Poor”. White Paper on International Development, London. http://www.official-documents.gov.uk/document/cm68/6876/6876.pdf (January 2014).

United Nations Development Programme (2007/8). “Human Development Report 2007/08 – Fighting Climate Change: Human Solidarity in a Divided World”. United Nations, New York. http://hdr.undp.org/en/reports/global/hdr2007-8/ (December 2013).

United Nations Environment Programme and UNAIDS (2008). “Climate Change and AIDS: A Joint Working Paper”. UNAIDS, Geneva. http://data.unaids.org/Pub/basedocument/2008/20081223_unep_unaids_joint_working_paper_on_cca_en.pdf (December 2013).

United Nations Framework Convention on Climate Change (1992). “Full Text of the Convention”. FCCC/INFORMAL/84. http://unfccc.int/resource/docs/convkp/conveng.pdf (December 2013).

United Nations Framework Convention on Climate Change (2009). "Decisions Adopted by the Conference of the Parties". Report of the Conference of the Parties on its 15th session, Copenhagen. http://unfccc.int/resource/docs/2009/cop15/eng/11a01.pdf (January 2014).

United Nations Framework Convention on Climate Change (2010). "Decisions Adopted by the Conference of the Parties". Report of the Conference of the Parties on its 16th session, Cancun. http://unfccc.int/resource/docs/2010/cop16/eng/07a01.pdf (January 2014).

United Nations Framework Convention on Climate Change (2011). "Decisions Adopted by the Conference of the Parties". Report of the Conference of the Parties on its 17th session, Durban. http://unfccc.int/resource/docs/2011/cop17/eng/09a02.pdf (January 2014).

United Nations Framework Convention on Climate Change (2012). "Decisions Adopted by the Conference of the Parties". Report of the Conference of the Parties on its 18th session, Doha. http://unfccc.int/resource/docs/2012/cop18/eng/08a01.pdf (January 2014).

United Nations Framework Convention on Climate Change (2013). "National Adaptation Programmes of Action". Bonn. http://unfccc.int/adaptation/workstreams/national_adaptation_programmes_of_action/items/7567.php (December 2013).

World Bank (2010). "World Development Report 2010: Development and Climate Change". Washington DC. http://siteresources.worldbank.org/INTWDR2010/Resources/5287678-1226014527953/WDR10-Full-Text.pdf (January 2014).

World Food Programme (2009). "Climate Change and Hunger: Responding to the Challenge". Rome. http://documents.wfp.org/stellent/groups/public/documents/newsroom/wfp212536.pdf (January 2014).

World Health Organization (1997). "Health and Environment in Sustainable Development: Five Years after the Earth Summit". Geneva. http://whqlibdoc.who.int/hq/1997/WHO_EHG_97.12_eng.pdf (December 2013).

World Health Organization (2005). "Health and the Millennium Development Goals". Geneva. http://www.who.int/hdp/publications/mdg_en.pdf (December 2013).

World Health Organization (2008). "Climate Change and Health: Report by the Secretariat". A61/14, March 20, Geneva. http://apps.who.int/gb/ebwha/pdf_files/A61/A61_14-en.pdf (December 2013).

World Meteorological Organization (2007). "Report by the Task Team on Definitions of Extreme Weather and Climate Events". Geneva.

World Meteorological Organization (2013). "The Global Climate 2001–2010: A Decade of Climate Extremes". Geneva. http://library.wmo.int/pmb_ged/wmo_1103_en.pdf (January 2014).

Chapter 12

Connecting Climate Change and Health: The Global Governance Gap

John J. Kirton and Jenilee Guebert

Global health challenges are growing in frequency, intensity, scale, and scope, and in their comprehensiveness, interconnectedness, complexity, and uncertainty as well. Issues once conveniently categorized under the singular, siloed headings of the economy, security, trade, and the environment are now seen as integrally connected to, and thus inherently part of, global health (Fidler 2007; Blouin 2007; Hsu and White 2007; Smith and Martínez Álvarez 2008; Gostin 2012; Rogelj et al. 2013; Kirton and Guebert 2013). Intellectual property, bioterrorism, education, food and nutrition, zoonotic disease transmission, migration, and virus sharing are leading examples of these connections. Global health challenges thus now need to be examined not only in a cross-border context, but in a cross-sector and cross-disciplinary manner as well.

Of the many clear and compelling connections, climate change could well be the "biggest global health threat of the 21st century" (Costello et al. 2009). The effects of climate change will be increasingly devastating, particularly in Africa (Ramin 2009). It will intensify as populations become increasingly urbanized (Sclar and Volavka-Close 2013). The impacts of climate change on human health will be severe without a significant and effective policy intervention. Management of this interconnected challenge "will require … new ways of international cooperation that have hitherto eluded us" (Costello et al. 2009). The current segmented system of global governance is dominated by the long-established system of the heavily legalized United Nations galaxy, with several, separate specialized institutions for climate and for health, and by nongovernmental organizations (NGOs) focused solely on either environmental or health problems and national governments that have separate ministries and agencies for health and the environment. As such, the system is ill equipped to deal with the interlinked challenge, especially without the required institutionalized connections.

Effective global governance for climate and health requires collaboration and coherence. This chapter examines the current climate–health connection, various actors' increasing recognition of these connected challenges, and the recent and inadequate global governance response. It assesses who has reacted most effectively to the interconnected challenges. It suggests several innovative and integrated approaches available to help fill the existing governance gaps. As an inherently global problem that will have more severe effects in different parts of the world, this analysis is directly relevant to Africa's future.

This chapter argues that the climate–health connection will become stronger in the scientific, political, and policy realms. However, the currently inadequate governance response to this challenge will only become more effective if global, regional, and national institutions increasingly acknowledge its severity, comprehensiveness, and complexity, and work together across the health–climate divide in a mutually beneficial way. Several leading cross-sectoral institutions such as the Group of Eight (G8), the Organisation for Economic Co-operation and Development (OECD), and the African Union (AU) are best positioned to overcome the divide. These institutions have a history of dealing with both climate change and health. They convene high-level politicians and policy makers, who are experienced in dealing with a wide range of issues in mutually supportive and collectively coherent ways. They have successfully governed challenging interlinked issues in the past. Responses will also improve as climate and health actors realize that they can help each other produce more positive outcomes for both the climate and for human health.

The Inherent Climate–Health Connection

It has become increasingly clear that there is a close, compounding, and complex link between climate change and human health (Steiner 2009; Sturchio 2009; Walpole et al. 2009; Friel et al. 2008; Costello et al. 2009; World Health Organization 2009b; Rogelj et al. 2013). In 2008, the World Health Organization (WHO) reported that "a warmer and more variable climate threatens to lead to higher levels of some air pollutants, increase transmission of diseases through unclean water and through contaminated food, to compromise agricultural production in some of the least developed countries, and to increase the hazards of extreme weather" (WHO 2008e, 2). Since the 1990s, the direct and indirect climate–health connections have risen in number and intensity (Haines et al. 2000). In 2011, UNEP director Achim Steiner (2011) noted, "the Earth's changing climate has profound implications for global stability and security". Africa is particularly vulnerable (Gottwald 2012). For instance, climate change "drives competition for access to water and arable land in Darfur … [By 2020] crop yields in some parts of Africa are expected to drop by 50 per cent, and water stress could affect as many as 250 million Africans" (Orbinski and Guebert 2010).

Citizens are concerned about the impact of climate change on human health more than any other area. In 2001, a leading 32 per cent of global respondents said they were concerned by the health impacts of climate change (Leiserowitz 2007). This was followed, after a great gap, by the related effect of droughts and water shortages (17 per cent), species loss (15 per cent), extreme weather (13 per cent), economic costs (6 per cent) and sea-level rise (4 per cent).

To date, most of the emphasis on the climate–health connection has been on how climate change affects human health. Here, the evidence – from heat-wave deaths, the increasing number and severity of extreme weather events and storms, and the increasing spread of infectious vectors such as malaria, West Nile Virus, and dengue fever – has been abundant and increasing, even if some of the specific pathways and particular impacts, especially at the regional and local levels, remain under debate within the scientific and policy communities (see Appendices B–G; see also Holmes 2008; Costello et al. 2009; WHO Regional Office for Europe 2009; Parry et al. 2007).

More recently there has been increasing attention paid to the reciprocal relationship of how human health affects climate change (WHO and Health Care Without Harm 2009; Walpole et al. 2009; WHO 2009f). Research has focused on the large carbon footprints of hospitals, the co-benefits from active transportation, and the link between healthy populations and higher greenhouse gas emissions. This research has helped underscore that the climate–health link flows both ways. Much work still needs to be done to explore this health-first side of the climate–health connection. But already it is clear that both issues can serve as a cause and solution to the challenges in the other area. Human health is affected by climate change. Climate change is affected by human health. Thus, both issues can gain from collaboration and both will lose if none takes place (Walpole et al. 2009).

The Health Community's Increasing Response

Because actors that work in the health and climate change sectors tend to operate separately, most of the responses to this increasingly accepted and understood connected challenge have been independent. Climate and health actors have both responded, but not in an integrated and collaborative way (WHO 2009e).

The health community has increasingly drawn the climate–health link, emphasizing that climate change harms human health in many ways (WHO 2009e; Chan 2008). At the global level, WHO, the leading international institution dedicated to health, has acknowledged the climate–health link since the 1990s.[1] The first available document on this topic, in 1990, examined the scientific aspects of climate change, and its potential direct and indirect effects on health and concluded with several recommendations for policy makers (WHO 1990).

In 1996 and 2000, WHO produced additional reports (McMichael et al. 1996; WHO 2000). In 2005, a factsheet on climate–health links was published (WHO 2005a). In 2008, World Health Day focused on the adverse health affects of climate change and WHO director general Margaret Chan (2008) made a statement outlining the five major health consequences of climate change. On May 24, 2008,

1 Some even suggest that WHO's very definition of health indicates that environmental law must seek to protect it (see Onzivu 2012; Gostin 2008).

the World Health Assembly issued resolution 61.19 on climate change and health. It urged member states to take action to mitigate the health impacts of climate change (World Health Organization 2008b, 2008d, 2008e, 2008f, 2008g) In the lead-up to the Conference of the Parties (COP) to the United Nations Framework Convention on Climate Change (UNFCCC) in Copenhagen in December 2009, WHO published a brochure and background report on how climate change affects health (World Health Organization 2009e, 2009b). Indeed, since 2009 it has planned events to take place on the side lines of the climate community's annual COP meetings, in order to "facilitate the inclusion of health concerns in the new agreement, decision-making, resource allocation and outreach activities ... [and] to facilitate information exchange and mutually beneficial interactions amongst the stakeholders for raising awareness and actively involving the health sector in responding to the climate change challenge" (WHO 2009c). Furthermore, WHO has provided expert input on climate change to other agencies, such as the UNFCCC's Subsidiary Body of Scientific and Technological Advice and the Nairobi Work Programme (Onzivu 2012). Thus, WHO has played an active role in influencing climate change by providing scientific evidence, participating in negotiations and helping draft international environmental laws (Onzivu 2012).

Regional bodies such as WHO's regional offices for South-East Asia and Europe and the Pan American Health Organization and national governments from Canada, France, Sweden, and the Czech Republic have also acknowledged the climate–health connection (WHO 2014; Kintzele 2012; Health Canada 2013). WHO's Regional Office for Africa (AFRO) established a program for the environment-health link, but by 2013 had not created one dedicated specifically to the climate–health link (Onzivu 2012; WHO Regional Office for Africa undated-a).[2] However, the subject has been discussed in other regional forums. In most cases, these regional and national bodies have followed WHO's lead.

Beyond international, regional, and national bodies, other actors have mobilized to advance the climate–health cause. Nongovernmental organizations (NGOs), foundations and public–private partnerships have played a role (Cooper and Kirton 2009; Kirton 2009). In 2002, the International Federation of Red Cross and Red Crescent Societies (2012) established a climate centre, which deals with the humanitarian consequences, including addressing health concerns and providing health care. The Global Fund to Fight AIDS, Tuberculosis, and Malaria (2004a) found in 2004 that "more than 41% of the world's population is at risk of acquiring malaria, and the proportion increases yearly due to deteriorating health systems, growing drug and insecticide resistance, climate change, and war". The Rockefeller Foundation (2014) supported the establishment of the Asian Cities Climate Change Resilience Network in 2008 to focus on the impacts that climate change has on various sectors including health. In 2009, Save the

2 However, under its Protection of the Human Environment Program, vector-borne diseases such as malaria and schistosomiasis are identified as major health problems due in part to the proliferation of climate change (WHO for the African Region undated-b).

Children (2009) published a report entitled, "Feeling the Heat: Child Survival in a Changing Climate".

The Climate Community's Increasing Response

Climate actors have also acknowledged the climate–health challenge. As the leading international agreement on climate change, UNFCCC and its COPs and Meetings of the Parties (MOPs) have sought to govern the climate–health connection. In the 1990s, the UNFCCC set the overarching framework for the international community to tackle climate change. It was adopted on May 9, 1992, opened for signature in June 1992 and entered into force on March 21, 1994. The climate–health connection was present in this "constitutional" document from the start. Articles 1 and 4 declared, as the core connecting principle, that climate change caused "significant deleterious effects" for public health and that the signatories should "take climate change considerations into account, to the extent feasible, in their relevant social, economic and environmental policies and actions, and employ appropriate methods, for example impact assessments, formulated and determined nationally, with a view to minimizing adverse effects on the economy, on public health and on the quality of the environment, of projects or measures undertaken by them to mitigate or adapt to climate change" (UN 1992). Also identified were several climate–health pathways such as drought, food, agriculture, water, natural disasters, and other social consequences (Smith and Martínez Álvarez 2008; Kirton and Guebert 2009a).

Since this strong start, however, the recognition of the climate–health connection in the UNFCCC process has varied, and most recently has declined (Onzivu 2012). A direct climate–health connection was made at the COP in 1996 and those from 1999 to 2003, and at the MOPs in 2005, 2010, and 2011. At these meetings, several key links were identified, including how climate change, extreme weather events, and ozone-affecting chemicals were causing health problems, and how these health impacts were significant, harmful, adverse, and potentially irreversible. The members recognized that developing countries, small island states, Central America, and Africa were being affected the most. Also specified were principles and instruments for preventing and minimizing the adverse effects, such as the expression of regret, adaptation, the monitoring of debt relief finance, climate funds, forecasting, early warning, prevention, the setting of integrative objectives, technology transfer, afforestation, reforestation, and carbon dioxide capture and storage. However, no real link between climate change and health was made at either the COPs or MOPs in 2012 or 2013.

Parties to the UNFCCC thus made an early effort to govern the climate–health link by acknowledging the connections. However, WHO has never been explicitly recognized as a relevant international organization in the UNFCCC documentation, even though several other UN bodies, such as the Food and Agriculture Organization and International Energy Agency have been (Kirton and Guebert 2009a). It has never been included in the process. This has remained the case, despite WHO's increased lobbying to be included since 2009 (Singh 2012). The UNFCCC process has failed to encourage member countries to address these serious climate–health challenges. And while the scientific evidence supporting the climate–health link has increased – particularly in the late 2000s – attention to the issue has remained limited within the climate change negotiations, unlike within WHO. In Cancun in 2010, the delegates "acknowledged that human health *should* be an important factor in the UNFCCC negotiations" (Singh et al. 2011). However, they went no further. At the 2011 meeting in Durban, despite it having "the largest health presence in a UNFCCC conference to date", the health perspective remained on the side lines (Singh 2012).

In addition, even when there has been a recognition of the link, it has had little impact (Onzivu 2012). There has been "increasing concern that international and national environmental law have not been emphasized to advance the protection of public health" (Onzivu 2012, 301). More specifically, there has been an acknowledgement that the legal regimes under the UNFCCC and Kyoto Protocol are centred on mitigation and energy and not human health (Onzivu 2012, 302). Health has remained at the periphery of both the UNFCCC and Kyoto Protocol.

The neglect of the politically driven UNFCCC process is all the more surprising given the accumulating findings of the scientifically based Intergovernmental Panel on Climate Change (IPCC).[3] The scientific case for forging the climate–health connection, and doing so fast and in full, is not in doubt. Since soon after the IPCC was established, the comprehensive, complex, direct climate–health connections have been consistently clear and compelling. The climate–health connection and WHO as a relevant actor were identified as important as early as the IPCC's Second Assessment Report in 1995 (IPCC 1995). Both were identified again in the Third Assessment Report in 2001 (see IPCC 2001b). The IPCC's attention to health then increased (see IPCC 2007c). A detailed analysis was presented in the IPCC's Working Group II Report, "Impacts, Adaption and Vulnerability" (IPCC 2007a). The executive summary of Chapter Eight, which was dedicated exclusively to human health, noted 15 specific climate–health challenges (see Appendix 12-D). The IPCC's attention to health has been supported and driven by partnerships and collaboration with various stakeholders, including WHO, WHO sits on the IPCC and has published a series of reports on the health risks of climate change since 1990.

States that are parties to other international environmental processes have also been made aware of the climate–health link. In a 2010 policy brief, the COHAB Initiative (2010) urged "the parties to the Convention on Biological Diversity and the member states of the World Health Organisation to build a closer collaboration on these issues, in order to mainstream biodiversity concerns and conservation strategies into local, national and global policy and action to mitigate and adapt to

3 The IPCC was identified as the key actor responsible for carrying out the UNFCCC's work (see article 21, UN 1992).

the health implications of climate change". Major environmental NGOs, including the David Suzuki Foundation, Pollution Probe, and AcidRain.org, have also identified climate–health challenges. Several development-based organizations, such as World Neighbors, have too. However, there has been no major move to collaborate on the topic in response (Kirton and Guebert 2009a).

The Inadequate Climate–Health Global Governance Response

Outside the UN galaxy, other global and regional institutions have governed both health and climate, and have done so in an increasingly integrated but still inadequate way.

Major Economies Meeting and Forum

The Major Economies Meeting on Energy Security and Climate Change ([MEM], later known as the Major Economies Forum [MEF]), which was created by the United States in mid 2007 to advance global discussions on climate change and prepare for the UNFCCC's Copenhagen conference in December 2009. It did not acknowledge the health–climate connection at its first two officials-level meetings (Major Economies Meeting on Energy Security and Climate Change 2007, 2008b). However, when France hosted the third meeting in April 2008, President Nicolas Sarkozy (2008) stated: "The situation is urgent, since climate change already poses a major security challenge … Together we must immediately grasp the magnitude of the tragedies experienced by the countries of the South, where there is increasing demand for food but shrinking food supplies and worsening health conditions".

At its first leaders' level meeting, taking place as part of the G8 summit in 2008, the leaders stated: "conscious of our leadership role in meeting such challenges, we, the leaders of the world's major economies, both developed and developing, commit to combat climate change in accordance with our common but differentiated responsibilities and respective capabilities and confront the interlinked challenges of sustainable development, including energy and food security, and human health" (MEM 2008a).

The G8

At the global level, the G8 has been governing health and climate change in parallel since 1979 (Kirton and Guebert 2009b, 2009c). In 1997, when the Kyoto Protocol was concluded with no attention to the climate–health connection, the G7/8 made the link for the first time. At its American-hosted Denver Summit, the leaders declared:

> Overwhelming scientific evidence links the build-up of greenhouse gasses in the atmosphere to changes in the global climate system. If current trends continue

> into the next century, unacceptable impacts on human health and the global environment are likely. Reversing these trends will require a sustained global effort over several decades, with the involvement of all our citizens, and changes in our patterns of consumption and production (G8 1997).

The leaders thus declared that climate change was a major challenge: it affected human health, did so in unacceptable, harmful ways, and required an immediate response.

After an absence of several years, during which time the COP's attention to the connection flourished, the G8 returned to the connection in 2003, just as the COP's emphasis faded (G8 2003b). The climate–health connection, missing from the 2004 American-hosted Sea Island Summit, came back at the British-hosted G8 Gleneagles Summit in 2005 (G8 2005c, 2005b). There the G8 identified the specific impacts of climate change on respiratory disease and healthcare costs. In doing so, for the first time, it made the trilateral link among climate change, health, and the economy.[4] After an absence at the Russian-hosted St. Petersburg Summit in 2006, from 2007 to 2012 the connection was forged (G8 2007, 2008, 2009, 2010, 2011b, 2011a, 2012). The G8 thus gave increasing attention to the climate–health connection. Its attention was strongest when its summits had climate change as a priority, as in 1997, 2003, 2005, 2007, 2008, and 2009, in contrast to health, which was a priority only in 2006 and 2010. It has also been stronger when the summits have been more closely and directly connected to Africa, and thus to the acute health challenges there (Cooper et al. 2007).

Other Institutions

Additional multi-issue international institutions have forged the link. In 2006, at the meeting of OECD's (2006) Development Assistance Committee and Environment Policy Committee, participating ministers concluded that "global environmental challenges, such as climate change, biodiversity loss, and desertification, have important implications for the achievement of many development objectives: poverty alleviation, enhanced access to primary education, gender equity, reduced child mortality, improved maternal health, and the eradication of many diseases are closely linked to a healthy environment". The impacts of climate change on child and maternal health were very clear. Subsequently, secretary general Angel Gurría (2008) remarked, "climate change is the defining issue of our era. Our health, our security and our economies are being threatened by climate change. Although uncertain, the damage is likely to be unevenly distributed, with poorer

4 The economic impact of climate change will be severe in many parts of the world. For instance, Donald Spady (2012, 131) notes, "climate change costs for Canada are estimated to be $21–43 billion per year by 2050, and even higher beyond that if we do not quickly reduce carbon emissions".

economies and households incurring greater losses". The OECD thus merged climate and health with other important areas, such as the economy, food and agriculture, and security. In particular, it showed how health could benefit from supporting and advocating climate change control (OECD 2009).

Regional organizations that deal with a wide range of issues at the leaders and ministerial levels, such as the European Council, the Asia Pacific Economic Cooperation (APEC) forum, the Arctic Council and the AU have also acknowledged the climate–health link (European Council 2001; APEC 1997; Arctic Council 1997, 2006, 2009; Gore and Støre 2009; AU 2008). The AU dealt with both climate change and health for many years, but only recently with the issues in a combined manner (AU 2011). In 2011, the theme of the fifth session of the AU Conference of Ministers of health was "The Impact of Climate Change on Health and Development in Africa" (AU 2011). However, for the most part these regional bodies have not shown that they are well positioned or determined to govern climate–health challenges (Kirton and Guebert 2009a). For instance, William Onzivu (2012) notes, "despite [European Commission] collaboration with WHO on issues such as climate change … the limited integration of public health concerns across EC environmental law has undermined the efficacy of the strategy of health protection". This is not surprising given the fact that these are truly global challenges. Regional organizations, such as the AU and Arctic Council, where member states are feeling the impacts disproportionately, may be able to help raise awareness of these concerns. However, in order to be effective, the response needs to be global in scope (Kintzele 2012).

The Critical Gaps

While occasional efforts have been made to forge the climate–health connection at the global and regional governance levels, much more could and should be done. In the physical world, the direct and indirect climate–health connections continue to expand. It is becoming clearer that the link flows two ways, as both areas are suffering from the harmful impacts of the other and could help each other. More institutions have acknowledged that the connection is physically real and a cause for policy concern. However, the global or regional governance response required to deal with the interconnected challenge effectively has not yet been established. Indeed, climate researchers have suggested that inadequate governance is the biggest hurdle to addressing the challenge (Rogelj et al. 2013). The health–climate link has fallen in importance in some institutions, while it has risen on others, in a fitful fashion overall. Meanwhile, the harmful impacts will only get more severe as time goes on (Parry et al. 2007; Costello et al. 2009).

Several gaps exist that should be addressed in the following ways. First, in the scientific world more research needs to be undertaken to show how the climate–health connection is growing, and to identify and communicate the complex causal pathways that connect the two (IPCC 2007c; Parry et al. 2007).

This is critical if politicians and policy makers are to address the challenges significantly. The scientific case for the close climate–health connection must continue to be built, in a way that resonates with actors in both the health and climate communities, and with the public at large. This scientific program should flow from long-established, cumulative findings of the IPCC, with WHO equally involved.

Second, health actors need to focus on their own impact on climate change. This will help ensure that the health community not only emphasizes shaming the climate community into action by highlighting the health costs of not dealing with climate change, but that it also takes action to contribute positively to climate change control. The health community can take ownership and responsibility, and be part of the solution, rather than simply decry its role as a victim. Health actors can advance the climate agenda in its vision, mitigation, adaptation, reduction targets and timetables, sectoral actions, finance, investment, and technology in order to achieve better, synergistic, simultaneous outcomes for both climate change and public health.

One such mutually beneficial tactic is to identify the climate mitigation links. Here climate change and heath can both benefit from specific activities that can be readily reduced – as would happen with the reduction of the use of coal. As German chancellor Helmut Schmidt recognized as long ago as 1979, the use of coal causes global warming and harms human heath throughout its full life cycle, from deaths in mining accidents and black lung disease, through to mercury emissions and ambient air emissions from sulphur dioxide and carbon dioxide when it is burned. More broadly, mitigation depends on addressing the supply of energy that has well-established direct and indirect climate and health effects. A systematic study can identify where both the climate and health benefits are greatest, throughout its full lifespan and across all energy sources – from wood, peat, and coal, through oil and gas in various forms, to nuclear, hydroelectricity, wind, geothermal, solar and tidal power. The results would help guide efforts in health and climate, but also in the more broadly connected areas of finance, investment, and technology. In the meantime, the Group of 20 ([G20] 2009) should fulfil its commitment to eliminate inefficient fossil fuel subsidies worldwide, as this would reduce carbon emissions, save more than half a trillion dollars in government spending and reduce ill health from the use of wood and coal in cooking and heating in poor households.

In the realm of adaptation, a premium should be placed on well-known deadly diseases, such as malaria and dengue fever, that global warming brings to new locales (Berrang-Ford et al. 2009). Action on these diseases in the areas where they are prevalent will help prevent their spread to uninfected areas. Another target is any process that directly causes death in large volume: natural disasters, drought, desertification, famine, and water contamination are at the core here. There is also the new and growing challenge, including in a moving Africa, of “climate refugees” (including those who bring diseases with them), and the expensive development and humanitarian efforts that such mobile people create.

Other connections should be drawn. The economic link stands out, but other links such as food and agricultural and traditional security concerns are important too. In the realm of finance and economics, the task is to mobilize the established international financial institutions, national governments, NGOs, and businesses to finance activities that simultaneously enhance climate change control and health. One priority is to get the climate institutions to systematically identify and assess ex ante the health impacts of their programs and proposals and then use the results as criteria in funding allocations. The converse is true for the health organizations, starting with WHO. Another priority is to have the major international financial institutions, starting with the International Monetary Fund and the Financial Stability Board, as well as the World Bank and regional development banks, routinely identify the climate and health impacts of their activities as well as the threats to those activities, and to privilege those activities where the climate–health co-benefits are most pronounced (McInerney-Lankford et al. 2011). Financing healthy and clean energy alternatives and reducing energy subsidies, as the G20 leaders initially agreed to do at their Pittsburgh Summit in 2009, show how this approach might work (Kirton and Koch 2009; Kirton and Guebert 2009a).

Investment incentives could be used, focused on areas where the climate–health co-benefits loom largest. This could include providing financing incentives for investments in new green infrastructure that have a health component, such as energy-efficient buildings that are designed and built in ways that do not harm and that enhance human health (WHO and Health Care Without Harm 2009). The construction of carbon-reducing hospitals is another obvious place to start. Also useful would be ensuring that health investments, such as the development and production of pharmaceuticals, do not contribute to climate change. Curbing obesity through the promotion of consuming more sustainable agricultural crops, such as pulses, in place of climate-harmful animal products may also help (Gottwald 2012).

In the political realm of global governance, climate and health actors need to work together in a more convergent, collaborative, coordinated way. Here, closer cooperation at the international level is most important between the leading international climate institution in the form of the UNFCCC secretariat and its COPs/MOPs and the leading global health institution in the form of WHO. In 2001, a WHO (2001c) report on climate change and human health noted that "intersectoral and interagency collaboration is essential to address climate related health problems and maximize effective resource use. Capacity building at all levels was agreed to be an important component among measures needed to reduce vulnerability to climate variability and change". However, while WHO has worked with the UN Environment Programme and World Meteorological Organization, direct participation in the UNFCCC process has remained absent. WHO has yet to be recognized as a relevant international organization in COP and MOP decisions, even though several other UN bodies have been.

Comprehensive, concerned, multi-issue global governors and others with the capacity to govern multiple issues should be encouraged to address the climate–health challenge. Such governors include the G8, which has a strong history of governing climate and health and other important issues such as the economy and security, and the G20. Leaders who convene at G8 and G20 summits have the authority and capability to forge the connection between climate change and health, and do so in the context of the predominant concern with the economy (Kirton and Guebert 2009a). This is also true at the national level, especially where leaders have priorities on, or experience in climate, health or both. One example is the declaration by US president Barack Obama just before the opening of the 2009 UNFCCC Copenhagen Conference on Climate Change that greenhouse gases are a health hazard (Reguly 2009). Opportunities for others arise at meetings of national leaders of consequential countries, which have become far more frequent in recent decades (Anderson and Sands 2009).

Conclusions

It has become increasingly clear that climate and health are connected in many close and complex ways. The links that can be drawn between the two are compounding. Numerous climate and health actors from the scientific, political, policy, and civil society spheres have acknowledged this connection at the national, regional, and global levels. Broader, more multi-issue global governance institutions, led by the G8 and OECD, have too. However, the global governance response to these interconnected challenges has remained fitful and fragile. There is still no clearly defined core leader to address this challenge. Climate and health actors have not been able to collaborate and cooperate in the way necessary to produce an effective response. Both sides now need to make a better effort to engage each other and act together.

The recent surge of information, analysis, and attention to the climate–health connection suggests that a positive change could come soon. However, this will require a major effort from climate and health actors from all communities, and from all levels of governance. This will not be easy. It will require fresh thinking, innovation, and perseverance. But a successful and effective response is critical, not only for health and climate change, but also for global governance more broadly – as it becomes evident that the leading global challenges are no longer separate. They are interconnected and interdependent. They need to be governed in such a way.

References

African Union (2008). "Decisions, Declarations, Tribute, and Resolution". June 30–July 1, Sharm El-Sheikh. http://www.africa-union.org/root/au/Conferences/2008/june/summit/dec/ASSEMBLY%20DECISIONS%20193%20-%20207%20(XI).pdf (December 2013).

African Union (2011). "Theme: The Impact of Climate Change on Health and Development in Africa". April 17–21, Windhoek. http://www.au.int/en/sites/default/files/OVERVIEW_OF_THE_THEME_EN_17_21_APRIL_2011_SA_MINISTERS_MEETING_FIFTH_SESSION_AFRICAN_UNION_CONFERENCE_MINISTERS_HEALTH_WINDHOEK_NAMIBIA.doc (December 2013).

Anderson, Greg and Christopher Sands (2009). "The Summit Pandemic". *Edmonton Journal*, August 8. http://www.hudson.org/index.cfm?fuseaction=publication_details&id=6402 (December 2013).

Arctic Council (1997). "Alta Declaration". June 13, Alta, Norway. http://library.arcticportal.org/1271/1/The_Alta_Declaration.pdf (December 2013).

Arctic Council (2006). "Salekhard Declaration". October 26, Salekhard, Russia. http://www.arctic-council.org/index.php/en/document-archive/category/5-declarations?download=39:salekhard-declaration-2006 (December 2013).

Arctic Council (2009). "Tromsø Declaration". April 29, Tromsø. http://www.arctic-council.org/index.php/en/document-archive/category/53-final-reports-and-statements?download=222:the-tromso-declaration (December 2013).

Asia-Pacific Economic Cooperation (1997). "Vancouver Declaration: Connecting the APEC Community". November 27, Vancouver. http://www.apec.org/Meeting-Papers/Leaders-Declarations/1997/1997_aelm.aspx (December 2013).

Berrang-Ford, Lea, J.D. MacLean, Theresa W. Gyorkos, et al. (2009). "Climate Change and Malaria in Canada: A Systems Approach". *Interdisciplinary Perspectives on Infectious Diseases* 2009. Article ID 385487. doi: 10.1155/2009/385487.

Blouin, Chantal (2007). "Can the World Trade Organization Help Achieve the Health Millennium Development Goals?". In *Governing Global Health: Challenge, Response, Innovation*, Andrew F. Cooper, John J. Kirton, and Ted Schrecker, eds. Aldershot: Ashgate, pp. 87–100.

Chan, Margaret (2008). "The Impact of Climate Change on Human Health". World Health Organization, April 7. http://www.who.int/mediacentre/news/statements/2008/s05/en/index.html (December 2013).

COHAB Initiative (2010). "The Health Effects of Climate Change Impacts on Biodiversity". UN CBD COP 10 Policy Brief: Biodiversity and Global Health 3, October, Galway. http://www.cbd.int/doc/health/cohab-policy-brief3-en.pdf (December 2013).

Cooper, Andrew F. and John J. Kirton, eds. (2009). *Innovation in Global Health Governance: Critical Cases*. Farnham: Ashgate.

Cooper, Andrew F., John J. Kirton, and Ted Schrecker, eds. (2007). *Governing Global Health: Challenge, Response, Innovation*. Aldershot: Ashgate.

Costello, Anthony, Mustafa Abbas, Adriana Allen, et al. (2009). "Managing the Health Effects of Climate Change: Lancet and University College London Institute for Global Health Commission". *Lancet* 373(9676): 1693–733.

http://www.ucl.ac.uk/global-health/project-pages/lancet1/ucl-lancet-climate-change.pdf (October 2013).
European Council (2001). "Presidency Conclusions". SN 2001/1/01 REV 1, June 15–16, Göteborg. http://ec.europa.eu/smart-regulation/impact/background/docs/goteborg_concl_en.pdf (December 2013).
Fidler, David P. (2007). "A Pathology of Public Health Securitism: Approaching Pandemics as Security Threats". In *Govern"g Global Health: Challenge, Response, Innovation*, Andrew F. Cooper, John J. Kirton, and Ted Schrecker, eds. Aldershot: Ashgate, pp. 41–64.
Friel, Sharon, Michael Marmot, Anthony J. McMichael, et al. (2008). "Global Health Equity and Climate Stabilisation: A Common Agenda". *Lancet* 372(9650): 1677–83.
G8 (1997). "Communiqué". June 22, Denver. http://www.g8.utoronto.ca/summit/1997denver/g8final.htm (December 2013).
G8 (2003). "Science and Technology for Sustainable Development: A G8 Action Plan". Evian, June 2. http://www.g8.utoronto.ca/summit/2003evian/sustainable_development_en.html (December 2013).
G8 (2005a). "Climate Change, Clean Energy, and Sustainable Development". Gleneagles, July 8. http://www.g8.utoronto.ca/summit/2005gleneagles/climatechange.html (December 2013).
G8 (2005b). "Gleneagles Plan of Action: Climate Change, Clean Energy, and Sustainable Development". Gleneagles, July 8. http://www.g8.utoronto.ca/summit/2005gleneagles/climatechangeplan.html (December 2013).
G8 (2007). "Growth and Responsibility in Africa". Heiligendamm, June 7. http://www.g8.utoronto.ca/summit/2007heiligendamm/g8-2007-africa.html (December 2013).
G8 (2008). "Development and Africa". Hokkaido, July 8. http://www.g8.utoronto.ca/summit/2008hokkaido/2008-africa.html (December 2013).
G8 (2009). "Responsible Leadership for a Sustainable Future". L'Aquila, Italy, July 8. http://www.g8.utoronto.ca/summit/2009laquila/2009-declaration.html (December 2013).
G8 (2010). "G8 Muskoka Declaration: Recovery and New Beginnings". Huntsville, Canada, June 26. http://www.g8.utoronto.ca/summit/2010muskoka/communique.html (December 2013).
G8 (2011a). "G8 Declaration: Renewed Commitment for Freedom and Democracy". Deauville, May 27. http://www.g8.utoronto.ca/summit/2011deauville/2011-declaration-en.html (December 2013).
G8 (2011b). "G8/Africa Joint Declaration: Shared Values, Shared Responsibilities". Deauville, May 27. http://www.g8.utoronto.ca/summit/2011deauville/2011-africa-en.html (December 2013).
G8 (2012). "Camp David Declaration". Camp David, May 19. http://www.g8.utoronto.ca/summit/2012campdavid/g8-declaration.html (December 2013).

G20 (2009). "G20 Leaders Statement: The Pittsburgh Summit". Pittsburgh, September 25. http://www.g20.utoronto.ca/2009/2009communique0925.html (July 2012).

Global Fund to Fight AIDS, Tuberculosis, and Malaria (2004). "The Malaria Epidemic". Geneva. http://www.globalfundatm.org/journalists/fsheets/malaria.htm (December 2013).

Gore, Al and Jonas Gahr Støre (2009). "Co-chair's Summary – Melting Ice: Regional Dramas, Global Wake-Up Call". April 29, Tromsø. http://www.arctic-council.org/index.php/en/document-archive/category/53-final-reports-and-statements?download=213:co-chars-summary-meeting-ice-conferance

Gostin, Lawrence O. (2008). "Meeting Basic Survival Needs of the World's Least Healthy People: Toward a Framework Convention on Global Health". *Georgetown Law Journal* 96(2): 331–92. http://georgetownlawjournal.org/files/pdf/96-2/Gostin-Article.PDF (December 2013).

Gostin, Lawrence O. (2012). "Conclusion". In *Human Health and Ecological Integrity: Ethics, Law, and Human Rights*, Laura Westra, Colin L. Soskolne, and Donald W. Spady, eds. Abdingdon: Routledge, pp. 335–8.

Gottwald, Franz-Theo (2012). "Are Cows 'Climate Killers'?". In *Human Health and Ecological Integrity: Ethics, Law, and Human Rights*, Laura Westra, Colin L. Soskolne, and Donald W. Spady, eds. Abdingdon: Routledge, pp. 277–88.

Gurría, Angel (2008). "The OECD: An Active Player in Building Global Governance". In *Growth, Innovation, Inclusion: The G20 at Ten*, John J. Kirton and Madeline Koch, eds. London: Newsdesk, pp. 45–6. http://www.g8.utoronto.ca/newsdesk/G20at10.pdf (December 2013).

Haines, Andrew, Anthony J McMichael, and Paul R. Epstein (2000). "Environment and Health: 2. Global Climate Change and Health". *Canadian Medical Association Journal* 163(6): 729–34. http://www.cmaj.ca/content/163/6/729.full (December 2013).

Health Canada (2013). "Climate Change and Health". Ottawa. http://www.hc-sc.gc.ca/ewh-semt/pubs/climat/index-eng.php (December 2013).

Holmes, John (2008). "More Help Now, Please: How to Tackle Tomorrow's Disasters". In *The World in 2009*, Daniel Franklin, ed. London: The Economist. http://www.economist.com/node/12494621 (December 2013).

Hsu, Lee-Nah and Jessica White (2007). "Partnerships for Health, the Environment, and Governance". In *Governing Global Health: Challenge, Response, Innovation*, Andrew F. Cooper, John J. Kirton, and Ted Schrecker, eds. Aldershot: Ashgate, pp. 101–12.

Intergovernmental Panel on Climate Change (1995). "IPCC Second Assessment: Climate Change 1995". Geneva. http://www.ipcc.ch/ipccreports/tar/wg2/ (December 2013).

Intergovernmental Panel on Climate Change (2001). "Climate Change 2001: Synthesis Report. Summary for Policymakers". Geneva. http://www.ipcc.ch/pdf/climate-changes-2001/synthesis-spm/synthesis-spm-en.pdf (December 2013).

Intergovernmental Panel on Climate Change (2007a). *Climate Change 2007: Impacts, Adaptation, and Vulnerability. Contribution of Working Group II to the Fourth Assessment Report of the Intergovernmental Panel on Climate Change.* Cambridge: Cambridge University Press. http://www.ipcc-wg2.gov/publications/AR4/index.html (December 2013).

Intergovernmental Panel on Climate Change (2007b). "Climate Change 2007: Synthesis Report". Geneva. http://www.ipcc.ch/pdf/assessment-report/ar4/syr/ar4_syr.pdf (December 2013).

International Federation of Red Cross and Red Crescent Societies (2012). "Annual Report 2012. Towards Climate-Smart Resilience: A Year of Engagement". Geneva. http://www.climatecentre.org/downloads/File/reports/Annual%20Reports/RCCC_AR_2012%20web.pdf (December 2013).

Kintzele, Kathryn (2012). "Ethical Principles on the Environment and Human Health in State Statutes". In *Human Health and Ecological Integrity: Ethics, Law, and Human Rights*, Laura Westra, Colin L. Soskolne, and Donald W. Spady, eds. Abdingdon: Routledge, pp. 20–31.

Kirton, John J., ed. (2009). *Global Health.* Farnham: Ashgate.

Kirton, John J. and Jenilee Guebert (2009a). "Bringing Health into the Climate Change Regime: The Opportunity for Copenhagen 2009 and Muskoka 2010". Paper prepared for the Learning Forum on Global Health Research of the Canadian Coalition for Global Health Research, October 25, Ottawa. http://www.g8.utoronto.ca/scholar/kirton-guebert-health-climate-2009.pdf (December 2013).

Kirton, John J. and Jenilee Guebert (2009b). "Canada's G8 Global Health Diplomacy: Lessons for 2010". *Canadian Foreign Policy* 15(3): 85–105.

Kirton, John J. and Jenilee Guebert (2009c). "Climate Change Accountability: The G8's Compliance Record from 1975 to 2009". November 28, G8 Research Group. http://www.g8.utoronto.ca/scholar/kirton-guebert-climate-091128.pdf (December 2013).

Kirton, John J. and Jenilee Guebert (2013). "Global Environmental Diplomacy: Comparing and Sharing". In *Global Health Diplomacy: Concepts, Issues, Actors, Instruments, Fora, and Cases*, Ilona Kickbusch, Graham Lister, Michaela Told, et al., eds. New York: Springer, pp. 141–54.

Kirton, John J. and Madeline Koch, eds. (2009). *The G20 Pittsburgh Summit 2009.* London: Newsdesk. http://www.g8.utoronto.ca/newsdesk/pittsburgh.html (December 2013).

Leiserowitz, Anthony (2007). "International Public Opinion, Perception, and Understanding of Global Climate Change". Yale University. http://environment.yale.edu/climate-communication/files/IntlPublicOpinion.pdf (December 2013).

Major Economies Meeting on Energy Security and Climate Change (2007). "Final Chairman's Summary: First Major Economies Meeting on Energy Security and Climate Change". Washington DC, September 27–8. http://www.g8.utoronto.ca/mem/mem-070927.html (December 2013).

Major Economies Meeting on Energy Security and Climate Change (2008a). "Declaration of Leaders Meeting of Major Economies on Energy Security and Climate Change". Hokkaido, Japan, July 9. http://www.g8.utoronto.ca/summit/2008hokkaido/2008-mem.html (December 2013).

Major Economies Meeting on Energy Security and Climate Change (2008b). "Final Chairman's Summary: Second Major Economies Meeting on Energy Security and Climate Change". Honolulu, January 31. http://2001-2009.state.gov/g/oes/rls/or/2008/99953.htm (December 2013).

McInerney-Lankford, Siobhán, Mac Darrow, and Lavanya Rajamani (2011). "Human Rights and Climate Change: A Review of the International Legal Dimensions". World Bank, Washington DC. http://siteresources.worldbank.org/INTLAWJUSTICE/Resources/HumanRightsAndClimateChange.pdf (December 2013).

McMichael, Anthony J., Andrew Haines, Rudolf Slooff, et al. (1996). "Climate Change and Human Health". World Health Organization, Geneva. http://whqlibdoc.who.int/hq/1996/WHO_EHG_96.7.pdf (December 2013).

Onzivu, William (2012). "Re-examining Health Protection in International Environmental Regulation". In *Human Health and Ecological Integrity: Ethics, Law, and Human Rights*, Laura Westra, Colin L. Soskolne, and Donald W. Spady, eds. Abdingdon: Routledge, pp. 301–14.

Orbinski, James and Jenilee Guebert (2010). "Climate Change and Global Health: The Time Is Now". In *G8 & G20: The 2010 Canadian Summits*, John J. Kirton and Madeline Koch, eds. London: Newsdesk, pp. 286–7. http://www.g8.utoronto.ca/newsdesk/g8g20/g8g20-2010.pdf (December 2013).

Organisation for Economic Co-operation and Development (2006). "Meeting of the OECD Development Assistance Committee (DAC) and the Environment Policy Committee (EPOC) at Ministerial Level". Paris, April 4. http://web.archive.org/web/20080117163820/http://www.oecd.org/document/38/0,3343,en_21571361_36099755_36099814_1_1_1_1,00.html (December 2013).

Organisation for Economic Co-operation and Development (2009). "Health: Improving Policy Coherence for Development". Policy Brief, OECD Observer, October, Paris.

Parry, Martin, Osvaldo Canziani, Jean Palutikof, et al., eds. (2007). *Climate Change 2007: Impacts, Adaptation, and Vulnerability. Contribution of Working Group II to the Fourth Assessment Report of the Intergovernmental Panel on Climate Change.* Cambridge: Cambridge University Press. http://www.ipcc.ch/publications_and_data/publications_ipcc_fourth_assessment_report_wg2_report_impacts_adaptation_and_vulnerability.htm (October 2013).

Ramin, Brodie (2009). "Slums, Climate Change, and Human Health in Sub-Saharan Africa". *Bulletin of the World Health Organization* 87: 886–886. doi: 10.2471/BLT.09.073445.

Reguly, Eric (2009). "U.S. Makes First Move at Copenhagen". *Globe and Mail*, December 7. http://www.theglobeandmail.com/news/world/climate-change/us-makes-first-move-at-copenhagen/article1391958 (December 2013).

Rockefeller Foundation (2014). "Asian Cities Climate Change Resilience Network (ACCCRN)". New York. http://www.rockefellerfoundation.org/our-work/current-work/climate-change-resilience/asian-cities-climate-change-resilience (January 2014).

Rogelj, Joeri, David L. McCollum, Andy Reisinger, et al. (2013). "Probabilistic Cost Estimates for Climate Change Mitigation". *Nature* 493: 79–83. doi: 10.1038/nature11787.

Sarkozy, Nicolas (2008). "Third Major Economies Meeting on Energy and Climate Change: Speech". Paris, April 18. http://www.ambafrance-ca.org/spip.php?page=mobile_art&art=2191 (December 2013).

Save the Children (2009). "Feeling the Heat: Child Survival in a Changing Climate". London. https://www.savethechildren.org.uk/sites/default/files/docs/Feeling_the_Heat_composite_low_res_1.pdf (December 2013).

Sclar, Elliott D. and Nicole Volavka-Close (2013). "Understanding the Twenty-First Century Urban Transformation: A Global South Perspective". In *The Urban Transformation: Health, Shelter, and Climate Change*, Elliott D. Sclar, Nicole Volavka-Close, and Peter Brown, eds. London: Routledge, pp. 1–14.

Singh, Jerome Amir (2012, June 5). "Why Human Health and Health Ethics Must Be Central to Climate Change Deliberations". *PLoS Medicine* 9(6). doi: 10.1371/journal.pmed.1001229.

Singh, Sudhvir, Usman Mushtaq, Charlotte Holm-Hansen, et al. (2011). "The Importance of Climate Change to Health". *Lancet* 378(9785): 29–30. doi: 10.1016/S0140-6736(11)61018-0.

Smith, Richard and Melisa Martínez Álvarez (2008). "Global Change and Health: Mapping the Challenges of Global Non-healthcare Influences on Health". World Health Organization, Geneva.

Spady, Donald W. (2012). "Public Healthcare in the Time of Transition: The Need to Revert to Basics". In *Human Health and Ecological Integrity: Ethics, Law, and Human Rights*, Laura Westra, Colin L. Soskolne, and Donald W. Spady, eds. Abdingdon: Routledge, pp. 121–31.

Steiner, Achim (2009). "The Environment-Health Axis". In *The G8 2009: From La Maddalena to L'Aquila*, John J. Kirton and Madeline Koch, eds. London: Newsdesk, pp. 65–6. http://www.g8.utoronto.ca/newsdesk/G8-2009.pdf (December 2013).

Steiner, Achim (2011). "UNEP Chief Addresses UN Security Council Debate on Climate Change and Security". United Nations Environment Programme, July 20. http://www.unep.org/newscentre/default.aspx?DocumentID=2646&ArticleID=8817 (December 2013).

Sturchio, Jeff (2009). "Health Security from Economic and Environmental Innovation". In *The G20 Pittsburgh Summit 2009: Sustaining Global Recovery*, John J. Kirton and Madeline Koch, eds. London: Newsdesk, pp. 163–5. http://www.g8.utoronto.ca/newsdesk/pittsburgh/sturchio.html (December 2013).

United Nations (1992). "United Nations Framework Convention on Climate Change". FCCC/INFORMAL/84. http://unfccc.int/resource/docs/convkp/conveng.pdf (December 2013).

Walpole, Sarah Catherine, Kumanan Rasanathan, and Diarmid Campbell-Lendrum (2009). "Natural and Unnatural Synergies: Climate Change Policy and Health Equity". *Bulletin of the World Health Organization* 87: 799–801. doi: 10.2471/BLT.09.067116.

World Health Organization (1990). "Potential Health Effects of Climatic Change: Report of a WHO Task Group". WHO/PEP/90/10, Geneva. http://whqlibdoc.who.int/hq/1990/WHO_PEP_90_10.pdf (December 2013).

World Health Organization (2000). "Climate Change and Human Health: Impact and Adaptation". Geneva. http://whqlibdoc.who.int/hq/2000/WHO_SDE_OEH_00.4.pdf (December 2013).

World Health Organization (2001). "Report on WHO Activities on Climate Change and Human Health". Statement to the 15th session of the Subsidiary Body of Scientific and Technological Advice, October, Marrakesh. http://web.archive.org/web/20050611235935/http://www.euro.who.int/document/gch/actrep_sbsta15.pdf (December 2013).

World Health Organization (2005). "Climate and Health". Fact sheet, Geneva, July. http://www.who.int/globalchange/news/fsclimandhealth/en/index.html (December 2013).

World Health Organization (2008a). "Climate Change Will Erode Foundations of Health". Geneva, April 8. http://www.who.int/mediacentre/news/releases/2008/pr11/en/ (December 2013).

World Health Organization (2008b). "New World Health Assembly Resolution on Climate Change and Health". Geneva, May. http://www.who.int/globalchange/climate/EB_CChealth_resolution/en/ (December 2013).

World Health Organization (2008c). "Protecting Health from Climate Change: World Health Day 2008". Geneva. http://www.who.int/world-health-day/toolkit/report_web.pdf (December 2013).

World Health Organization (2008d). "WHO Event on Climate Change and Health at UNFCCC Conference". Poznan, Poland, December 1–12. http://www.who.int/mediacentre/events/meetings/climatechange/en (December 2013).

World Health Organization (2008e). "World Health Assembly Sets Bold New Action for WHO". Geneva, May 24. http://www.who.int/mediacentre/news/releases/2008/wha02/en (December 2013).

World Health Organization (2009a). "Climate Change Is Affecting Our Health: Something Should Be Done Now". Geneva. http://www.who.int/entity/globalchange/publications/factsheets/Climate_change_and_health_brochure.pdf (December 2013).

World Health Organization (2009b). "COP15 United Nations Climate Change Conference 2009". Copenhagen, December 7–18. http://www.who.int/globalchange/news/2009/climatechange_conference_7122009/en/ (December 2013).

World Health Organization (2009c). "Protecting Health from Climate Change: Global Research Priorities". Geneva. http://www.who.int/globalchange/publications/9789241598187/en/ (October 2013).

World Health Organization (2009d). "WHO Carbon Footprint Study FY2008". Final Report V2, October, Geneva. http://www.who.int/globalchange/health_policy/WHO_Carbon_study.pdf (December 2013).

World Health Organization (2014). "Climate Change and Human Health: Publications". Geneva. http://www.who.int/globalchange/publications/en/ (January 2014).

World Health Organization and Health Care Without Harm (2009). "Healthy Hospitals, Healthy Planet, Healthy People: Addressing Climate Change in Healthcare Settings". Geneva. http://www.who.int/entity/globalchange/publications/climatefootprint_report.pdf (December 2013).

World Health Organization Regional Office for Africa (undated-a). "Clusters and Programs of WHO in the African Region". http://www.afro.who.int/en/clusters-a-programmes.html (December 2013).

World Health Organization Regional Office for Africa (undated-b). "Protection of the Human Environment: Overview". http://www.afro.who.int/en/clusters-a-programmes/hpr/protection-of-the-human-environment/overview.html (December 2013).

World Health Organization Regional Office for Europe (2009). "EuroHEAT: Improving Public Health Responses to Extreme Weather/Heat-Waves". Copenhagen. http://www.euro.who.int/__data/assets/pdf_file/0009/95913/E92473.pdf (December 2013).

Appendix 12-A Health–Climate Change in G8 Leaders' Documents, 1975–2008

Year	Total Health–Climate Change Mentions	Total Health–Climate Change Sentences	Total Health–Climate Change Paragraphs
1975	0	0	0
1976	0	0	0
1977	0	0	0
1978	0	0	0
1979	0	0	0
1980	0	0	0
1981	0	0	0
1982	0	0	0
1983	0	0	0
1984	0	0	0
1985	0	0	0
1986	0	0	0
1987	0	0	0
1988	0	0	0
1989	0	0	0
1990	0	0	0
1991	0	0	0
1992	0	0	0
1993	0	0	0
1994	0	0	0
1995	0	0	0
1996	0	0	0
1997	1	1	1
1998	0	0	0
1999	0	0	0
2000	0	0	0
2001	0	0	0
2002	0	0	0
2003	1	1	1
2004	0	0	0
2005	3	2	3
2006	0	0	0

Appendix 12-A continued

Year	Total Health-Climate Change Mentions	Total Health–Climate Change Sentences	Total Health–Climate Change Paragraphs
2007	1	1	1
2008	2	1	2
Total	8	5	8
Average	24%	15%	24%

Notes:
The chart accounts for all official documents. Only documents with an English version were included in the calculations.
"Total Health–Climate Change Mentions" refers to the number of times climate change and health, or cognate terms of climate change and health, were mentioned simultaneously in the official documents for the year specified. The words are calculated by sentence and paragraph because the sentence/paragraph is the unit of analysis.
"Total Health–Climate Change Sentences" refers to the number of sentences that climate change and health, or cognate terms of climate change and health, were mentioned simultaneously in the official documents for the year specified.
"Total Health–Climate Change Paragraphs" refers to the number of paragraphs that climate change and health, or cognate terms of climate change and health, were mentioned simultaneously in the official documents for the year specified.

Appendix 12-B Number of Natural Disasters, 1975–2013

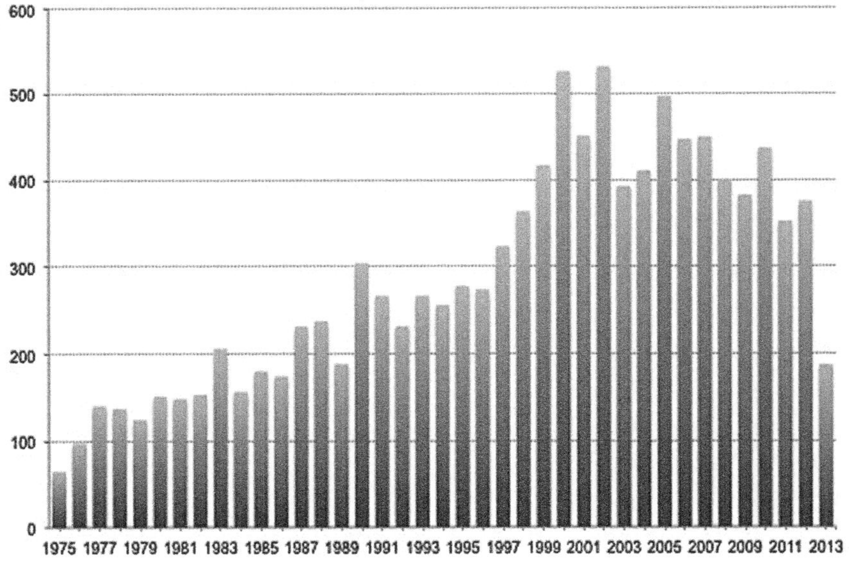

Source: EM-DAT: The OFDA/CRED International Disaster Database – www.emdat.be – Université Catholique de Louvain – Brussels – Belgium.

Appendix 12-C People Affected in Disasters, 1975–2013, millions

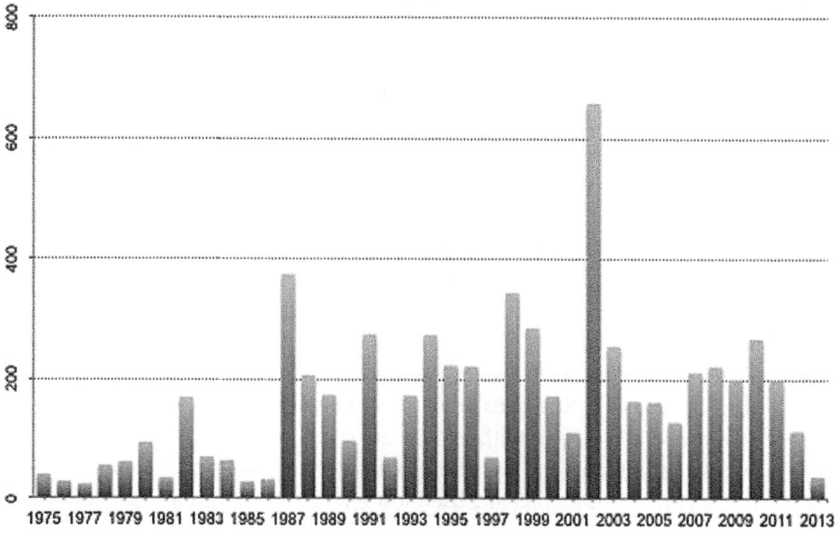

Source: EM-DAT: The OFDA/CRED International Disaster Database – www.emdat.be – Université Catholique de Louvain – Brussels – Belgium.

Appendix 12-D IPCC Health-Climate Challenges, by Varying Confidence

Very High Confidence

- Climate change currently contributed to the global burden of disease and premature deaths.
- Projected trends in climate change-related exposures of importance to human health will have mixed effects on malaria: in some places the geographical range will contract, elsewhere the geographical range will expand and the transmission season may be changed.
- Economic development is an important component of adaptation, but on its own will not insulate the world's population from disease and injury due to climate change.

High Confidence

- Emerging evidence of climate change effects on human health shows that climate change has altered the seasonal distribution of some allergenic pollen species.
- Projected trends in climate change-related exposures of importance to human health will increase malnutrition and consequent disorders, including those relating to child growth and development.

- Projected trends in climate change-related exposures of importance to human health will increase the number of people suffering from death, disease and injury from heat waves, floods, storms, fires and droughts.
- Projected trends in climate change-related exposures of importance to human health will continue to change the range of some infectious disease vectors.
- Projected trends in climate change-related exposures of importance to human health will increase cardio-respiratory morbidity and mortality associated with ground-level ozone.
- Projected trends in climate change-related exposures of importance to human health will bring some benefits to health, including fewer deaths from cold, although it is expected that these will be outweighed by the negative effects of rising temperatures worldwide, especially in developing countries.
- Adaptive capacity needs to be improved everywhere; impacts of recent hurricanes and heat waves show that even high-income countries are not well prepared to cope with extreme weather events.
- Adverse health impacts will be greatest in low-income countries. Those at greater risk include, in all countries, the urban poor, the elderly and children, traditional societies, subsistence farmers and coastal populations.

Medium Confidence

- Emerging evidence of climate change effects on human health shows that climate change has altered the distribution of some infectious disease vectors.
- Emerging evidence of climate change effects on human health shows that climate change has increased heat wave-related deaths.
- Projected trends in climate change-related exposures of importance to human health will increase the burden of diarrheal diseases.

Low Confidence

- Projected trends in climate change-related exposures of importance to human health will increase the number of people at risk of dengue.

PART V
Conclusion

Chapter 13
Conclusion

John J. Kirton

The movement of pathogens, people, and the processes that propel them have added new dimensions to the profound health challenges that Africans have long faced. The response by national governments and international organizations, premised on the classic Westphalian concepts of sovereignty and citizenship, appears increasingly inadequate to accurately account for and effectively address the proliferating problems that result (Kirton 2009). There is thus an urgent need to develop and apply innovative concepts, policies, instruments, and institutions to comprehend and cope with the basic health problems afflicting Africans and their fellow humans in the global community beyond (Cooper and Kirton 2009).

To help meet this need, this book has been designed with three central purposes in mind. Its first purpose is to chart the challenges brought by the clash between the new world of moving people and pathogens and the old world of static sovereign governance, as the clash affects the health needs of Africans and others. Its second purpose is to assess the existing and emerging governance responses – in ideas, instruments, and institutions – of the authorities that are most responsible, affected, and concerned. Its third purpose is to identify the innovations introduced, needed, and available to improve African's health.

This book thus began by adapting the earlier basic challenge-response-innovation model of global health governance in three central ways (Cooper et al. 2007). It added movement – in pathogens, people, and broader processes – as a central component and cross-cutting dimension of the already formidable health challenge facing Africans. It added sovereignty, in classic, contested, and changing forms, as the core if contested concept guiding the governance response (Ruggie 1993). And it applied these enhanced concepts to Africa, as the region of the world where they were most advanced, and had them addressed by authors who were largely Africans themselves.

The resulting analyses presented in these chapters have generated considerable consensus and ongoing differences on the key questions and component issues addressed in this book. Together they show the usefulness of the enhanced challenge-response-innovation model of global health in its application to Africa, with movement and sovereignty as central concepts now built in, and how the model can and should be further enriched by changing concepts and characteristics of movement, sovereignty, and the innovations that they breed and need in a globalizing region and world.

Central Challenges for Africans' Health

The first component, at the centre of the challenge-response-innovation model, consists of the global health challenges generated by globalization, as it affects Africa and Africans' health. Here there is a strong consensus among many contributors that health is a central challenge for Africa amid the many afflictions it must address and that a top health challenge is the crisis of HIV/AIDS, a pandemic that affects the economy, society, and polity alike. Many contributors also emphasize the challenges of malaria and tuberculosis, two opportunistic diseases that often render HIV more lethal. Also identified are several other infectious diseases that present challenges to global and African health – cholera and diarrheal diseases, the H5N1 and H1N1 viruses, neglected tropical diseases, and transmitted zoonotic diseases.

Yet an additional challenge arises from chronic, noncommunicable diseases (NCDs). Obijiofor Aginam and Siphamandla Zondi stress the importance of addressing the burdens posed by obesity, hypertension, diabetes, heart disease, and cancer. More broadly, health security is a new challenge. Pieter Fourie and John Kirton and Jenilee Guebert list bioweapons and bioterrorism as major threats to health. Obijiofor Aginam and Dennis Willms highlight vulnerable children and orphans as those who are most assaulted by global and continental health challenges. And many authors emphasize or acknowledge climate change and its health connection as a challenge assuming centre stage.

Underlying Causes of Africans' Health Challenges

There is also considerable consensus on the second component – the major causes of these health challenges. Leading the list of salient common causes are expensive and unavailable drugs; a lack of access to preventive tools, information, and education; food insecurity; and inadequate or unsafe water. Nelson Sewankambo, James K. Tumwine, and Hany Besada add exposure to indoor smoke.

As the key causes for poor African health and health systems, most contributors identify poverty and inequality – the classic socioeconomic determinants of health. Other causes come from the political determinants of health – poor internal African governance, particularly poor health and climate change governance, compounded by corruption, lack of transparency and accountability, ineffective disease control systems, and lack of communication and coordination among actors. Aginam notes Africa's poor health infrastructure, and Rangarirai Machemedze emphasizes undefended health services. Oscar Picazo adds the slow diffusion of knowledge, technology, and good practices, and the small size of African countries, as factors that prevent them from developing their health systems to the full extent. Kirton and Guebert note stifled economic growth as a major contributing factor.

International factors join the internal ones as key causes. Both Aginam and Picazo list trade, a key component of globalization, as having deleterious effects on health. Aginam includes the globalization of food, tobacco, unhealthy lifestyles, and foreign direct investment. He stresses more generally the negative consequences of global interconnectedness, which prevents Africa as a continent from developing a unique perspective on public health. Foreign forces bred by imported globalization and neo-liberalism have the effect of concentrating power within the hands of market forces and external players, while diminishing the role of government within the health sector.

Other causes arise as the intersection of international and internal factors. Annamarie Bindenagel Šehović emphasizes competing local and global priorities, noting the erosion of South Africa's sovereignty and power in dealing with HIV/AIDS. While South Africa has faced international pressure to deal with issues such as poverty, malnutrition, and food security, little has been done to forward local, long-term HIV/AIDS solutions. Similarly, Zondi claims that neo-liberal interventions embed real power in external players or in market forces. African governments can therefore no longer assure the delivery of public goods, including health services.

Ecological causes of Africans' health challenges also have a prominent place. Sewankambo, Tumwine, and Besada suggest that the chief causes of health challenges are vulnerable ecosystems and reduced access to natural resources, including water, land, and vegetation. This is due to changes in the hydrologic cycle as a result of the build-up of greenhouse gasses and increasing global temperatures. Willms and Franklyn Lisk, as well as Kirton and Guebert, note climate change as a major cause of health challenges and insecurity. Lisk lists droughts, floods, and coastal storms as major climate change disasters that affect human health. These disasters have the power to reduce human capital through forced migration and mortality.

Taken together, the challenges and their causes are comprehensively multilevel and intersectoral. They embrace internal African, international, and intersecting forces. They span the biomedical, socioeconomic, political-security, and ecological dimensions and determinants of health.

The Multiplier of Mobility

On the third component of the enhanced challenge-response-innovation model – mobility – it is clear that movement matters. Almost all authors agree that the mobility of pathogens, people, pests, and processes have compounded African's health challenges a great deal. Picazo and Kirton and Guebert emphasize virus sharing and cross-border disease transmission as affecting global health and perpetuating HIV/AIDS and other diseases.

For other contributors, the movement of people takes pride of place. Many agree that increased international migration has compounded the health challenge. In particular, Zondi draws attention to the movement of vulnerable groups, comprising the sickly, trafficked individuals, and refugees. He also points to the processes of faster communication and international travel. Machemedze and Kirton and Guebert see the migration of scarce health workers to developed countries as problematic. Lisk addresses the impacts of climate change and natural disasters on forced migration and displacement of populations.

Sovereignty as an Inadequate and Adaptable Response

On the fourth component of the enhanced challenge-response-innovation model – sovereignty – classic and changing concepts and characteristics of sovereignty also have important effects. In the face of massive multifaceted movement, the classic Westphalian conception of sovereignty has been an inadequate and thus adaptable response as the core principle on which Africans' health governance does and should take place. Sovereignty implies the state's responsibility for territorial and physical security and the provision of that security; the protection of its citizens through the provision of health, welfare, and economic stability; the establishment and maintenance of effective government as the single source of legitimate authority; and accountability to citizens and the international community (Krasner 1999, 2001, 2009). Šehović and Fourie see the general classic concept of sovereignty being challenged and changed. Fourie notes three major ideological developments, starting with the establishment of the modern state through the Treaty of Westphalia, the French Revolution of 1789, which came to see the state as complementary to citizen interests, and, finally, the period following 1989, which saw the revision and reconsideration of notions of security.

The classic concept of sovereignty has been specifically challenged in its application to health. According to Machemedze, health sovereignty is defined by the power of a sovereign state to promote and protect public health through the provision of health services. Health sovereignty requires, in its international dimension, health diplomacy, because such protection and promotion in a world of movement require major action abroad as well as at home. There is a consensus among most authors that health challenges are no longer – and should no longer be – viewed as residing solely within the purview of sovereign states. Health issues do not respect territorial boundaries, resulting in the blurring of national health governance and global health governance. As a result, many important nonstate actors and transnational actors have penetrated the arenas of health and climate change governance.

Aginam interprets current global health diplomacy as isolationist, resulting in the marginalization of Africa within the international system. Šehović and Machemedze agree that African governments and their sovereignty have been bypassed by local and external actors in their provision of health services. Picazo examines the World Bank, while Machemedze focuses on trade policies imposed by the World Trade Organization (WTO). The presence of the World Bank and WTO in the domain of African health provision has resulted in the blurring of sovereignty.

Changing Concepts of Sovereignty

Even as classic conceptions and characteristics of sovereignty become increasingly inadequate, several components of the changing concept of sovereignty offer a promising foundation on which a more adequate African health diplomacy and governance response is being and can be built. Many contributors agree that addressing health challenges, many of which now transcend sovereign borders, requires a move from a state-centric approach to more global policy responses. In order for health governance to respond effectively to global health challenges, there must be sustained coordination and consensus among multiple actors including not just sovereign nation-states but also private actors, intergovernmental organizations, and civil society. Both national priorities and global standards should be married in order to improve Africans' health.

Such greater coordination among these different spheres of power does not mean that states should relinquish their traditional national sovereignty. There is overwhelming consensus among contributors that national governments should play an active role in redesigning global health.

Yet there is a reluctance to apply the hard core component of sovereignty – national security – to health. Fourie outlines some benefits of health securitization, such as the rapid mobilization of resources to defeat a common, identifiable threat. Yet he points to greater problems that accompany the securitization discourse. Health securitization can increase stigmatization by "othering" individuals with diseases such as HIV/AIDS. Most importantly, the securitization of HIV/AIDS specifically is problematic. There is a lack of association between HIV/AIDS and state fragility and collapse and no clear link between HIV/AIDS and military, political, social, and economic insecurity. Zondi, in contrast, asserts that diseases such as HIV/AIDS, malaria, and diarrheal diseases tend to break out in countries with weak political governance and in situations of political crises.

There is a similar reluctance to return to the closed sovereign polities of old, even in the face of devastating global financial and economic crises, such as that which erupted in 2008. According to Machemedze, the 2008 financial meltdown and accompanying rise in food and energy prices demonstrated the negative aspects of neo-liberalism. In order to successfully re-establish global financial and economic security, he suggests a move away from market fundamentalism and an end to the liberalization of financial services in order to reduce problems in public sectors such as health. Yet few other authors endorse such an approach.

Governance Responses

On the fifth component of the enhanced challenge-response-innovation model – the governance response – there is considerable consensus on the key actors at the global and national level, if not on how well they are responding and why. In the face of the new world of movement and shifting sovereignty, several existing intergovernmental health institutions have responded with old repertoires but have also adjusted through the innovative adoption of new principles, instruments, and designs.

At the centre stands the Global Fund to Fight AIDS, Tuberculosis, and Malaria, an international financing organization created by the G8 and the United Nations in 2000–01. Contributors agree that although the Global Fund is effective in disbursing money to African countries, it both weakens state sovereignty and fails to produce sustainable health solutions. Šehović and Zondi highlight health setbacks within African states and the Global Fund itself. According to Šehović, the presence of the Global Fund undermines long-term, state-led health governance, reducing the responsibility and accountability of African governments to their citizens. Zondi states that Global Fund investments do not produce successful outcomes due to weak health governance in African countries. In order to enhance health outcomes, states should improve internal governance. Meanwhile, Sewankambo, Tumwine, and Besada highlight critics' concerns that the Global Fund is too specialized and narrow. Some suggest that emphasis on specific diseases such as HIV/AIDS weakens the overall health system of African countries.

The World Health Organization (WHO), created in 1948, is another institution of great interest. According to Sewankambo, Tumwine, and Besada, WHO innovatively began to frame HIV/AIDS as a human rights issue in 1980. More recently it arranged a global workplan designed to assess the consequences of climate change for health systems within low- and middle-income countries and island states, which lack the ability to establish strategies designed to address issues of climate change. As Lisk and Kirton and Guebert highlighted, WHO concurrently launched a global campaign to highlight health consequences related to climate change. WHO has tried to improve the health outcomes of Africans by recommending the need for further research in climate change and its health-related impacts.

Beyond these health-specific institutions, those of more comprehensive policy scope have an important and adapting role as well. Here the World Bank, G8, the Organisation for Economic Co-operation and Development (OECD), and the WTO stand out.

Many authors highlight the World Bank's role as a socioeconomic driver of Africans' health. Zondi argues that, through its role in imposing structural adjustment programs, the World Bank has weakened African health sovereignty and the public sector in order to allow market forces to dictate public policies such as those affecting the health service delivery. The World Bank is thus seen to be undermining the capacity of states to respond and overcome the state-specific socioeconomic determinants of HIV/AIDS.

In contrast, Picazo emphasizes the World Bank's financial contributions. He highlights its major programs, such as the Multi-Country HIV/AIDS Program (MAP), the Booster Program for Malaria Control in Africa, the Africa Region Avian and Human Influenza Task Force, and the World Bank's Poverty Reduction Strategy Credit, as well as several country-specific projects. He argues that the MAP has contributed positively to regional initiatives in Africa through a multisectoral approach. Others, however, criticize it for not having African states as the primary designers and implementers of the program (Harman 2010).

In regard to the informal, plurilateral summit-level G8, John Kirton, Jenilee Guebert, and Julia Kulik highlight its role in establishing the Global Fund in 2001. They see the 2002 Kananaskis Summit and the 2010 Muskoka Summit significantly advancing African development and African health. They also see the 2005 Gleneagles Summit bringing the climate–health connection back to the forefront. In 2005, the G8 advanced health care, which provided grounds for the establishment of the climate-health-economy connection. Kirton, Guebert, and Kulik and Zondi also focus on the 2006 St. Petersburg Summit and its decision to place health as the top priority. Zondi acknowledges St. Petersburg for having increased general health awareness, and for having improved epidemiological surveillance and disease control of the avian influenza, which had that year become a global threat. He applauds the summit for bringing together various stakeholders such as the World Bank, WHO, UNAIDS, and ministers from various countries. Kirton, Guebert, and Kulik approve of the 2010 Muskoka Summit for producing the Muskoka Initiative for Maternal, Newborn, and Child Health. G8 leaders have consistently emphasized private-public partnerships and multistakeholder approaches to public health governance.

Also relevant is the formal, plurilateral, ministerial level OECD. Kirton and Guebert note its contribution to forging the climate-health-economy link. The OECD has also connected climate change and health with security, food, and agriculture. Sewankambo, Tumwine, and Besada include the financial contributions of OECD members to countries and organizations that seek, or require, assistance in adapting to the impacts of climate change.

The WTO and its General Agreement on Trade in Services and Agreement on Trade-Related Aspects of Intellectual Property (TRIPS) loom large here, as they do in analyses of global health governance elsewhere. Machemedze criticizes both agreements for increasing the liberalization of the services sector and the privatization of health services. Machemedze claims that the liberalization of the health sector leads to disastrous effects and removes government responsibility to its citizens. He believes that the WTO and its application of neo-liberal economic policies cannot be counted on to provide health services to African states.

Among the formal regional intergovernmental institutions of relevance that are reforming, the African Union (AU) stands out as the major body designed to address health needs on the continent. Zondi and Kirton, Guebert, and Kulik highlight its inability to establish successful health governance on its own. Zondi addresses organizational shortcomings, which prevent African states from developing common policy positions and engaging with global actors. African states have focused on national interests instead of working on the development of a collective health agenda. Other contributors refer to particular responses, at times innovative, that the AU has made in terms of health contributions. Having identified the root cause of poor African health governance, AU ministers developed the African Health Strategy in order to implement a comprehensive program of action. Sewankambo, Tumwine, and Besada, as well as Kirton and Guebert, also note climate change advances made by the AU. Sewankambo, Tumwine, and Besada highlight AU discussions that called for a consistent African position on climate change. Kirton and Guebert note its acknowledgement of the link between climate change and health.

Also relevant as a regional body is the African Development Bank, which was designed to promote economic and social development in Africa. According to Lisk, it has demonstrated that it recognizes Africa's vulnerability to climate change impacts, through its provision of financial assistance to several countries and its creation of projects such as the climate risk management approach, and through its Clean Energy Investment Framework.

Still, the greatest institutional inadequacy comes in regard to the climate change–health link. Sewankambo, Tumwine, and Besada identify the negative effects of climate change that will likely affect Africa the most. In order for Africans to cope well with these health impacts and adapt to other consequences, they stress the need for health and climate change governance to incorporate indigenous knowledge and best practices by working with local communities. Due to the close connection between climate change and health, Kirton and Guebert propose increased governance and coherence among climate change and health actors and institutions in order to reduce governance gaps.

Instruments

Beyond the ongoing work of these international institutions lie the more specific instruments they use. Continuity, as well as change and iteration, and innovation are evident here as well.

Šehović argues that national governments have the right and responsibility to protect citizens. However, if state sovereignty erodes, and governments are either unwilling or unable to provide protection, then such state responsibility and accountability should be transferred elsewhere.

Sewankambo, Tumwine, and Besada see official development assistance as the primary instrument for coping with HIV/AIDS in the long run. Picazo, however, sees further innovative governance structures and instruments as required to improve the results of grant funding, as well as financial and technical assistance. Sewankambo, Tumwine, and Besada identify community mobilization, education, social justice, and equity considerations as major instruments in combating the spread of HIV/AIDS.

Institutional Innovation

On the sixth and final component of the enhanced challenge-response-innovation model – innovation – there is considerable consensus. It arises most strongly on how governance arrangements can and should innovate to adjust to the new conceptions of sovereignty and the new physical world of movement that lies behind.

At the state level, most contributors emphasize innovative African leadership and greater transparency, accountability, and responsibility, in order to reflect new conceptions of sovereignty. They argue that health issues cannot be tackled by sovereign states alone. They agree that engagement with different levels of society, such as civil society organizations and the private sector, are needed in order to deal effectively with globalized health problems. There must be decentralization, a greater appreciation of the effects of globalization, and an understanding of the principal socioeconomic causes of sickness, such as poverty and underdevelopment. At the same time, there is general agreement that African states must retain their sovereignty in order to negotiate in the international realm.

Intergovernmental institutions must also innovate in order to reflect new conceptions of sovereignty. Contributors agree that intergovernmental institutions need to implement long-term commitments in order to advance development in the health sector. Picazo argues that the World Bank has made several steps to innovate. It created adaptable program lending, designed to deal with long-term needs of health system. The World Bank has also taken steps to improve health systems as a whole, rather than focusing on individual health components. Another major innovation development by the World Bank has been health systems strengthening to provide long-term technical assistance to African health systems. With regards to climate change specifically, Lisk believes that the UN Framework Convention on Climate Change (UNFCCC) should innovate by incorporating elements of human development such as health, human, and food security into its agreement, rather than simply focusing on avoiding the negative consequences of climate change. The UNFCCC should therefore emphasize the fundamental tie between climate change, health, and development. Lisk believes that it should still recognize individual state sovereignty.

Civil society must innovate as well. Zondi argues that the neo-liberal nongovernmental organizations (NGOs) and civil society of today have come to undermine African states' sovereignty, development, and governance. He believes that civil society has generally ignored comprehensive African health reform, preferring to focus on specific issues like HIV/AIDS, as a result of its surrounding hype. The delivery of essential health services to the poor has therefore not been promoted by NGOs and civil society. Emphasis must be placed on improving African health governance so that long-term comprehensive health services can be provided to African citizens. Kirton, Guebert, and Kulik acknowledge the importance of NGOs collaborating among themselves and with national governments and their international institutions in order to implement effective responses to major infectious diseases and maternal, newborn, and child health. Kirton and Guebert emphasize an innovative approach on how health harms and helps climate change control.

Recommendations

From this analysis and the consensus that arises, several major recommendations stand out for addressing African and global health challenges.

The first and most important is the adoption of a globalized policy response. Contributors recommend greater consensus, coordination, and participation among all parties within and related to the realm of health in order to achieve sustainable development. External organizations such as the US President's Emergency Plan for AIDS Relief, WHO, the Global Fund, the World Bank, G8 and G20 members, the OECD, and the AU, as well as internal and external civil society and NGOs, must work alongside African states in order to produce a common global health agenda.

The second recommendation deals with African leadership and the use of indigenous African knowledge. This begins with producing an African perspective on global health challenges in order to address the myriad of external health-related impacts. To do so, African health governance must be strengthened in order to generate coherent, proactive responses that focus on the causes of sickness. As Willms and others emphasize, improvements must come in interacting with local communities, using indigenous knowledge such as local concepts, dialogues, languages, healers, technologies, and programs in order to respond to health challenges.

The third recommendation calls for long-term thinking and planning as crucial to guarantee improved African health services in future years. Current health governance relies heavily on short-term solutions. The international community has emphasized the securitization of HIV/AIDS, which fails to provide the basis for long-term change. It has employed international instruments such as the World Bank's MAP and the WTO's TRIPS Agreement – neither of which emphasize long-term solutions. This requires reforms within international organizations along with the active assertion of state power so that African states may regain some of their health sovereignty, in order to identify socioeconomic determinants of health and implement long-term policies accordingly. In order to successfully implement long-term solutions, African health and climate change systems require improved legislation and policies plus better internal coordination and management.

The fourth recommendation is to link health more closely, coherently, and comprehensively with climate change. There is an increasing need to tackle both issues concurrently, as climate change has proven to pose threats to human health and development. The UNFCCC, along with other global, regional, and national institutions, must work together to reduce the divide between health and climate change.

The fifth recommendation is for African states themselves to adopt a culture of responsibility. African leaders must cease to assume that African countries are naturally susceptible to disease, and must actively deal with the health challenges Africans confront.

The sixth recommendation is to increase the use of two short-term instruments of proven effectiveness. Lisk emphasizes the need for developed countries to increase development assistance. Šehović argues for greater provision of anti-retroviral drugs.

The seventh recommendation concerns the many African states that experience insecurity and that may thus need to activate a version of the international responsibility to protect. According to Šehović, if a sovereign state is unable to provide security and protection to its citizens, provisions should be made for other actors to fill the resulting vacuum in order to ensure continued survival. This suggestion points to the need to create, in both principle and practice, a clear international responsibility to protect human health.

References

Cooper, Andrew F. and John J. Kirton, eds. (2009). *Innovation in Global Health Governance: Critical Cases*. Farnham: Ashgate.

Cooper, Andrew F., John J. Kirton, and Ted Schrecker, eds. (2007). *Governing Global Health: Challenge, Response, Innovation.* Aldershot: Ashgate.

Harman, Sophie (2010). *The World Bank and HIV/AIDS: Setting a Global Agenda.* Abdingdon: Routledge.

Kirton, John J., ed. (2009). *Global Health.* Farnham: Ashgate.

Krasner, Stephen (1999). *Sovereignty: Organized Hypocrisy.* Princeton: Princeton University Press.

Krasner, Stephen (2001). *Problematic Sovereignty: Contested Rules and Political Possibilities.* New York: Columbia University Press.

Krasner, Stephen (2009). *Power: The State, and Sovereignty: Essays on International Relations.* Abdingdon: Routledge.

Ruggie, John G. (1993). "Territoriality and Beyond: Problematizing Modernity in International Relations". *International Organization* 47(1): 139–74.

Bibliography

Africa Adaptation Programme (2010). "Africa Adaptation Programme: An Insight into AAP and Country Project Profiles". United Nations Development Programme. http://www.undp.org/content/dam/undp/library/Environment%20and%20Energy/Climate%20Change/UNDP_GOJ_HR.pdf (January 2014).

African Development Bank (2008). "Integrating Climate Change Adaptation into AfDB Group Operations". Internal memo, Tunis.

African Development Bank, Asian Development Bank, United Kingdom. Department for International Development, et al. (2003). "Poverty and Climate Change: Reducing the Vulnerability of the Poor through Adaptation". World Bank, Washington DC. http://www.unpei.org/sites/default/files/publications/Poverty-and-Climate-Change.pdf (January 2014).

African Union (2008). "Decisions, Declarations, Tribute, and Resolution". June 30–July 1, Sharm El-Sheikh. http://www.africa-union.org/root/au/Conferences/2008/june/summit/dec/ASSEMBLY%20DECISIONS%20193%20-%20207%20(XI).pdf (December 2013).

African Union (2011). "Theme: The Impact of Climate Change on Health and Development in Africa". April 17–21, Windhoek. http://www.au.int/en/sites/default/files/OVERVIEW_OF_THE_THEME_EN_17_21_APRIL_2011_SA_MINISTERS_MEETING_FIFTH_SESSION_AFRICAN_UNION_CONFERENCE_MINISTERS_HEALTH_WINDHOEK_NAMIBIA.doc (December 2013).

African Union Conference of Ministers of Health (2007). "Johannesburg Declaration of the 3rd Ordinary Session of the African Union Conference of Ministers of Health". Johannesburg, April 9–13. http://www.africa-union.org/root/UA/Conferences/2007/avril/SA/9-13%20avr/doc/en/SA/DECLARATION_OF_JOHGANNESBURG.pdf (September 2013).

Aginam, Obijiofor (2002). "From the Core to the Peripheries: Multilateral Governance of Malaria in a Multi-Cultural World". *Chicago Journal of International Law* 3(1): 87–103.

Aginam, Obijiofor (2004). "Between Isolationism and Mutual Vulnerability: A South–North Perspective on Global Governance of Epidemics in an Age of Globalization". *Temple Law Review* 77: 297–312. http://www.temple.edu/lawschool/iilpp/Docs/Aginam,%20Final%20to%20Publisher,%2011-23-04.pdf (January 2013).

Aginam, Obijiofor (2005). *Global Health Governance: International Law and Public Health in a Divided World*. Toronto: University of Toronto Press.

Aginam, Obijiofor (2007). "Diplomatic Rhetoric or Rhetorical Diplomacy: The G8 and Global Health Governance". In *Governing Global Health: Challenge, Response, Innovation*, Andrew F. Cooper and John J. Kirton, eds. Aldershot: Ashgate, pp. 147–55.

Aginam, Obijiofor (2010). "Health or Trade? A Critique of Contemporary Approaches to Global Health Diplomacy". *Asian Journal of WTO and International Health Law and Policy* 5(2): 355–80.

Agrawal, Arun (2008). "The Role of Local Institutions in Adaptation to Climate Change and Conflict in Africa". Paper prepared for the Social Dimensions of Climate Change, Social Development Department, World Bank, March 5–6, Washington DC. http://www.icarus.info/wp-content/uploads/2009/11/agrawal-adaptation-institutions-livelihoods.pdf (October 2013).

Agrawala, Shardul, ed. (2005). *Bridge Over Troubled Waters: Linking Climate Change and Development*. Paris: Organisation for Economic Co-operation and Development.

ALive Partnership for Livestock Development, Poverty Alleviation and Sustainable Growth (2013). "About ALive". http://www.alive-online.org/web/page/521/sectionid/339/pagelevel/2/interior.asp (September 2013).

Altman, Dennis (1999). "AIDS and Questions of Global Governance". *Pacifica Review* 11(2): 195–211.

Altman, Dennis (2003). "AIDS and Security". *International Relations* 17(4): 417–27.

Altman, Dennis and Kent Buse (2012). "Thinking Politically about HIV: Political Analysis and Action in Response to AIDS". *Contemporary Politics* 18(2): 127–40. doi: 10.1080/13569775.2012.674334.

American College of Chest Physicians (1995). "Smoking and Health: Physician Responsibility". *Chest* 108(4): 118–1121. doi: 10.1378/chest.108.4.1118.

amfAR (2013). "Statistics: Worldwide". New York. http://www.amfar.org/about-hiv-and-aids/facts-and-stats/statistics--worldwide/ (November 2013).

Anderson, Greg and Christopher Sands (2009). "The Summit Pandemic". *Edmonton Journal*, August 8. http://www.hudson.org/index.cfm?fuseaction=publication_details&id=6402 (December 2013).

Angola Press Agency (2012). "Africa: Communicable Diseases Leading Causes of Deaths in the Continent – WHO Official". *All Africa*, November 12. http://allafrica.com/stories/201211200297.html (January 2014).

Arctic Council (1997). "Alta Declaration". June 13, Alta, Norway. http://library.arcticportal.org/1271/1/The_Alta_Declaration.pdf (December 2013).

Arctic Council (2006). "Salekhard Declaration". October 26, Salekhard, Russia. http://www.arctic-council.org/index.php/en/document-archive/category/5-declarations?download=39:salekhard-declaration-2006 (December 2013).

Arctic Council (2009). "Tromsø Declaration". April 29, Tromsø. http://www.arctic-council.org/index.php/en/document-archive/category/53-final-reports-and-statements?download=222:the-tromso-declaration (December 2013).

Asia-Pacific Economic Cooperation (1997). "Vancouver Declaration: Connecting the APEC Community". November 27, Vancouver. http://www.

apec.org/Meeting-Papers/Leaders-Declarations/1997/1997_aelm.aspx (December 2013).

Barnett, Tony (2006). "A Long-Wave Event. HIV/AIDS, Politics, Governance, and 'Security': Sundering the Intergenerational Bond?" *International Affairs* 82(2): 297–313.

Barnett, Tony and Gwyn Prins (2006). "HIV/AIDS and Security: Fact, Fiction, and Evidence: A Report to UNAIDS". *International Affairs* 82(2): 359–68.

Baruchel, Hanae and Steve Dasilva (2005). "Global Civil Society Action at the 2005 G8 Gleneagles Summit". G8 Research Group, Toronto. http://www.g8.utoronto.ca/evaluations/csed/csed2005.pdf (December 2013).

Bates, Bryson, Zbigniew W. Kundzewicz, Shaohong Wu, et al. (2008). "Climate Change and Water: Technical Paper VI". Intergovernmental Panel on Climate Change, Geneva. https://www.ipcc.ch/publications_and_data/publications_and_data_technical_papers.shtml (December 2013).

Bayne, Nicholas (1999). "Continuity and Leadership in an Age of Globalisation". In *The G8's Role in the New Millennium*, Michael R. Hodges, John J. Kirton, and Joseph P. Daniels, eds. Aldershot: Ashgate, pp. 21–44.

Bayne, Nicholas (2005). *Staying Together: The G8 Summit Confronts the 21st Century*. Aldershot: Ashgate.

Bayne, Nicholas (2011). "Plurilateralism and Multilateralism: Comparing Institutions". In *The New Economic Diplomacy: Decision-Making and Negotiation in International Relations*, Nicholas Bayne and Stephen Woolcock, eds. Aldershot: Ashgate, pp. 205–29.

Behrman, Greg (2004). *The Invisible People: How the United States Has Slept through the Global AIDS Pandemic, the Greatest Humanitarian Catastrophe of Our Time*. New York: Free Press.

Bell, Clive, Shantayanan Devarajan, and Hans Gersbach (2003). "The Long-Run Economic Costs of AIDS: Theory and an Application to South Africa". World Bank, Washington DC. doi: 10.1596/1813-9450-3152.

Benatar, Solomon (2001). "South Africa's Transition in a Globalizing World: HIV/AIDS as a Window and a Mirror". *International Affairs* 77(2): 347–75.

Benatar, Solomon (2005). "The HIV/AIDS Pandemic: A Sign of Instability in a Complex Global System". In *Ethics and AIDS in Africa: The Challenge to Our Thinking*, Anton A. van Niekerk and Loretta M. Kopelman, eds. Claremont, South Africa: David Philip Publishers, pp. 71–83.

Berrang-Ford, Lea, J.D. MacLean, Theresa W. Gyorkos, et al. (2009). "Climate Change and Malaria in Canada: A Systems Approach". *Interdisciplinary Perspectives on Infectious Diseases* 2009. Article ID 385487. doi: 10.1155/2009/385487.

Besada, Hany (2009). "Coming to Terms with Southern Africa's HIV/AIDS Epidemic". In *Innovation in Global Health Governance: Critical Cases*, Andrew F. Cooper and John J. Kirton, eds. Farnham: Ashgate, pp. 155–78.

Bloom, David, Lakshmi Reddy Bloom, and Mark Weston (2006). "Business and Malaria: A Neglected Threat?". World Economic Forum, Davos. http://www.weforum.org/pdf/MalariaReport.pdf (July 2013).
Blouin, Chantal (2007). "Can the World Trade Organization Help Achieve the Health Millennium Development Goals?". In *Governing Global Health: Challenge, Response, Innovation*, Andrew F. Cooper, John J. Kirton, and Ted Schrecker, eds. Aldershot: Ashgate, pp. 87–100.
Blouin, Chantal, Mark Pearcey, and Valerie Percival (2013). "Instruments for Global Health Diplomacy in the UN System Beyond the WHO". In *Global Health Diplomacy: Concepts, Issues, Actors, Instruments, Fora, and Cases*, Ilona Kickbusch, Graham Lister, Michaela Told, et al., eds. New York: Springer, pp. 199–212.
Bradford, Colin I. (2007). "Reaching the Millennium Development Goals". In *Governing Global Health: Challenge, Response, Innovation*, Andrew F. Cooper and John J. Kirton, eds. Aldershot: Ashgate, pp. 79–86.
Brühl, Tanja and Volker Rittberger (2001). "From International to Global Governance: Actors, Collective Decision-Making, and the United Nations in the World of the Twenty-First Century". In *Global Governance and the United Nations System*, Volker Rittberger, ed. Tokyo: United Nations University Press, pp. 1–47.
Brundtland, Gro Harlem (2000). "Address at the Opening Dinner of the Massive Effort Advocacy Meeting". Winterthur, October 3. http://www.who.int/director-general/speeches/2000/english/20001003_massive_effort.html (December 2013).
Brundtland, Gro Harlem (2001). "Globalization as a Force for Better Health". Lecture presented in the Global Dimensions program, March 16, London School of Economics and Political Science. http://www.who.int/director-general/speeches/2001/english/20010316_lselecturelondon.en.html (January 2014).
Brundtland, Gro Harlem (2003). "Global Health and International Security". *Global Governance* 9(4): 417–23.
Brushett, Stephen and John Stephen Osika (2005). "Lessons Learned to Date from HIV/AIDS Transport Corridor Projects". World Bank Global HIV/AIDS Program Discussion Paper, August, World Bank, Washington DC. http://siteresources.worldbank.org/INTHIVAIDS/Resources/375798-1103037153392/Transport.pdf (September 2013).
Bryant, Leo, Louise Carver, Colin D. Butler, et al. (2009). "Climate Change and Family Planning: Least-Developed Countries Define the Agenda". *World Health Bulletin* 87(11): 852–7. http://www.who.int/bulletin/volumes/87/11/08-062562.pdf.
Burke, Marshall B., Edward Miguel, Shanker Satyanath, et al. (2009, 23 November). "Warming Increases the Risk of Civil War in Africa". *Proceedings of the National Academy of Sciences*. doi: 10.1073/pnas.0907998106.
Buzan, Barry and Ole Wæver (2003). *Regions and Powers: The Structure of International Security*. Cambridge: Cambridge University Press.

Byass, Peter (2009, 11 November). "Climate Change and Population Health in Africa: Where Are the Scientists?". *Global Health Action*. doi: 10.3402/gha.v2i0.2065.

Byass, Peter (2009). "The Unequal World of Health Data". *PLoS Medicine* 6(11). doi: 10.1371/journal.pmed.1000155.

Cabral, Amilcar (1966). "The Weapon of Theory". Address delivered to the first Tricontinental Conference of the Peoples of Asia, Africa and Latin America, Havana, January. http://www.marxists.org/subject/africa/cabral/1966/weapon-theory.htm (September 2013).

Callahan, Daniel and Angela A. Wasunna (2006). *Medicine and the Market: Equity v. Choice*. Baltimore: Johns Hopkins University Press.

Cameron, David (2013). "Prime Minister's Letter to G8 Leaders". London, January 2. http://www.g8.utoronto.ca/summit/2013lougherne/130102-cameron.html (December 2013).

Campbell-Lendrum, Diarmid, Carlos Corvalán, and Maria Neira (2007). "Global Climate Change: Implications for International Public Health Policy". *World Health Bulletin* 85(3): 161–244. http://www.who.int/bulletin/volumes/85/3/06-039503/en/ (October 2013).

Campbell-Lendrum, Diarmid and Manjula Lusti-Narasimhan (2009). "Taking the Heat Out of the Population and Climate Debate". *World Health Bulletin* 87(11): 807. http://www.who.int/bulletin/volumes/87/11/09-072652/en/ (October 2013).

Carment, David (2003). "Assessing State Failure: Implications for Theory and Policy". *Third World Quarterly* 24(3): 407–27.

Centers for Disease Control and Prevention (1998, September 11). "Preventing Emerging Infectious Diseases: A Strategy for the 21st Century". *Morbidity and Mortality Weekly Report* 47(RR-15). Overview of the Updated CDC plan. http://www.cdc.gov/mmwr/PDF/rr/rr4715.pdf (January 2013).

Chan, Margaret (2008). "The Impact of Climate Change on Human Health". World Health Organization, April 7. http://www.who.int/mediacentre/news/statements/2008/s05/en/index.html (December 2013).

Chand, Sudeep, J. Stephen Morrison, Peter Piot, et al. (2010, 23 June). "From G8 to G20, Is Health Next in Line?" *Lancet*. Published online. http://c657621.r21.cf2.rackcdn.com/commissioners/lancetg8g20.pdf (January 2014).

Coghlan, Benjamin, Richard J. Brennan, Pascal Ngoy, et al. (2006). "Morality in the Democratic Republic of Congo: A Nationwide Survey". *Lancet* 367(9504): 44–51.

Coghlan, Benjamin, Pascal Ngoy, Flavien Mulumba, et al. (2008). "Mortality in the Democratic Republic of Congo: An Ongoing Crisis". International Rescue Committee, New York. http://www.rescue.org/sites/default/files/migrated/resources/2007/2006-7_congomortalitysurvey.pdf (October 2013).

COHAB Initiative (2010). "The Health Effects of Climate Change Impacts on Biodiversity". UN CBD COP 10 Policy Brief: Biodiversity and Global

Health 3, October, Galway. http://www.cbd.int/doc/health/cohab-policy-brief3-en.pdf (December 2013).

Commission for Africa (2005). "Our Common Interest". Report of the Commission for Africa, London. http://www.commissionforafrica.info/2005-report (October 2012).

Commission for Africa (2010). "Still Our Common Interest". London. http://www.commissionforafrica.info/wp-content/uploads/2010/09/cfa-report-2010-full-version.pdf (October 2013).

Commission on Macroeconomics and Health (2001). "Macroeconomics and Health: Investing in Health for Economic Development". World Health Organization, Geneva. http://www.cid.harvard.edu/archive/cmh/cmhreport.pdf (October 2012).

Commission on Social Determinants of Health (2008). "Closing the Gap in a Generation: Health Equity through Action on the Social Determinants of Health. Final Report of the Commission on Social Determinants of Health". World Health Organization, Geneva. http://www.who.int/social_determinants/thecommission/finalreport/en/index.html (December 2013).

Connolly, Gregory N. (1992). "Worldwide Expansion of Transnational Tobacco Industry". *Journal of the National Cancer Institute* 12: 29–35.

Cook, Alethia H. (2010). "Securitization of Disease in the United States: Globalization, Public Policy, and Pandemics". *Risks, Hazards and Crisis in Public Policy* 1(1): 10–30.

Cooper, Andrew F. (2013). "The G8/G20 and Global Health Governance". In *Global Health Diplomacy: Concepts, Issues, Actors, Instruments, Fora, and Cases*, Ilona Kickbusch, Graham Lister, Michaela Told, et al., eds. New York: Springer, pp. 243–52.

Cooper, Andrew F. and John J. Kirton, eds. (2009). *Innovation in Global Health Governance: Critical Cases*. Farnham: Ashgate.

Cooper, Andrew F., John J. Kirton, Franklyn Lisk, et al., eds. (2013). *Africa's Health Challenges: Sovereignty, Mobility of People, and Healthcare Governance*. Farnham: Ashgate.

Cooper, Andrew F., John J. Kirton, and Ted Schrecker, eds. (2007). *Governing Global Health: Challenge, Response, Innovation*. Aldershot: Ashgate.

Cooper, Richard N. (1989). "International Cooperation in Public Health as a Prologue to Macroeconomic Cooperation". In *Can Nations Agree? Issues in International Economic Cooperation*, Richard Cooper, Barry Eichengreen, Gerald Holtham, et al., eds. Washington DC: Brookings Institution, pp. 178–254.

Cornia, Giovanni Andrea and Germano Mwabu (1997). "Health Status and Health Policy in Sub-Saharan Africa: A Long-Term Perspective" Working Paper 1997/141, United Nations University World Institute for Development Economics Research. http://www.wider.unu.edu/publications/working-papers/previous/en_GB/wp-141 (July 2013).

Correa, Carlos M. (2000). *Intellectual Property Rights, the WTO, and Developing Countries: The TRIPS Agreement and Policy Options*. London: Zed Books.

Costello, Anthony, Mustafa Abbas, Adriana Allen, et al. (2009). "Managing the Health Effects of Climate Change: Lancet and University College London Institute for Global Health Commission". *Lancet* 373(9676): 1693–733. http://www.ucl.ac.uk/global-health/project-pages/lancet1/ucl-lancet-climate-change.pdf (October 2013).

Costello, Anthony, Mark Maslin, Hugh Montgomery, et al. (2011). "Global Health and Climate Change: Moving from Denial and Catastrophic Fatalism to Positive Action". *Philosophical Transactions of the Royal Society* 369(1942): 1866–82. http://rsta.royalsocietypublishing.org/content/369/1942/1866.full (October 2013).

Davies, Sara (2013). "Securitizing Infectious Disease". *International Affairs* 84(2): 295–313.

De Coning, Cedric and Fanie Cloete (2000). "Theories and Models for Analyzing Public Policy". In *Improving Public Policy: From Theory to Practice*, Fanie Cloete and Cedric De Coning, eds. Pretoria: Van Schaik.

de Schutter, Jacqueline and Manuel Riemer (2009). "Participatory Decision-Making Models in the Context of Environmental Justice: Are They Working?" Paper prepared for "Earth System Governance: People, Places and the Planet", 2009 Amsterdam Conference on the Human Dimensions of Global Environmental Change, December 2–4, Amsterdam. http://www.earthsystemgovernance.org/ac2009/papers/AC2009-0151.pdf (October 2013).

de Waal, Alex (2003). "Human Rights Organizations and the Political Imagination: How the West and Africa Have Diverged". *Journal of Human Rights* 2(4): 475–94.

de Waal, Alex (2006). *AIDS and Power: Why There Is No Political Crisis – Yet*. New York: Zed Books.

De Wet, Phillip (2014). "Big Pharma's 'Satanic' Plot Is Genocide, Mtsoaledi Rages". *Mail and Guardian*, January 17. http://mg.co.za/article/2014-01-16-motsoaledi-big-pharmas-satanic-plot-is-genocide (January 2014).

Deribe, Shewaye (2007). "Wichi Integrated Wetland-Watershed Management Project". Presentation prepared for the International Conference on Population, Health, and Environment: Integrated Development for East Africa, 14–16 November, Addis Ababa. http://www.ehproject.org/PDF/phe/deribe-wichi.pdf (October 2012).

Diamond, Jared (2005). *Collapse: How Societies Choose to Fail or Succeed*. revised edn. New York: Penguin.

Dibua, J.I. (1998). "Journey to Nowhere: Neo-liberalism and Africa's Development Crisis". *Comparative Studies of South Asia, Africa, and the Middle East* 18(2): 119–30.

Ebi, Kristie L. and Jan C. Semenza (2008). "Community-Based Adaptation to the Health Impacts of Climate Change". *American Journal of Preventive Medicine* 35(5): 501–7.

Economist (2008). “Redesigning Global Finance”. November 13. http://www.economist.com/node/12599261 (October 2013).

Eizenstat, Stuart E., John Edward Porter, and Jeremy Weinstein (2005). “Rebuilding Weak States”. *Foreign Affairs* 84(134): 134–46.

Elbe, Stefan (2006). “Should HIV/AIDS Be Securitized? The Ethical Dilemmas of Linking HIV/AIDS and Security”. *International Studies Quarterly* 50(1): 119–44.

Elbe, Stefan (2009). *Virus Alert: Security, Governmentality, and the AIDS Pandemic*. New York: Columbia University Press.

Emmelin, Anders, Mesganaw Fantahun, Yemane Berhane, et al. (2008, December 16). “Vulnerability to Episodes of Extreme Weather: Butajira, Ethiopia, 1998–1999”. *Global Health Action* 2. http://www.globalhealthaction.net/index.php/gha/article/view/1829/2088 (October 2013).

Epstein, Helen (2007). *The Invisible Cure: Africa, The West, and the Fight against AIDS*. New York: Farrar, Straus and Giroux.

Equinet (2007). “Reclaiming the Resources for Health: A Regional Analysis of Equity in Health in East and Southern Africa”. Harare. http://www.equinetafrica.org/bibl/docs/EQUINET%20Reclaiming%20the%20Resources%20for%20Health%20in%20ESA.pdf (October 2013).

Equinet and Southern and Eastern African Trade Information and Negotiations Institute (SEATINI) (2007). “Trade and Health in East and Southern Africa”. Policy Series No. 18, July, Equinet, Harare. http://www.equinetafrica.org/bibl/docs/POLBRIEF18%20trade.pdf (October 2013).

Escobar, Arturo (1995). *Encountering Development: The Making and Unmaking of the Third World*. Princeton: Princeton University Press.

Ethiopia. Ministry of Water Resources and Ethiopia. National Meteorological Agency (2007). “Climate Change Adaptation Programme of Action (NAPA) of Ethiopia”. Addis Ababa. http://unfccc.int/resource/docs/napa/eth01.pdf (October 2012).

European Council (2001). “Presidency Conclusions”. SN 2001/1/01 REV 1, June 15–16, Göteborg. http://ec.europa.eu/smart-regulation/impact/background/docs/goteborg_concl_en.pdf (December 2013).

Evans, Tim (2004). “The G20 and Global Public Health”. Paper prepared for the conference on The G20 at Leaders’ Level? organized by the International Development Research Centre, February 29, Ottawa. http://www.l20.org/publications/25_63_g20_ottawa_evans.pdf (January 2014).

Evans, Tim and Carla AbouZahr (2008, November 14). “INDEPTH @ 10: Celebrate the past and illuminate the future”. *Global Health Action* 1. http://www.globalhealthaction.net/index.php/gha/article/view/1899/2003 (October 2013).

Falola, Toyin and Matthew M. Heaton, eds. (2007). *HIV/AIDS, Illness, and African Well-Being*. Rochester NY: University Rochester Press.

Faris, Stephen (2007). “The Real Roots of Darfur”. *Atlantic Monthly*, pp. 67–9. http://www.theatlantic.com/magazine/archive/2007/04/the-real-roots-of-darfur/305701/ (January 2014).

Farmer, Paul (1992). *AIDS and Accusation: Haiti and the Geography of Blame*. 1st edn. Berkeley CA: University of California Press.

Farmer, Paul (1999). *Infections and Inequalities: The Modern Plagues*. Berkeley: University of California Press.

Fassin, Didier (2007) *When Bodies Remember: Experiences and Politics of AIDS in South Africa*. Berkeley: University of California Press.

Fidler, David P. (1997). "The Globalization of Public Health: Emerging Infectious Diseases and International Relations". *Indiana Journal of Global Legal Studies* 5(1): 11–51.

Fidler, David P. (1999). *International Law and Infectious Diseases*. Oxford: Oxford University Press.

Fidler, David P. (2001). "The Globalization of Public Health: The First 100 Years of International Health Diplomacy". *Bulletin of the World Health Organization* 79(9): 742–849. http://www.who.int/bulletin/archives/79(9)842.pdf (January 2014).

Fidler, David P. (2004). "Constitutional Outlines of Public Health's 'New World Order'". *Temple Law Review* 77(247): 247–89.

Fidler, David P. (2007). "A Pathology of Public Health Securitism: Approaching Pandemics as Security Threats". In *Governing Global Health: Challenge, Response, Innovation*, Andrew F. Cooper, John J. Kirton, and Ted Schrecker, eds. Aldershot: Ashgate, pp. 41–64.

Fidler, David P. and Laurence O. Gostin (2006). "The New International Health Regulations: An Historic Development for International Law and Public Health". *Journal of Law, Medicine, and Ethics* 34(1): 85–94.

Founou-Tchuigou, Bernard (1996). "Africa Confronted with the Ravages of Neo-liberalism". *Africa Development* 21(2–3): 5–24.

Fourie, Pieter (2006). *The Political Management of HIV and AIDS in South Africa: One Burden Too Many?* London: Palgrave Macmillan.

Fourie, Pieter (2007) "The Relationship between the AIDS Pandemic and State Fragility". *Global Change, Peace, and Security* 19(3): 281–300.

Fourie, Pieter and Melissa Meyer (2010). *The Politics of Aids Denialism: South Africa's Failure to Respond*. Farnham: Ashgate.

Fourie, Pieter and Martin Schönteich (2001). "Africa's New Security Threat". *African Security Review* 10(4): 29–42.

Friel, Sharon, Alan D. Dangour, Tara Garnett, et al. (2009). "Public Health Benefits of Strategies to Reduce Greenhouse-Gas Emissions: Food and Agriculture". *Lancet* 374(9706): 2016–25.

Friel, Sharon, Michael Marmot, Anthony J. McMichael, et al. (2008). "Global Health Equity and Climate Stabilisation: A Common Agenda". *Lancet* 372(9650): 1677–83.

Frumkin, Howard, Anthony J. McMichael, and Jeremy J. Hess (2008). "Climate Change and the Health of the Public". *American Journal of Preventive Medicine* 35(5): 401–2.

G7 (1980). "Declaration". Venice, June 23. http://www.g8.utoronto.ca/summit/1980venice/communique (December 2013).
G7 (1987). "Chairman's Statement on AIDS". Venice, June 10. http://www.g8.utoronto.ca/summit/1987venice/aids.html (December 2013).
G7 (1996). "Chairman's Statement [Political Declaration]: Toward Greater Security and Stability in a More Cooperative World". June 29, Lyon. http://www.g8.utoronto.ca/summit/1996lyon/chair.html (December 2013).
G8 (1997). "Communiqué". June 22, Denver. http://www.g8.utoronto.ca/summit/1997denver/g8final.htm (December 2013).
G8 (1998). "Communiqué". Birmingham, May 15. http://www.g8.utoronto.ca/summit/1998birmingham/finalcom.htm (December 2013).
G8 (2002). "G8 Africa Action Plan". Kananaskis, June 27. http://www.g8.utoronto.ca/summit/2002kananaskis/africaplan.html (December 2013).
G8 (2003). "Health: A G8 Action Plan". Evian, June 2. http://www.g8.utoronto.ca/summit/2003evian/health_en.html (December 2013).
G8 (2003). "Science and Technology for Sustainable Development: A G8 Action Plan". Evian, June 2. http://www.g8.utoronto.ca/summit/2003evian/sustainable_development_en.html (December 2013).
G8 (2005). "Africa". Gleneagles, July 8. http://www.g8.utoronto.ca/summit/2005gleneagles/africa.html (December 2013).
G8 (2005). "Climate Change, Clean Energy, and Sustainable Development". Gleneagles, July 8. http://www.g8.utoronto.ca/summit/2005gleneagles/climatechange.html (December 2013).
G8 (2005). "Gleneagles Plan of Action: Climate Change, Clean Energy, and Sustainable Development". Gleneagles, July 8. http://www.g8.utoronto.ca/summit/2005gleneagles/climatechangeplan.html (December 2013).
G8 (2006). "Fight against Infectious Disease". St. Petersburg, July 16. http://www.g8.utoronto.ca/summit/2006stpetersburg/infdis.html (September 2013).
G8 (2007). "Growth and Responsibility in Africa". Heiligendamm, June 7. http://www.g8.utoronto.ca/summit/2007heiligendamm/g8-2007-africa.html (December 2013).
G8 (2008). "Development and Africa". Hokkaido, July 8. http://www.g8.utoronto.ca/summit/2008hokkaido/2008-africa.html (December 2013).
G8 (2009). "Responsible Leadership for a Sustainable Future". L'Aquila, Italy, July 8. http://www.g8.utoronto.ca/summit/2009laquila/2009-declaration.html (December 2013).
G8 (2010). "G8 Muskoka Declaration: Recovery and New Beginnings". Huntsville, Canada, June 26. http://www.g8.utoronto.ca/summit/2010muskoka/communique.html (December 2013).
G8 (2011). "G8 Declaration: Renewed Commitment for Freedom and Democracy". Deauville, May 27. http://www.g8.utoronto.ca/summit/2011deauville/2011-declaration-en.html (December 2013).

G8 (2011). "G8/Africa Joint Declaration: Shared Values, Shared Responsibilities". Deauville, May 27. http://www.g8.utoronto.ca/summit/2011deauville/2011-africa-en.html (December 2013).

G8 (2012). "Camp David Declaration". Camp David, May 19. http://www.g8.utoronto.ca/summit/2012campdavid/g8-declaration.html (December 2013).

G20 (2009). "G20 Leaders Statement: The Pittsburgh Summit". Pittsburgh, September 25. http://www.g20.utoronto.ca/2009/2009communique0925.html (July 2012).

Gambia (2008). "Climate Change in the Gambia". Department of State for Forestry and the Environment, Banjul.

Garrett, Laurie (2005). "Lessons of HIV/AIDS". *Foreign Affairs* 84(51): 51–64.

Garrett, Laurie (2007). "The Challenge of Global Health". *Foreign Affairs* 86(1): 14–38. http://www.foreignaffairs.com/articles/62268/laurie-garrett/the-challenge-of-global-health (January 2014).

Garrett, Laurie (2009). "Global Health Update". December 23, Council on Foreign Relations, New York. http://www.cfr.org/content/thinktank/GlobalHealth/GHU_Copenhagen_Dec2309.pdf (July 2013).

German Presidency of the G8 (2006). "Focuses of the G8 Presidency". October 18. http://www.g8.utoronto.ca/summit/2007heiligendamm/2007focus.html (December 2013).

Global Fund to Fight AIDS, Tuberculosis, and Malaria (2004). "The Malaria Epidemic". Geneva. http://www.globalfundatm.org/journalists/fsheets/malaria.htm (December 2013).

Global Fund to Fight AIDS, Tuberculosis, and Malaria (2004). "Report of the Executive Director". Ninth board meeting, Arusha, Geneva, November 18–19. http://www.theglobalfund.org/documents/board/09/BM09_03ExecutiveDirector_Report_en (September 2013).

Global Fund to Fight AIDS, Tuberculosis, and Malaria (2012). "Global Fund Support Extends Antiretroviral Treatment to 4.2 Million People". Geneva, November 29. http://www.theglobalfund.org/en/mediacenter/newsreleases/2012-11-29_Global_Fund_support_extends_antiretroviral_treatment_to_4,2_million_people/ (October 2012).

Global Fund to Fight AIDS, Tuberculosis, and Malaria (2012). "Strategic Investments for Impact: Global Fund Results Report 2012". Geneva. http://www.theglobalfund.org/documents/publications/progress_reports/Publication_2012Results_Report_en/ (September 2013).

Global Fund to Fight AIDS, Tuberculosis, and Malaria (2013). "Fighting AIDS, Tuberculosis, and Malaria". Geneva. http://www.theglobalfund.org/en/about/diseases/ (September 2013).

Global Markets Institute (2006). "G8 Summit in St. Petersburg". Goldman Sachs, New York.

Godlee, Fiona (1994). "WHO in Retreat: Is It Losing Its Influence?" *British Medical Journal* 309(6967): 1491–5.

Goodhart, Michael and Stacy Bondanella Taninchev (2011). "The New Sovereigntist Challenge for Global Governance: Democracy without Sovereignty". *International Studies Quarterly* 55(4): 1047–68. doi: 10.1111/j.1468-2478.2011.00691.x.

Gore, Al and Jonas Gahr Støre (2009). "Co-chair's Summary – Melting Ice: Regional Dramas, Global Wake-Up Call". April 29, Tromsø. http://www.arctic-council.org/index.php/en/document-archive/category/53-final-reports-and-statements?download=213:co-chars-summary-meeting-ice-conferance

Gostin, Lawrence O. (2008). "Meeting Basic Survival Needs of the World's Least Healthy People: Toward a Framework Convention on Global Health". *Georgetown Law Journal* 96(2): 331–92. http://georgetownlawjournal.org/files/pdf/96-2/Gostin-Article.PDF (December 2013).

Gostin, Lawrence O. (2012). "Conclusion". In *Human Health and Ecological Integrity: Ethics, Law, and Human Rights*, Laura Westra, Colin L. Soskolne, and Donald W. Spady, eds. Abdingdon: Routledge, pp. 335–8.

Gottwald, Franz-Theo (2012). "Are Cows 'Climate Killers'?". In *Human Health and Ecological Integrity: Ethics, Law, and Human Rights*, Laura Westra, Colin L. Soskolne, and Donald W. Spady, eds. Abdingdon: Routledge, pp. 277–88.

Grosfoguel, Ramón (2009). "A Decolonial Approach to Political-Economy: Transmodernity, Border Thinking, and Global Coloniality". *Kult* 6 (Special Issue): 10–38. http://postkolonial.dk/artikler/GROSFOGUEL.pdf (January 2014).

Guebert, Jenilee (2012). "Global Health at the G8: Integration, In Decline or Simply Stalled?". Global Health Governance (Blog). 11 June. http://blogs.shu.edu/ghg/2012/06/11/global-health-at-the-g8-integration-in-decline-or-simply-stalled-jenilee-m-guebert/ (December 2013).

Gurría, Angel (2008). "The OECD: An Active Player in Building Global Governance". In *Growth, Innovation, Inclusion: The G20 at Ten*, John J. Kirton and Madeline Koch, eds. London: Newsdesk, pp. 45–6. http://www.g8.utoronto.ca/newsdesk/G20at10.pdf (December 2013).

Haffajee, Ferial (2007). "Not in My Father's House: Trevor Manuel". *Mail and Guardian*, December 13.

Haines, Andrew, Anthony J McMichael, and Paul R. Epstein (2000). "Environment and Health: 2. Global Climate Change and Health". *Canadian Medical Association Journal* 163(6): 729–34. http://www.cmaj.ca/content/163/6/729.full (December 2013).

Haines, Andy, Sari Kovats, Diarmid Campbell-Lendrum, et al. (2006). "Climate Change and Human Health: Impacts, Vulnerability, and Mitigation". *Lancet* 367(9528): 2101–9. http://dx.doi.org/10.1001/jama.291.1.99.

Haines, Andy, Paul Wilkinson, Cathryn Tonne, et al. (2009). "Aligning Climate Change and Public Health Policies". *Lancet* 374(9707): 2035–8.

Hajnal, Peter I. (1999). *The G7/G8 System: Evolution, Role, and Documentation*. Aldershot: Ashgate.

Hajnal, Peter I., ed. (2002). *Civil Society in the Information Age*. Aldershot: Ashgate.

Hales, Simon, Neil de Wet, John Maindonald, et al. (2002). "Potential Effect of Population and Climate Changes on Global Distribution of Dengue Fever: An Empirical Model". *Lancet* 2002(360): 9336. 830–34.

Harman, Sophie (2010). *The World Bank and HIV/AIDS: Setting a Global Agenda*. Abdingdon: Routledge.

Health Canada (2013). "Climate Change and Health". Ottawa. http://www.hc-sc.gc.ca/ewh-semt/pubs/climat/index-eng.php (December 2013).

Hein, Wolfgang, Sonja Bartsch, and Lars Kohlmorgen, eds. (2007). *Global Health Governance and the Fight Against HIV/AIDS*. New York: Palgrave Macmillan.

Held, David and Anthony McGrew (2002). "Introduction". In *Governing Globalization: Power, Authority, and Global Governance*, David Held and Anthony McGrew, eds. Cambridge: Polity Press.

Helleiner, Eric and Geoffrey Cameron (2006). "Another World Order? The Bush Administration and HIPC Debt Cancellation". *New Political Economy* 11(1): 125–40. doi: 10.1080/13563460500494958.

High-Level Panel on Threats, Challenges, and Change (2004). "A More Secure World: Our Shared Responsibility". United Nations, New York. http://www.un.org/secureworld/ (July 2013).

Hogan, Barbara (2008). "Speech by the Minister of Health at the HIV Vaccine Research Conference". Cape Town, October 13. http://www.tac.org.za/community/node/2421 (July 2013).

Holbrooke, Richard and Laurie Garrett (2008). ""Sovereignty" That Risks Global Health". *Washington Post*, August 10. http://www.washingtonpost.com/wp-dyn/content/article/2008/08/08/AR2008080802919.html (December 2013).

Holdren, John P. (2008). "Science and Technology for Sustainable Well-Being". *Science*, pp. 424–34. http://www.sciencemag.org/content/319/5862/424.full (October 2013).

Holmes, John (2008). "More Help Now, Please: How to Tackle Tomorrow's Disasters". In *The World in 2009*, Daniel Franklin, ed. London: *The Economist*. http://www.economist.com/node/12494621 (December 2013).

Hösle, Vittorio (2004). *Morals and Politics*. Translated by Steven Rendall. Notre Dame, IN: University of Notre Dame Press.

Howard, Lee (1989). "The Evolution of Bilateral and Multilateral Cooperation for Health in Developing Countries". In *International Cooperation for Health: Problems, Prospects, and Priorities*. Michael R. Reich and Eiji Marui, eds. Dover MA: Auburn House.

Howard-Jones, Norman (1975). *The Scientific Background of the International Sanitary Conferences, 1851–1938*. Geneva: World Health Organization.

Hsu, Lee-Nah and Jessica White (2007). "Partnerships for Health, the Environment, and Governance". In *Governing Global Health: Challenge, Response, Innovation*, Andrew F. Cooper, John J. Kirton, and Ted Schrecker, eds. Aldershot: Ashgate, pp. 101–12.

Hunter, Susan (2003). *Black Death: AIDS in Africa*. New York: Palgrave Macmillan.

Huq, Saleemul (2005). "Adaptation to Climate Change: A Paper for the International Climate Change Taskforce". Institute for Public Policy Research, London. http://www.ippr.org/ecomm/files/adaptation.pdf (January 2014).

Huq, Saleemul, Hannah Reid, and Laurel A. Murray (2006). "Climate Change and Development Links". International Institute for Environment and Development, London. http://pubs.iied.org/14516IIED.html?k=climate%20change%20and%20development%20links (January 2014).

Ikenberry, G. John (2001). *After Victory: Institutions, Strategic Restraint, and the Rebuilding of Order after Major Wars*. Princeton: Princeton University Press.

Iliffe, John (2006). *The African AIDS Epidemic: A History*. Athens, OH: Ohio University Press.

Ingram, Alan (2007). "HIV/AIDS, Security and the Geopolitics of US–Nigerian Relations". *Review of International Political Economy* 14(3): 510–34.

Institute for Development Studies and Tearfund (2006). "Overcoming the Barriers: Mainstreaming Climate Change Adaptation in Developing Countries". Tearfund Climate Change Briefing Paper 1, Tearfund, London. http://www.tearfund.org/webdocs/website/Campaigning/Policy%20and%20research/Overcoming%20the%20barriers%20briefing%20paper.pdf (December 2013).

Institute for Health Metrics and Evaluation (2013). "GBD Data". Database, Seattle WA. http://www.healthmetricsandevaluation.org/search-gbd-data (September 2013).

Intergovernmental Panel on Climate Change (1995). "IPCC Second Assessment: Climate Change 1995". Geneva. http://www.ipcc.ch/ipccreports/tar/wg2/ (December 2013).

Intergovernmental Panel on Climate Change (1997). *The Regional Impacts of Climate Change: An Assessment of Vulnerability*. Geneva: http://www.ipcc.ch/ipccreports/sres/regional/index.php?idp=0 (December 2013).

Intergovernmental Panel on Climate Change (2001). *Climate Change 2001: Impacts, Adaptation, and Vulnerability. Contribution of Working Group II to the Third Assessment Report of the Intergovernmental Panel on Climate Change*. Cambridge: Cambridge University Press. http://www.ipcc.ch/ipccreports/tar/wg2/ (December 2013).

Intergovernmental Panel on Climate Change (2001). "Climate Change 2001: Synthesis Report. Summary for Policymakers". Geneva. http://www.ipcc.ch/pdf/climate-changes-2001/synthesis-spm/synthesis-spm-en.pdf (December 2013).

Intergovernmental Panel on Climate Change (2007). *Climate Change 2007: Impacts, Adaptation, and Vulnerability. Contribution of Working Group II to the Fourth Assessment Report of the Intergovernmental Panel on Climate Change*. Cambridge: Cambridge University Press. http://www.ipcc-wg2.gov/publications/AR4/index.html (December 2013).

Intergovernmental Panel on Climate Change (2007). *Climate Change 2007: Mitigation. Contribution of Working Group III to the Fourth Assessment Report of the Intergovernmental Panel on Climate Change*. Cambridge: Cambridge University Press. http://www.ipcc.ch/publications_and_data/publications_

ipcc_fourth_assessment_report_wg3_report_mitigation_of_climate_change.htm (December 2013).

Intergovernmental Panel on Climate Change (2007). "Climate Change 2007: Synthesis Report". Geneva. http://www.ipcc.ch/pdf/assessment-report/ar4/syr/ar4_syr.pdf (December 2013).

Intergovernmental Panel on Climate Change (2007). *Climate Change 2007: The Physical Science Basis. Contribution of Working Group I to the Fourth Assessment Report of the Intergovernmental Panel on Climate Change.* Cambridge: Cambridge University Press. http://www.ipcc.ch/publications_and_data/publications_ipcc_fourth_assessment_report_wg1_report_the_physical_science_basis.htm (December 2013).

International Commission on Intervention and State Sovereignty (2001). "The Responsibility to Protect: Report of the International Commission on Intervention and State Sovereignty". December. http://responsibilitytoprotect.org/ICISS%20Report.pdf (December 2013).

International Conference on Primary Health Care and Health Systems in Africa (2008). "Ouagadougou Declaration on Primary Health Care and Health Systems in Africa: Achieving Better Health for Africa in the New Millennium". Ouagadougou, April 28–30. http://www.who.int/management/OuagadougouDeclarationEN.pdf (September 2013).

International Federation of Red Cross and Red Crescent Societies (2012). "Annual Report 2012. Towards Climate-Smart Resilience: A Year of Engagement". Geneva. http://www.climatecentre.org/downloads/File/reports/Annual%20Reports/RCCC_AR_2012%20web.pdf (December 2013).

International Monetary Fund (2013). "Regional Economic Outlook: Sub-Saharan Africa Keeping the Pace". October, Washington DC. https://www.imf.org/external/pubs/ft/reo/2013/afr/eng/sreo1013.pdf (January 2014).

International Monetary Fund (2013). "World Economic Outlook Database". Washington DC, October. http://www.imf.org/external/pubs/ft/weo/2013/01/weodata/index.aspx (October 2013).

Janzen, John M. (1978). *The Quest for Therapy in Lower Zaire.* Berkeley: University of California Press.

Japan. Ministry of Foreign Affairs (2000). "Summit Meeting in Tokyo among President Olusegun Obasanjo of the Federal Republic of Nigeria, President Thabo Mbeki of the Republic of South Africa, President Abdelaziz Bouteflica of the Democratic People's Republic of Algeria, Prime Minister Chuan Leekpai of the Kingdom of Thailand and G8 Leaders". Tokyo, July 20. http://www.g8.utoronto.ca/summit/2000okinawa/devs.htm (December 2013).

Jarman, Melanie (2007). *Climate Change.* London: Pluto Press.

Joint Learning Initiative (2004). "Human Resources for Health: Overcoming the Crisis". Harvard University, Cambridge MA. http://www.who.int/hrh/documents/JLi_hrh_report.pdf (October 2012).

Kaberuka, Donald (2013). "Africa Can Give the World the Economic Pulse It Needs". In *The Russia G20 Summit: St Petersburg 2013*, John J. Kirton and

Madeline Koch, eds. London: Newsdesk, pp. 124–6. http://www.g8.utoronto.ca/newsdesk/stpetersburg.

Kaplan, Robert D. (2000). *The Coming Anarchy: Shattering the Dreams of the Post Cold War*. New York: Random House.

Kasun, Jacqueline (1999). *The War Against Population: The Economics and Ideology of World Population Control*. 2nd ed. San Francisco: Ignatius Press.

Kategekwa, Joy (2008). "Liberalization of Trade in Health Services: Balancing Mode 4 Interests with Obligations to Provide Universal Access to Basic Services". July, South Centre. http://www.southcentre.int/wp-content/uploads/2013/05/RP16_Liberalization-of-Trade-in-Health-Services_EN.pdf (October 2013).

Kaubab, Rashid (2005). *Benchmarking Development for Hong Kong and Beyond: Strengthening Africa in World Trade*. Harare: Southern and Eastern African Trade Information and Negotiations Institute (SEATINI).

Kelle, Alexander (2007). "Securitization of International Public Health: Implications for Global Health Governance and the Biological Weapons Prohibition Regime'", *Global Governance* 13(2007): 217–35.

Kickbusch, Ilona, Graham Lister, Michaela Told, et al., eds. (2013). *Global Health Diplomacy: Concepts, Issues, Actors, Instruments, Fora, and Cases*. New York: Springer.

King, Nicholas (2002). "Security, Disease, Commerce: Ideologies of Postcolonial Global Health". *Social Studies of Science* 32(5–6): 763–89.

Kintzele, Kathryn (2012). "Ethical Principles on the Environment and Human Health in State Statutes". In *Human Health and Ecological Integrity: Ethics, Law, and Human Rights*, Laura Westra, Colin L. Soskolne, and Donald W. Spady, eds. Abdingdon: Routledge, pp. 20–31.

Kirton, John J. (1989). "Contemporary Concert Diplomacy: The Seven-Power Summit and the Management of International Order". Paper presented at the annual convention of the International Studies Association, March 29–April 1, London. http://www.g8.utoronto.ca/scholar/kirton198901 (July 2010).

Kirton, John J. (1993). "The Seven Power Summits as a New Security Institution". In *Building a New Global Order: Emerging Trends in International Security*, David Dewitt, David Haglund, and John J. Kirton, eds. Toronto: Oxford University Press, pp. 335–57.

Kirton, John J. (2005). "Gleneagles G8 Boosts Blair at Home". Toronto, August 1. http://www.g8.utoronto.ca/evaluations/2005gleneagles/coverage.html (December 2013).

Kirton, John J., ed. (2009). *Global Health*. Farnham: Ashgate.

Kirton, John J. (2013). *G20 Governance for a Globalized World*. Farnham: Ashgate.

Kirton, John J. and Jenilee Guebert (2009). "Bringing Health into the Climate Change Regime: The Opportunity for Copenhagen 2009 and Muskoka 2010". Paper prepared for the Learning Forum on Global Health Research of the Canadian Coalition for Global Health Research, October 25, Ottawa.

http://www.g8.utoronto.ca/scholar/kirton-guebert-health-climate-2009.pdf (December 2013)

Kirton, John J. and Jenilee Guebert (2009). "Canada's G8 Global Health Diplomacy: Lessons for 2010". *Canadian Foreign Policy* 15(3): 85–105.

Kirton, John J. and Jenilee Guebert (2009). "Climate Change Accountability: The G8's Compliance Record from 1975 to 2009". November 28, G8 Research Group. http://www.g8.utoronto.ca/scholar/kirton-guebert-climate-091128.pdf (December 2013).

Kirton, John J. and Jenilee Guebert (2010). "North American Health Governance: Shocks, Summitry, and Societal Support". *Revista Norteamericana* 5(1): 221–44. http://www.scielo.org.mx/scielo.php?script=sci_arttext&pid=S1870-35502010000100008 (July 2012).

Kirton, John J. and Jenilee Guebert (2013). "Global Environmental Diplomacy: Comparing and Sharing". In *Global Health Diplomacy: Concepts, Issues, Actors, Instruments, Fora, and Cases*, Ilona Kickbusch, Graham Lister, Michaela Told, et al., eds. New York: Springer, pp. 141–54.

Kirton, John J. and Madeline Koch, eds. (2009). *The G20 Pittsburgh Summit 2009*. London: Newsdesk. http://www.g8.utoronto.ca/newsdesk/pittsburgh.html (December 2013).

Kirton, John J. and Ella Kokotsis (2007). "Keeping Faith with Africa's Health: Catalysing G8 Compliance". In *Governing Global Health: Challenge, Response, Innovation*, Andrew F. Cooper, John J. Kirton, and Ted Schrecker, eds. Aldershot: Ashgate, pp. 157–80.

Kirton, John J. and Julia Kulik (2012). "A Summit of Significant Success: G20 Los Cabos Leaders Deliver the Desired Double Dividend". June 19. http://www.g20.utoronto.ca/analysis/120619-kirton-success.html (December 2013).

Kirton, John J., Marina Larionova, and Paolo Savona, eds. (2010). *Making Global Economic Governance Effective: Hard and Soft Law Institutions in a Crowded World*. Farnham: Ashgate.

Kirton, John J. and Jenevieve Mannell (2007). "The G8 and Global Health Governance". In *Governing Global Health: Challenge, Response, Innovation*, Andrew F. Cooper, John J. Kirton, and Ted Schrecker, eds. Aldershot: Ashgate, pp. 115–46.

Kirton, John J., Nikolai Roudev, and Laura Sunderland (2007). "Making G8 Leaders Deliver: An Analysis of Compliance and Health Commitments, 1996–2006". *Bulletin of the World Health Organization* 85(3): 192–9.

Kirton, John J., Nikolai Roudev, Laura Sunderland, et al. (2009). "Explaining Compliance with G8 Leaders' Health Commitments, 1996–2006". In *Innovation in Global Health Governance: Critical Cases*, Andrew F. Cooper and John J. Kirton, eds. Farnham: Ashgate, pp. 257–84.

Kirton, John J. and Junichi Takase, eds. (2002). *New Directions in Global Political Governance: The G8 and International Order in the Twenty-First Century*. Aldershot: Ashgate.

Kirton, John J. and Michael J. Trebilcock, eds. (2004). *Hard Choices, Soft Law: Voluntary Standards in Global Trade, Environment, and Social Governance.* Aldershot: Ashgate.

Kjellstrom, Tord (2009, March 6). "Climate Change, Direct Heat Exposure, Health, and Well-Being in Low and Middle Income Countries". *Global Health Action* 2. http://www.globalhealthaction.net/index.php/gha/article/view/1958/2183 (October 2013).

Krasner, Stephen (1999). *Sovereignty: Organized Hypocrisy.* Princeton: Princeton University Press.

Krasner, Stephen (2001). *Problematic Sovereignty: Contested Rules and Political Possibilities.* New York: Columbia University Press.

Krasner, Stephen (2009). *Power: The State, and Sovereignty: Essays on International Relations.* Abdingdon: Routledge.

Krasner, Stephen and Carlos Pascual (2005). "Addressing State Failure". *Foreign Affairs* 84(4): 153–63.

Krueger, Anne O. (1998). "Introduction". In *The WTO as an International Organization,* Anne O. Krueger, ed. Chicago: University of Chicago Press.

Kulik, Julia (2013). "Reducing the Economic Burden of Non-communicable Diseases in the BRICS: Lessons from Brazil". January 25, BRICS Research Group, Toronto. http://www.brics.utoronto.ca/biblio/Kulik-NCDs-Brazil.html (December 2013).

Labonté, Ronald, Ted Schrecker, David Sanders, et al. (2004). *Fatal Indifference: The G8, Africa, and Global Health.* Ottawa: International Development Research Centre.

Lee, Kelley (2001). "Globalization: A New Agenda for Health?" In *International Cooperation and Health,* Martin McKee, Paul Adrian Garner, and Robin Stott, eds. Vol. 1. Oxford: Oxford University Press, pp. 19–28.

Lee, Kelley, Kent Buse, and Suzanne Fustukian, eds. (2002). *Health Policy in a Globalising World.* Cambridge: Cambridge University Press.

Lee, Kelley and Richard Dodgson (2000). "Globalization and Cholera: Implications for Global Governance". *Global Governance* 6(2): 213–36.

Lee, Kelley, Suzanne Fustukian, and Kent Buse (2002). "An Introduction to Global Health Policy". In *Health Policy in a Globalising World,* Kelley Lee, Kent Buse, and Suzanne Fustukian, eds. Cambridge: Cambridge University Press, pp. 3–17.

Leiserowitz, Anthony (2007). "International Public Opinion, Perception, and Understanding of Global Climate Change". Yale University. http://environment.yale.edu/climate-communication/files/IntlPublicOpinion.pdf (December 2013).

Lewis, Stephen (2005). *Race Against Time: Searching for Hope in AIDS-Ravaged Africa.* Toronto: House of Anansi.

Lifson, Alan R. (1996). "Mosquitoes, Models, and Dengue". *Lancet* 347(9010): 1201–2. doi: 10.1016/S0140-6736(96)90730-8.

Lindsay, Steve and Pim Martens (1998). "Malaria in the African Highlands: Past, Present, and Future". *World Health Bulletin* 76(1): 33–45. http://whqlibdoc.who.int/bulletin/1998/Vol76-No1/bulletin_1998_76(1)_33-45.pdf (October 2013).

Linklater, Andrew (2007). *Critical Theory and World Politics: Citizenship, Sovereignty, and Humanity*. Abdingdon: Routledge.

Lisk, Franklyn (2010). *Global Institutions and the HIV/AIDS Epidemic: Responding to an International Crisis*. London: Routledge.

Lown, Bernard, James Muller, Eric Chivian, et al. (1981). "The Nuclear-Arms Race and the Physician". *New England Journal of Medicine* 304(12): 726–9.

Machemedze, Rangarirai (2003). "Trade Related Aspects of Intellectual Property Rights (TRIPs Agreement)". Fact Sheet. http://www.seatini.org/publications/factsheets/trips.htm (October 2013).

MacKellar, Landis (2005). "Priorities in Global Health Assistance for Health, Aids, and Population (HAP)". OECD Development Centre Working Papers No. 244, Organisation for Economic Co-operation and Development, Paris. http://www.oecd-ilibrary.org/content/workingpaper/725643456002 (November 2013).

MacLeod, Roy and Milton Lewis, eds. (1988). *Disease, Medicine, and Empire: Perspectives on Western Medicine and the Experience of European Expansion*. London: Routledge.

Major Economies Meeting on Energy Security and Climate Change (2007). "Final Chairman's Summary: First Major Economies Meeting on Energy Security and Climate Change". Washington DC, September 27–8. http://www.g8.utoronto.ca/mem/mem-070927.html (December 2013).

Major Economies Meeting on Energy Security and Climate Change (2008). "Declaration of Leaders Meeting of Major Economies on Energy Security and Climate Change". Hokkaido, Japan, July 9. http://www.g8.utoronto.ca/summit/2008hokkaido/2008-mem.html (December 2013).

Major Economies Meeting on Energy Security and Climate Change (2008). "Final Chairman's Summary: Second Major Economies Meeting on Energy Security and Climate Change". Honolulu, January 31. http://2001-2009.state.gov/g/oes/rls/or/2008/99953.htm (December 2013).

Malunga, Chiku (2009). *Understanding Organizational Leadership through Ubuntu*. London: Adonis and Abbey Publishers.

Mannak, Miriam (2009). "Climate Change Threatens Livelihoods Along Africa's Coast". *Inter Press Service*, February 19. http://www.ipsnews.net/2009/02/environment-climate-change-threatens-livelihoods-along-africa39s-coast (December 2013).

Markandya, Anil, Ben G. Armstrong, Simon Hales, et al. (2009). "Public Health Benefits of Strategies to Reduce Greenhouse-Gas Emissions: Low-Carbon Electricity Generation". *Lancet* 374(9706): 2006–15.

Matovu, George (2011). "New Participatory Instruments in Local Governance: Cases from Rwanda, South Africa, and Uganda". Paper presented at the Commonwealth Local Government Research Colloquium, March 13–15,

Cardiff. http://www.lgma.org.au/downloads/File/Matovu%20-%20New%20Participatory%20Instruments1-1%20-%20African%20Case%20Studies.pdf (October 2013).

Mayaki, Ibrahim Assane and Michel Sidibé (2013). "Advancing the Africa-G8 Partnership: Towards an AIDS-Free Generation". In *The UK Summit: The G8 at Lough Erne 2013*, John J. Kirton and Madeline Koch, eds. London: Newsdesk, pp. 188–9. http://www.g8.utoronto.ca/newsdesk/stpetersburg.

McCoy, David, Gayatri Kembhavi, Jinesh Patel, et al. (2009). "The Bill and Melinda Gates Foundation's Grant-Making Programme for Global Health". *Lancet* 373(9675): 1645–53.

McInerney-Lankford, Siobhán, Mac Darrow, and Lavanya Rajamani (2011). "Human Rights and Climate Change: A Review of the International Legal Dimensions". World Bank, Washington DC. http://siteresources.worldbank.org/INTLAWJUSTICE/Resources/HumanRightsAndClimateChange.pdf (December 2013).

McInnes, Colin (2006). "HIV/AIDS and Security". *International Affairs* 82(2): 315–26.

McMichael, Anthony J., Diarmid Campbell-Lendrum, Carlos Corvalán, et al., eds. (2003). *Climate Change and Human Health: Risks and Responses*. Geneva: World Health Organization. http://whqlibdoc.who.int/publications/2003/924156248X_eng.pdf (October 2013).

McMichael, Anthony J., Diarmid Campbell-Lendrum, Sari Kovats, et al. (2004). "Global Climate Change". In *Comparative Quantification of Health Risks: Global and Regional Burden of Disease Attributable to Selected Major Risk Factors*, Majid Ezzati, Alan D. Lopez, Anthony Rodgers, et al., eds. Vol. 1. Geneva: World Health Organization, pp. 1543–650.

McMichael, Anthony J., Andrew Haines, Rudolf Slooff, et al. (1996). "Climate Change and Human Health". World Health Organization, Geneva. http://whqlibdoc.who.int/hq/1996/WHO_EHG_96.7.pdf (December 2013).

Medical News Today (2006). "Canadian Health Minister Clement Notes Progress At G8 Health Ministers Meeting". April 30. http://www.medicalnewstoday.com/releases/42487.php (September 2013).

Menne, Bettina, Nino Kunzli, and Roberto Bertollini (2002). "The Health Impacts of Climate Change and Variability in Developing Countries". *International Journal of Global Environmental Issues* 2(3/4): 181–205. doi: 10.1504/IJGENVI.2002.002399.

Mhone, Guy (2003). "The Challenges of Governance, Public Sector Reform, and Public Administration in Africa: Some Research Issues". *DPMN Bulletin* 10(3). http://www.dpmf.org/images/challenges-governance-guy.html (July 2013).

MicrobiologyBytes (2009). "Malaria". April 8. http://www.microbiologybytes.com/introduction/Malaria.html (September 2013).

Mitchell, Tom and Thomas Tanner (2006). "Adapting to Climate Change: Challenges and Opportunities for the Development Community". Tearfund, London. http://www.tearfund.org/webdocs/website/Campaigning/policy%20

and%20research/Adapting%20to%20climate%20change%20discussion%20paper.pdf (December 2013).

Morris, Kelly (2009). "USA Failing on HIV/AIDS Accountability and Action". *Lancet Infectious Diseases* 9(1): 14.

Mugambe, Lydia (2002). The Exceptions to Patent Rights under the WTO-TRIPS Agreement: Where Is the Right to Health Guaranteed?, LLM thesis, Community Law Centre, University of the Western Cape, Cape Town.

Munyuki, Elijah and Shorai Jasi (2009). "Capital Flows in the Health Care Sector in Zimbabwe: Trends and Implications for the Health System". Discussion Paper 79, August, Equinet, Harare. http://www.equinetafrica.org/bibl/docs/DIS79pppMUNYUKI.pdf (October 2013).

Munyuki, Elijah, Rangarirai Machemedze, and Helene Bank (2005). "WTO Systems and Processes: Making People Understand the Impact". Issue 1-2005, Occasional Paper Series, Southern African People's Solidarity Network.

Murray, Jessica, Busani Tshabangu, and Natasha Erlank (2010). "Enhancing Participatory Governance and Fostering Active Citizenship: An Overview of Local and International Best Practices". *Politikon: South African Journal of Political Studies* 37(1): 45–66.

Myers, Norman (1997). "Environmental Refugees". *Population and Environment* 19(2): 167–82.

Najam, Adil, Saleemul Huq, and Youba Sokona (2003). "Climate Negotiations beyond Kyoto: Developing Countries Concerns and Interests". *Climate Policy* 3(3): 221–31. doi: 10.1016/S1469-3062(03)00057-3.

Nattrass, Nicoli (2007). *Mortal Combat: AIDS Denialism and the Struggle for Antiretrovirals in South Africa.* Scottsville, South Africa: University of KwaZulu-Natal Press.

Nature (2009, July 2). "Time for Early Action". 460(12). Editorial. doi: 10.1038/460012a.

Nduru, Moyiga (2004). "The Mandela Charm Glistens AIDS Conference". *Common Dreams*, July 15. http://www.commondreams.org/headlines04/0715-03.htm (January 2014).

Neira, Maria (2009). "Foreword". *Global Health Action* 2. http://www.globalhealthaction.net/index.php/gha/article/view/2109/2545

Netherlands Ministry of Foreign Affairs (2005). "AIDS, Security, and Conflict Initiative". Summary of briefing, Netherlands Mission, New York, June 3.

Nilsson, Maria, Robert Beaglehole, and Rainer Sauerborn (2009). "Climate Policy: Lessons from Tobacco Control". *Lancet* 374(9706): 1955–6.

Nilsson, Maria, Birgitta Evengård, Rainer Sauerborn, et al. (2012). "Connecting the Global Climate Change and Public Health Agendas". *PLoS Med* 9(6): e1001227. doi: 10.1371/journal.pmed.1001227.

Nishtar, Sania and Ariel Pablos-Mendez (2009). "The Global Financial Downturn – Imperatives for the Health Sector". *Lancet* 373(9658): 124.

Nye, Joseph S. (2000). *Understanding International Conflicts*. 3rd edn. New York: Longman.

Nyong, Anthony, Francis Adesina, and Balgis Osman Elasha (2007). "The Value of Indigenous Knowledge in Climate Change Mitigation and Adaptation Strategies in the African Sahel". *Mitigation and Adaptation Strategies for Global Change* 12(5): 787–97. doi: 10.1007/s11027-007-9099-0. http://dx.doi.org/10.1007/s11027-007-9099-0.

Nzongola-Ntalaja, Georges (1987). *Revolution and Counter-Revolution in Africa: Essays in Contemporary Politics*. London: Zed Books.

O'Keefe, Michael (2012). "Lessons from the Rise and Fall of the Military AIDS Hypothesis: Politics, Evidence, and Persuasion". *Contemporary Politics* 18(2): 239–53. doi: 10.1080/13569775.2012.674340.

Obadina, Tunde (2008). "The Myth of Neo-colonialism". *Africa Economic Analysis*. http://www.africaeconomicanalysis.org/articles/55/1/Myths-about-globalisation/Page1.html (September 2013).

Onimode, Bade (1988). *A Political Economy of the African Crisis*. London: Zed Books.

Onzivu, William (2012). "Re-examining Health Protection in International Environmental Regulation". In *Human Health and Ecological Integrity: Ethics, Law, and Human Rights*, Laura Westra, Colin L. Soskolne, and Donald W. Spady, eds. Abdingdon: Routledge, pp. 301–14.

Orbinski, James (2008). *An Imperfect Offering: Humanitarian Action in the Twenty-First Century*. Toronto: Doubleday.

Orbinski, James and Jenilee Guebert (2010). "Climate Change and Global Health: The Time Is Now". In *G8 & G20: The 2010 Canadian Summits*, John J. Kirton and Madeline Koch, eds. London: Newsdesk, pp. 286–7. http://www.g8.utoronto.ca/newsdesk/g8g20/g8g20-2010.pdf (December 2013).

Organisation for Economic Co-operation and Development (2006). "Meeting of the OECD Development Assistance Committee (DAC) and the Environment Policy Committee (EPOC) at Ministerial Level". Paris, April 4. http://web.archive.org/web/20080117163820/http://www.oecd.org/document/38/0,3343,en_21571361_36099755_36099814_1_1_1_1,00.html (December 2013).

Organisation for Economic Co-operation and Development (2009). "Health: Improving Policy Coherence for Development". Policy Brief, OECD Observer, October, Paris.

Orlove, Ben, Carla Roncoli, Merit Kabugo, et al. (2010). "Indigenous Climate Knowledge in Southern Uganda: The Multiple Components of a Dynamic Regional System". *Climatic Change* 100(2): 243–65. doi: 10.1007/s10584-009-9586-2.

Ostergard, Robert L. and Crystal Barcelo (2005). "Personalist Regimes and the Insecurity Dilemma: Prioritizing AIDS as a National Security Threat in Uganda". In *The African State and the AIDS Crisis*, Amy Stephenson Patterson, ed. Aldershot: Ashgate, pp. 155–79.

Oxfam (2007). "Adapting to Climate Change: What's Needed in Poor Countries, and Who Should Pay". Oxfam Briefing Paper 104, May 29. http://www.oxfam.

org/sites/www.oxfam.org/files/adapting%20to%20climate%20change.pdf (January 2014).

Oxfam (2008). "Double Disaster: How Climate Change and HIV Are Twinning to Devastate Southern Africa's Poor". Oxfam Global Centre of Learning, Pretoria.

Parkhurst, Justin O. (2002). "The Ugandan Success Story? Evidence and Claims of HIV-1 Prevention". *Lancet* 360(9326): 78–80.

Parry, Martin, Osvaldo Canziani, Jean Palutikof, et al., eds. (2007). *Climate Change 2007: Impacts, Adaptation, and Vulnerability. Contribution of Working Group II to the Fourth Assessment Report of the Intergovernmental Panel on Climate Change.* Cambridge: Cambridge University Press. http://www.ipcc.ch/publications_and_data/publications_ipcc_fourth_assessment_report_wg2_report_impacts_adaptation_and_vulnerability.htm (October 2013).

Pascual, Mercedes, Jorge A. Ahumada, Luis Fernando Chaves, et al. (2006). "Malaria Resurgence in the East African Highlands: Temperature Trends Revisited". *Proceedings of the National Academy of Sciences* 103(15): 5829–34. doi: 10.1073/pnas.0508929103.

Patrick, Stewart (2006). "Weak States and Global Threats: Fact or Fiction?" *Washington Quarterly* 29(2): 27–33. http://www.cgdev.org/files/7034_file_06spring_patrickTWQ.pdf (July 2013).

Patrick, Stewart and Kaysie Brown (2006). "Fragile States and U.S. Foreign Assistance: Show Me the Money". Working Paper 96, Centre for Global Development, Washington DC. http://www.cgdev.org/publication/fragile-states-and-us-foreign-assistance-show-me-money-working-paper-96 (July 2013).

Patz, Jonathan A., Diarmid Campbell-Lendrum, Holly Gibbs, et al. (2008). "Health Impact Assessment of Global Climate Change: Expanding on Comparative Risk Assessment Approaches for Policy Making". *Annual Review of Public Health* 29: 27–39. doi: 10.1146/annurev.publhealth.29.020907.090750.

Patz, Jonathan A., Diarmid Campbell-Lendrum, Tracey Holloway, et al. (2005). "Impact of Regional Climate Change on Human Health". *Nature* 438(7066): 310–17. doi: 10.1038/nature04188.

Phaswana-Mafuya, Nancy and Dmitri Tassiopoulos, eds. (2001). *Non-Communicable Diseases (NCDs) in Developing Countries.* Hauppauge NY: Nova Publishers.

Pierce, David W., Tim P. Barnett, Benjamin D. Santer, et al. (2009). "Selecting Global Climate Models for Regional Climate Change Studies". *Proceedings of the National Academy of Sciences* 106(21): 8441–6. doi: 10.1073/pnas.0900094106.

Pirages, Dennis C. (2007). "Nature, Disease, and Globalization: An Evolutionary Perspective". *International Studies Review* 9(4): 616–28.

Poku, Nana K., Neil Renwick, and Joao Gomes Porto (2007). "Human Security and Development in Africa". *International Affairs* 83(6): 1155–70.

Poku, Nana K. and Alan Whiteside, eds. (2004). *The Political Economy of AIDS in Africa.* Aldershot: Ashgate.

Price-Smith, Andrew (2002). *The Health of Nations: Infectious Disease, Environmental Change, and Their Effects on National Security and Development*. Cambridge MA: MIT Press.

Raja, Kanaga (2010). "Trade: Concerns over Financial Crisis Surface at TNC Meeting". October 22, Third World Network. http://www.twnside.org.sg/title2/wto.info/twninfo20081010.htm (October 2013).

RamaRao, Saumaya, Marlina Lacuesta, Marilou Costello, et al. (2003). "The Link Between Quality of Care and Contraceptive Use". *International Family Planning Perspectives* 29(2). http://www.guttmacher.org/pubs/journals/2907603.html (October 2013).

Ramin, Brodie (2009). "Slums, Climate Change, and Human Health in Sub-Saharan Africa". *Bulletin of the World Health Organization* 87: 886–886. doi: 10.2471/BLT.09.073445.

Ramin, Brodie Morgan and Anthony J. McMichael (2009). "Climate Change and Health in Sub-Saharan Africa: A Case-Based Perspective". *EcoHealth* 6(1): 52–7. doi: 10.1007/s10393-009-0222-4.

Reguly, Eric (2009). "U.S. Makes First Move at Copenhagen". *Globe and Mail*, December 7. http://www.theglobeandmail.com/news/world/climate-change/us-makes-first-move-at-copenhagen/article1391958 (December 2013).

Reinicke, Wolfgang H. (1998). *Global Public Policy: Governing without Government*. Washington DC: Brookings Institution.

Renganathan, Elik (2013). "The World Health Organization as a Key Venue for Global Health Diplomacy". In *Global Health Diplomacy: Concepts, Issues, Actors, Instruments, Fora, and Cases*, Ilona Kickbusch, Graham Lister, Michaela Told, et al., eds. New York: Springer, pp. 173–87.

Reuveny, Rafael (2008). "Ecomigration and Violent Conflict: Case Studies and Public Policy Implications". *Human Ecology* 36(1): 1–13.

Richards, Michael (2003). "Poverty Reduction, Equity, and Climate Change: Global Governance Synergies or Contradictions?", Overseas Development Institute, London. http://www.odi.org.uk/sites/odi.org.uk/files/odi-assets/publications-opinion-files/2408.pdf (January 2014).

Risse, Thomas (2007). "Paradoxien der Souveränität". *Internationale Politik* 7/8: 40–47. https://zeitschrift-ip.dgap.org/de/ip-die-zeitschrift/archiv/jahrgang-2007/juli-august/paradoxien-der-souver%C3%A4nit%C3%A4t (July 2013).

Ritvo, Paul, Kumanan Wilson, Dennis Willms, et al. (2005). "Vaccines in the Public Eye". *Nature Medicine Supplement* 11(4): 520–24. http://www.canprep.ca/publications/ritvovaccines.pdf (September 2013).

Roberts, J. Timmons (2001). "Global Inequality and Climate Change". *Society and Natural Resources* 14(6): 501–9. doi: 10.1080/08941920118490.

Rockefeller Foundation (2014). "Asian Cities Climate Change Resilience Network (ACCCRN)". New York. http://www.rockefellerfoundation.org/our-work/current-work/climate-change-resilience/asian-cities-climate-change-resilience (January 2014).

Rogelj, Joeri, David L. McCollum, Andy Reisinger, et al. (2013). "Probabilistic Cost Estimates for Climate Change Mitigation". *Nature* 493: 79–83. doi: 10.1038/nature11787.

Roll Back Malaria (2012). "Key Malaria Facts". http://www.rollbackmalaria.org/keyfacts.html (September 2013).

Roll Back Malaria (undated). "Economic Costs of Malaria". Geneva. http://www.rbm.who.int/cmc_upload/0/000/015/363/RBMInfosheet_10.pdf (September 2013).

Rosenzweig, Cynthia, David Karoly, Marta Vicarelli, et al. (2008). "Attributing Physical and Biological Impacts to Anthropogenic Climate Change". *Nature* 453(7193): 353–7. doi: 10.1038/nature06937.

Ruggie, John G. (1993). "Territoriality and Beyond: Problematizing Modernity in International Relations". *International Organization* 47(1): 139–74.

Samuels, Fiona and Helen Spraos (2008). "HIV and Emergencies: Haiti". Overseas Development Institute, London. http://www.odi.org.uk/publications/3265-haiti-hiv-aids-emergencies (December 2013).

Santoro, Michael A. and Thomas M. Gorrie (2005). *Ethics and the Pharmaceutical Industry*. Cambridge: Cambridge University Press.

Sarkozy, Nicolas (2008). "Third Major Economies Meeting on Energy and Climate Change: Speech". Paris, April 18. http://www.ambafrance-ca.org/spip.php?page=mobile_art&art=2191 (December 2013).

Save the Children (2009). "Feeling the Heat: Child Survival in a Changing Climate". London. https://www.savethechildren.org.uk/sites/default/files/docs/Feeling_the_Heat_composite_low_res_1.pdf (December 2013).

Schrecker, Ted, Ronald Labonté, and David Sanders (2007). "Breaking Faith with Africa: The G8 and Population Health". In *Governing Global Health: Challenge, Response, Innovation*, Andrew F. Cooper and John J. Kirton, eds. Aldershot: Ashgate, pp. 181–205.

Sclar, Elliott D. and Nicole Volavka-Close (2013). "Understanding the Twenty-First Century Urban Transformation: A Global South Perspective". In *The Urban Transformation: Health, Shelter, and Climate Change*, Elliott D. Sclar, Nicole Volavka-Close, and Peter Brown, eds. London: Routledge, pp. 1–14.

Šehović, Annamarie Bindenagel (2014). *HIV/AIDS and the South African State*. Farnham: Ashgate.

Semenza, Jan C., Carol H. Rubin, Kenneth H. Falter, et al. (1996). "Heat-Related Deaths during the July 1995 Heat Wave in Chicago". *New England Journal of Medicine* 335(2): 84–90. doi: doi:10.1056/NEJM199607113350203.

Shaw, Timothy M., Sandra J. MacLean, and David R. Black (2006). "Introduction: A Decade of Human Security: What Prospects for Global Governance and New Multilateralisms?" In *Human Security: Global Governance and New Multilateralisms*, Sandra J. MacLean, David R. Black, and Timothy M. Shaw, eds. Aldershot: Ashgate, pp. 3–18.

Shivji, Issa G. (2006). "The Silences in the NGO Discourse: The Role and Future of NGOs in Africa". Special Report 14, Pambazuka News, Oxford. http://www.pambazuka.org/en/publications/pz_sr_14.pdf (July 2013).
Shope, Robert (1991). "Global Climate Change and Infectious Diseases". *Environmental Health Perspectives* 96: 171–4.
Simms, Andrew, Julian Oram, and Petra Kjell (2004). *The Price of Power: Poverty, Climate Change, the Coming Energy Crisis, and the Renewable Revolution.* London: New Economics Foundation.
Simms, Andrew and Hannah Reid (2005). "Africa: Up in Smoke? The Second Report from the Working Group on Climate Change and Development". New Economics Foundation and International Institute for Environment and Development, London. http://pubs.iied.org/9560IIED.html (December 2013).
Singh, Jerome Amir (2012, June 5). "Why Human Health and Health Ethics Must Be Central to Climate Change Deliberations". *PLoS Medicine* 9(6). doi: 10.1371/journal.pmed.1001229.
Singh, Sudhvir, Usman Mushtaq, Charlotte Holm-Hansen, et al. (2011). "The Importance of Climate Change to Health". *Lancet* 378(9785): 29–30. doi: 10.1016/S0140-6736(11)61018-0.
Smith, D. Mark (2006). *Just One Planet: Poverty, Justice, and Climate Change.* Warwickshire: Intermediate Technology Publications.
Smith, Kirk R. (1994). "Health, Energy, and Greenhouse-Gas Impacts of Biomass Combustion in Household Stoves". *Energy for Sustainable Development* 1(4): 23–9. http://www.whrc.org/policy/pdf/India/Smith_1994.pdf (October 2013).
Smith, Kirk R., Michael Jerrett, H. Ross Anderson, et al. (2009). "Public Health Benefits of Strategies to Reduce Greenhouse-Gas Emissions: Health Implications of Short-Lived Greenhouse Pollutants". *Lancet* 374(9707): 2091–103.
Smith, Richard and Melisa Martínez Álvarez (2008). "Global Change and Health: Mapping the Challenges of Global Non-healthcare Influences on Health". World Health Organization, Geneva.
Sohn, Jon, Smita Nakhood, and Kevin Baumert (2005). "Mainstreaming Climate Change Considerations at the Multilateral Development Banks". WRI Issue Brief, World Resources Institute, Washington DC. http://www.wri.org/sites/default/files/pdf/mainstreaming_climate_change.pdf (January 2014).
Sontag, Susan (2002). *Illness as Metaphor and Aids and Its Metaphors.* London: Penguin Classics.
South African Regional Programme on access to Medicines and Diagnostics (2012). "SADC Pooled Procurement Strategy for Essential Medicines and Health Commodities 2013–2017". http://www.sarpam.net/archives/2103 (September 2013).
Southern and Eastern African Trade Information and Negotiations Institute (SEATINI) and Equinet (2004). "The WTO Global Agreement on Trade in Services (GATS) and Health Equity in Southern Africa". Policy Paper

No. 12, February. http://www.equinetafrica.org/bibl/docs/POL12trade.pdf (October 2013).

Spady, Donald W. (2012). "Public Healthcare in the Time of Transition: The Need to Revert to Basics". In *Human Health and Ecological Integrity: Ethics, Law, and Human Rights*, Laura Westra, Colin L. Soskolne, and Donald W. Spady, eds. Abdingdon: Routledge, pp. 121–31.

Spiegel, Paul B., Anne Rygaard Bennedsen, Johanna Claas, et al. (2007). "Prevalence of HIV Infection in Conflict-Affected and Displaced People in Seven Sub-Saharan African Countries: A Systematic Review". *Lancet* 369(9580): 2187–95.

Spittal, Patricia, Janette Nakuti, Nelson Sewakambo, et al. (1997). "'We Are Dying and Getting Finished!': Linking an Ethnographic Research Design to an HIV/AIDS Participatory Approach in Uganda". In *Nurtured by Knowledge: Learning to Do Participatory Action-Research*, Susan E. Smith and Dennis Willms, eds. New York: Apex Press, pp. 86–110.

St. Louis, Michael E. and Jeremy J. Hess (2008). "Climate Change: Impacts on and Implications for Global Health". *American Journal of Preventive Medicine* 35(5): 527–38.

Steiner, Achim (2009). "The Environment-Health Axis". In *The G8 2009: From La Maddalena to L'Aquila*, John J. Kirton and Madeline Koch, eds. London: Newsdesk, pp. 65–6. http://www.g8.utoronto.ca/newsdesk/G8-2009.pdf (December 2013).

Steiner, Achim (2011). "UNEP Chief Addresses UN Security Council Debate on Climate Change and Security". United Nations Environment Programme, July 20. http://www.unep.org/newscentre/default.aspx?DocumentID=2646&ArticleID=8817 (December 2013).

Steiner, Sherrie (2012). "Faith-Based Accountability Mechanism Typology". *SAGE Open* 2(2). doi: 10.1177/2158244012450705.

Steiner, Sherrie (2012). "Religious Soft Power as Accountability Mechanism for Power in World Politics". *SAGE Open* 1(3). doi: 10.1177/2158244011428085.

Stern, Nicholas (2007). *The Economics of Climate Change: The Stern Review*. Cambridge: Cambridge University Press.

Sternberg, Steve (2004). "AIDS Discussion Focuses on Funds". *USA Today*, July 15. http://usatoday30.usatoday.com/news/health/2004-07-15-aids-conference_x.htm (September 2013).

Stuckler, David, Sanjay Basu, and Martin McKee (2011). "Global Health Philanthropy and Institutional Relationships: How Should Conflicts of Interest Be Addressed?". *PLoS Medicine* 8(4). doi: 10.1371/journal.pmed.1001020.

Sturchio, Jeff (2009). "Health Security from Economic and Environmental Innovation". In *The G20 Pittsburgh Summit 2009: Sustaining Global Recovery*, John J. Kirton and Madeline Koch, eds. London: Newsdesk, pp. 163–5. http://www.g8.utoronto.ca/newsdesk/pittsburgh/sturchio.html (December 2013).

Sullivan, Louis (1990). "An Opportunity to Oppose: Physicians' Role in the Campaign against Tobacco". *Journal of the American Medical*

Association 1990(264): 12. 1581–2. http://jama.jamanetwork.com/article.aspx?articleid=383349 (October 2013).
Suwanwela, Charas and Victor Neufeld (2001). "Health Research for Development: Realities and Challenges". In *Forging Links for Health Research: Perspectives from the Council on Health Research for Development*, Victor Neufeld and Nancy Johnson, eds. Ottawa: International Development Research Centre, pp. 241–66.
Swidler, Ann (2006). "Syncretism and Subversion in AIDS Governance: How Locals Cope with Global Demands". *International Affairs* 82(2): 269–84.
Tandon, Yash (2003). "Are There Alternatives To Neo-Liberalism? Yes There Are". Southern African and Eastern African Trade Information and Negotiations Institute (SEATINI). http://www.seatini.org/publications/epas/AlternativesToNeoliberalism.htm (October 2013).
Tumwine, James K. (1989). "Community Participation as Myth or Reality: A Personal Experience from Zimbabwe". *Health Policy and Planning* 4(2): 157–61. doi: 10.1093/heapol/4.2.157.
Tutu, Desmond (2008). "Responsibility to Protect". *International Herald Tribune*, February 20, p. 6.
UNAIDS (2008). "2008 Report on the Global AIDS Epidemic". Geneva. http://www.unaids.org/en/dataanalysis/knowyourepidemic/epidemiologypublications/2008reportontheglobalaidsepidemic/ (July 2013).
UNAIDS (2011). "UNAIDS World AIDS Day Report 2011: How to Get to Zero Faster". Geneva. http://www.unaids.org/en/media/unaids/contentassets/documents/unaidspublication/2011/jc2216_worldaidsday_report_2011_en.pdf (October 2013).
UNAIDS (2012). "Global Fact Sheet: World AIDS Day 2012". Geneva. http://www.unaids.org/en/media/unaids/contentassets/documents/epidemiology/2012/gr2012/20121120_FactSheet_Global_en.pdf (September 2013).
UNAIDS (2012). "Global Report: UNAIDS Report on the Global AIDS Epidemic 2012". Geneva. http://www.unaids.org/en/media/unaids/contentassets/documents/epidemiology/2012/gr2012/20121120_UNAIDS_Global_Report_2012_en.pdf (June 2013).
UNAIDS (2012). "Regional Fact Sheet 2012: Sub-Saharan Africa". Geneva. http://www.unaids.org/en/media/unaids/contentassets/documents/epidemiology/2012/gr2012/2012_FS_regional_ssa_en.pdf (September 2013).
UNAIDS (2012). "UNAIDS Global Report 2012: Epidemiology Slides". Geneva. http://www.unaids.org/en/resources/campaigns/20121120_globalreport2012/epislides/ (September 2013).
UNAIDS (2012). "UNAIDS World AIDS Day Report 2012: Results". Geneva. http://www.unaids.org/en/media/unaids/contentassets/documents/epidemiology/2012/gr2012/JC2434_WorldAIDSday_results_en.pdf (October 2013).
UNAIDS (2013). "AIDSinfo". Database, Geneva. http://www.unaids.org/en/dataanalysis/datatools/aidsinfo/ (September 2013).

UNAIDS (2013). "Global Report: UNAIDS Report on the Global AIDS Epidemic 2013". Geneva. http://www.unaids.org/en/media/unaids/contentassets/documents/epidemiology/2013/gr2013/UNAIDS_Global_Report_2013_en.pdf (January 2014).

United Kingdom. Department for International Development (2004). "Climate Change in Africa". Key Sheet 10. http://www.eldis.org/vfile/upload/1/document/0708/DOC15876.pdf (December 2013).

United Kingdom. Department for International Development (2006). "Eliminating World Poverty: Making Governance Work for the Poor". White Paper on International Development, London. http://www.official-documents.gov.uk/document/cm68/6876/6876.pdf (January 2014).

United Nations (1992). "United Nations Framework Convention on Climate Change". FCCC/INFORMAL/84. http://unfccc.int/resource/docs/convkp/conveng.pdf (December 2013).

United Nations Development Programme (2003). *Making Global Trade Work for People*. New York: Earthscan.

United Nations Development Programme (2007/8). "Human Development Report 2007/08 – Fighting Climate Change: Human Solidarity in a Divided World". United Nations, New York. http://hdr.undp.org/en/reports/global/hdr2007-8/ (December 2013).

United Nations Economic and Social Commission for Asia and the Pacific (2013). "What Is Good Governance?", Bangkok. http://www.unescap.org/pdd/prs/ProjectActivities/Ongoing/gg/governance.asp (October 2013).

United Nations Environment Programme and UNAIDS (2008). "Climate Change and AIDS: A Joint Working Paper". UNAIDS, Geneva. http://data.unaids.org/Pub/basedocument/2008/20081223_unep_unaids_joint_working_paper_on_cca_en.pdf (December 2013).

United Nations Framework Convention on Climate Change (1992). "Full Text of the Convention". FCCC/INFORMAL/84. http://unfccc.int/resource/docs/convkp/conveng.pdf (December 2013).

United Nations Framework Convention on Climate Change (2009). "Decisions Adopted by the Conference of the Parties". Report of the Conference of the Parties on its 15th session, Copenhagen. http://unfccc.int/resource/docs/2009/cop15/eng/11a01.pdf (January 2014).

United Nations Framework Convention on Climate Change (2010). "Decisions Adopted by the Conference of the Parties". Report of the Conference of the Parties on its 16th session, Cancun. http://unfccc.int/resource/docs/2010/cop16/eng/07a01.pdf (January 2014).

United Nations Framework Convention on Climate Change (2011). "Decisions Adopted by the Conference of the Parties". Report of the Conference of the Parties on its 17th session, Durban. http://unfccc.int/resource/docs/2011/cop17/eng/09a02.pdf (January 2014).

United Nations Framework Convention on Climate Change (2012). "Decisions Adopted by the Conference of the Parties". Report of the Conference of the

Parties on its 18th session, Doha. http://unfccc.int/resource/docs/2012/cop18/eng/08a01.pdf (January 2014).

United Nations Framework Convention on Climate Change (2013). "NAPAs Received by the Secretariat". Bonn. http://unfccc.int/adaptation/workstreams/national_adaptation_programmes_of_action/items/4585.php (November 2013).

United Nations Framework Convention on Climate Change (2013). "National Adaptation Programmes of Action". Bonn. http://unfccc.int/adaptation/workstreams/national_adaptation_programmes_of_action/items/7567.php (December 2013).

United Nations General Assembly (2007). "The State of South-South Cooperation". A/62/296, August 23, New York. http://daccess-dds-ny.un.org/doc/UNDOC/GEN/N07/488/80/PDF/N0748880.pdf (September 2013).

United Nations Population Fund (2012). "By Choice, Not By Chance: Family Planning, Human Rights, and Development". Geneva. http://www.unfpa.org/webdav/site/global/shared/documents/publications/2012/EN-SWP2012_Report.pdf (November 2013).

United States (2002). "The National Security Strategy of the United States". Washington DC, September 17. http://nssarchive.us/NSSR/2002.pdf (January 2014).

United States National Intelligence Council (2005). "Mapping Sub-Saharan Africa's Future". Discussion paper CR2005-02. http://www.au.af.mil/au/awc/awcgate/nic/africa_future.pdf. (July 2013).

United States President's Emergency Plan for AIDS Relief (2008). "Making a Difference: Funding". Washington DC. http://www.pepfar.gov/documents/organization/100073.pdf (November 2013).

United States President's Emergency Plan for AIDS Relief (2013). "Latest Results". Washington DC. http://www.pepfar.gov/funding/results/index.htm (November 2013).

Vallings, Claire and Magui Moreno-Torres (2005). "Drivers of Fragility: What Makes States Fragile?" PRDE Working Paper 7, Department for International Development, London. http://purl.umn.edu/12824 (July 2013).

van den Assum, Laetitia (2005). "Towards a UNAIDS Framework Agenda for AIDS and Security". Unpublished report produced for UNAIDS.

Vandemoortele, Jan (2003). "The MDGs and Pro-Poor Policies: Can External Partners Make a Difference?", December, United Nations Development Programme, New York. http://depot.gdnet.org/gdnshare/pdf2/gdn_library/annual_conferences/fifth_annual_conference/vandemoortele_paper.pdf

Vaughan, Megan (1991). *Curing Their Ills: Colonial Power and African Illness*. Stanford: Stanford University Press.

Vax (2004). "A Tale of Two Timeframes: Short- and Long-Term Agendas for the Response to AIDS". *Vax: The Bulletin on AIDS Vaccine Research* 2(7): 1–2. http://www.vaxreport.org/Back-Issues/Documents/IAVI_VAX_AUG_2004_ENG.pdf (January 2014).

Walpole, Sarah Catherine, Kumanan Rasanathan, and Diarmid Campbell-Lendrum (2009). "Natural and Unnatural Synergies: Climate Change Policy and Health Equity". *Bulletin of the World Health Organization* 87: 799–801. doi: 10.2471/BLT.09.067116.

Wehrwein, Peter (1998). "Jonathan Mann and Mary Lou Clements-Mann Killed in Airplane Crash". *Lancet* 352(9131): 888.

Wiggins, Sarah (2009). "CEDRA Climate Change and Environmental Degradation Risk and Adaptation Assessment". Tearfund. http://preventionweb.net/go/11964 (October 2013).

Wilkinson, Paul, Kirk R. Smith, Michael Davies, et al. (2009). "Public Health Benefits of Strategies to Reduce Greenhouse-Gas Emissions: Household Energy". *Lancet* 374(9705): 1917–29.

Willms, Dennis (2009). "Understanding Must Precede Behavioural Change". *Waterloo Record*, April 1.

Willms, Dennis, Maria-Ines Arratia, and Patrick Makondesa (2004). "Malawi Faith Communities Responding to HIV/AIDS: Preliminary Findings of a Knowledge Translation and Participatory-Action Research (PAR) Project". *African Journal of AIDS Research* 3(1): 23–32.

Willms, Dennis, Nancy Johnson, Alfred Chingono, et al. (2001). "AIDS Prevention in the *Matare* and the Community: A Training Strategy for Traditional Healers in Zimbabwe". In *Applying Health Social Science: The Best Practice in the Developing World*, Nick Higginbotham, Roberto Briceño-León, and Nancy Johnson, eds. London: Zed Books.

Willms, Dennis and Nelson Sewakambo (undated). "Title". Plattsville ON: Salama SHIELD Foundation. Unpublished.

Willms, Dennis and Karolina Werner (2009). "Climate Change and Conflict in Africa". In *Climate Change in Africa: Adaptation, Mitigation, and Governance Challenges*, Hany Besada and Nelson Sewankambo, eds. Waterloo ON: Centre for International Governance Innovation, pp. 26–30.

Woodcock, James, Phil Edwards, Cathryn Tonne, et al. (2009). "Public Health Benefits of Strategies to Reduce Greenhouse-Gas Emissions: Urban Land Transport". *Lancet* 374(9705): 1930–43.

Woodward, David, Nick Drager, Robert Beaglehole, et al. (2001). "Globalization and Health: A Framework for Analysis and Action". *World Health Bulletin* 79(9): 875–81. http://www.who.int/bulletin/archives/79%289%29875.pdf (July 2013).

Woodward, Susan L. (2004). "Fragile States: Exploring the Concept". Paper presented to the "States and Security" Learning Group at the Peace and Social Justice meeting of the Ford Foundation, November 29, Rio de Janeiro. http://statesandsecurity.org/_pdfs/Fragile%20States_Exploring%20the%20Concept.pdf (July 2013).

World Bank (1981). "Accelerated Development in Sub-Saharan Africa: An Agenda for Action". Washington DC. http://go.worldbank.org/6W8EDJW0T0 (September 2013).

World Bank (2000). "Health Expenditures, Services, and Outcomes in Africa". *Findings: Africa Region*, April, no. 157. https://openknowledge.worldbank.org/bitstream/handle/10986/9459/548070BRI0Box31570Apr0200001PUBLIC1.pdf (September 2013).
World Bank (2005). "Meeting the Challenge of Africa's Development: A World Bank Group Action Plan". Washington DC. http://siteresources.worldbank.org/INTAFRICA/Resources/aap_final.pdf (October 2013).
World Bank (2007). "World Development Report 2007: Development and the Next Generation". Washington DC. http://go.worldbank.org/Q42ZSKGOP0 (September 2013).
World Bank (2008). "The World Bank's Commitment to HIV/AIDS in Africa: Our Agenda for Action, 2007–2011". Washington DC. http://siteresources.worldbank.org/INTAFRREGTOPHIVAIDS/Resources/WB_HIV-AIDS-AFA_2007–2011_Advance_Copy.pdf (September 2013).
World Bank (2009). "World Bank: Avian and Human Influenza Operations (Status as of December 31, 2008)". Washington DC. http://siteresources.worldbank.org/EXTAVIANFLU/Resources/3124440-1208294248389/WB_AHI_Matrix_Apr09.pdf (September 2013).
World Bank (2010). "Cross-country Laboratory Network to Raise East Africa's Defenses Against Disease". Washington DC. http://go.worldbank.org/4WZODJ72I0 (September 2013).
World Bank (2010). "World Development Report 2010: Development and Climate Change". Washington DC. http://siteresources.worldbank.org/INTWDR2010/Resources/5287678-1226014527953/WDR10-Full-Text.pdf (January 2014).
World Bank (2011). "The Growing Danger of Non-Communicable Diseases: Acting Now to Reverse Course". Conference edition, September, Washington DC. http://siteresources.worldbank.org/HEALTHNUTRITIONANDPOPULATION/Resources/Peer-Reviewed-Publications/WBDeepeningCrisis.pdf (January 2013).
World Bank (2011). "Towards One Health: Interim Lessons from the Global Program on Avian and Human Pandemic Influenza". Washington DC. http://siteresources.worldbank.org/EXTARD/Resources/336681-1242670845332/TowardsOneHealth.pdf (September 2013).
World Bank (2013). "Booster Program for Malaria Control in Africa". Washington DC. http://go.worldbank.org/H31FEKFWE0 (September 2013).
World Bank (2013). "East Africa Public Health Laboratory Networking Project". Warsaw. http://www.worldbank.org/projects/P111556/east-africa-public-health-laboratory-networking-project?lang=en (September 2013).
World Bank (2013). "Great Lakes Initiative on HIV/AIDS (GLIA) Support". Washington DC. http://www.worldbank.org/projects/P080413/great-lakes-initiative-hivaids-glia-support?lang=en (September 2013).
World Bank (2013). "HIV/AIDS Project for Abidjan-Lagos Transport Corridor". Washington DC. http://www.worldbank.org/projects/P074850/hivaids-project-abidjan-lagos-transport-corridor?lang=en&tab=overview (September 2013).

World Bank (2013). "Meeting the Challenge: The World Bank and HIV/AIDS". Washington DC. http://www.worldbank.org/en/results/2013/04/03/hivaids-sector-results-profile (September 2013).

World Food Programme (2009). "Climate Change and Hunger: Responding to the Challenge". Rome. http://documents.wfp.org/stellent/groups/public/documents/newsroom/wfp212536.pdf (January 2014).

World Health Organization (1990). "Potential Health Effects of Climatic Change: Report of a WHO Task Group". WHO/PEP/90/10, Geneva. http://whqlibdoc.who.int/hq/1990/WHO_PEP_90_10.pdf (December 2013).

World Health Organization (1997). "Health and Environment in Sustainable Development: Five Years after the Earth Summit". Geneva. http://whqlibdoc.who.int/hq/1997/WHO_EHG_97.12_eng.pdf (December 2013).

World Health Organization (2000). "Climate Change and Human Health: Impact and Adaptation". Geneva. http://whqlibdoc.who.int/hq/2000/WHO_SDE_OEH_00.4.pdf (December 2013).

World Health Organization (2001). "Cholera in South Africa". Geneva, April 17. http://www.who.int/csr/don/2001_04_17/en/index.html (October 2013).

World Health Organization (2001). "Globalization, TRIPS, and Access to Pharmaceuticals". WHO Policy Perspectives on Medicines, No. 3, Geneva. http://apps.who.int/medicinedocs/en/d/Js2240e/ (October 2013).

World Health Organization (2001). "Report on WHO Activities on Climate Change and Human Health". Statement to the 15th session of the Subsidiary Body of Scientific and Technological Advice, October, Marrakesh. http://web.archive.org/web/20050611235935/http://www.euro.who.int/document/gch/actrep_sbsta15.pdf (December 2013).

World Health Organization (2005). "Climate and Health". Fact sheet, Geneva, July. http://www.who.int/globalchange/news/fsclimandhealth/en/index.html (December 2013).

World Health Organization (2005). "Health and the Millennium Development Goals". Geneva. http://www.who.int/hdp/publications/mdg_en.pdf (December 2013).

World Health Organization (2006). "The World Health Report 2006: Working Together for Health". World Health Organization, Geneva. http://www.who.int/whr/2006/en/ (October 2012).

World Health Organization (2007). "The World Health Report 2007 – A Safer Future: Global Public Health Security in the 21st Century". Geneva. http://www.who.int/whr/2007/en (October 2012).

World Health Organization (2008). "Climate Change and Health: Report by the Secretariat". EB124/11, November 20, Geneva. http://apps.who.int/gb/ebwha/pdf_files/EB124/B124_11-en.pdf (December 2013).

World Health Organization (2008). "Climate Change Will Erode Foundations of Health". Geneva, April 8. http://www.who.int/mediacentre/news/releases/2008/pr11/en/ (December 2013).

World Health Organization (2008). "The Kampala Declaration and Agenda for Global Action". Geneva. http://www.who.int/entity/workforcealliance/

Kampala%20Declaration%20and%20Agenda%20web%20file.%20FINAL.pdf (October 2013).
World Health Organization (2008). "New World Health Assembly Resolution on Climate Change and Health". Geneva, May. http://www.who.int/globalchange/climate/EB_CChealth_resolution/en/ (December 2013).
World Health Organization (2008). "Protecting Health from Climate Change: World Health Day 2008". Geneva. http://www.who.int/world-health-day/toolkit/report_web.pdf (December 2013).
World Health Organization (2008). "WHO Event on Climate Change and Health at UNFCCC Conference". Poznan, Poland, December 1–12. http://www.who.int/mediacentre/events/meetings/climatechange/en (December 2013).
World Health Organization (2008). "World Health Assembly Sets Bold New Action for WHO". Geneva, May 24. http://www.who.int/mediacentre/news/releases/2008/wha02/en (December 2013).
World Health Organization (2008). "The World Health Report 2008 – Primary Health Care (Now More Than Ever)". Geneva. http://www.who.int/whr/2008/en (October 2012).
World Health Organization (2008). "World Malaria Report 2008". Geneva. http://whqlibdoc.who.int/publications/2008/9789241563697_eng.pdf (September 2013).
World Health Organization (2009). "Cholera in Zimbabwe: Update 4". Geneva, June 9. http://www.who.int/csr/don/2009_06_09/en/index.html (September 2013).
World Health Organization (2009). "Climate Change Is Affecting Our Health: Something Should Be Done Now". Geneva. http://www.who.int/entity/globalchange/publications/factsheets/Climate_change_and_health_brochure.pdf (December 2013).
World Health Organization (2009). "COP15 United Nations Climate Change Conference 2009". Copenhagen, December 7–18. http://www.who.int/globalchange/news/2009/climatechange_conference_7122009/en/ (December 2013).
World Health Organization (2009). "Influenza A(H1N1): Update 42". Geneva, June 1. http://www.who.int/csr/don/2009_06_01a/en/index.html (September 2013).
World Health Organization (2009). "Protecting Health from Climate Change: Global Research Priorities". Geneva. http://www.who.int/globalchange/publications/9789241598187/en/ (October 2013).
World Health Organization (2009). "WHO Carbon Footprint Study FY2008". Final Report V2, October, Geneva. http://www.who.int/globalchange/health_policy/WHO_Carbon_study.pdf (December 2013).
World Health Organization (2010). "Health Coverage at the 16th Conference of the Parties to the UN Framework Convention on Climate Change". 29 November–10 December, Cancún, Mexico. http://www.wits.ac.za/files/res843b46a0ac83418f98d98ad8d8f3279c.pdf (October 2013).

World Health Organization (2010). "The World Health Report 2010 – Health Systems: The Path to Universal Coverage". Geneva. http://www.who.int/whr/2010/en/ (September 2013).

World Health Organization (2010). "World Health Statistics 2010". Geneva. http://www.who.int/entity/whosis/whostat/EN_WHS10_Full.pdf (January 2014).

World Health Organization (2011). "Global Status Report on Noncommunicable Diseases 2010". Geneva. http://www.who.int/nmh/publications/ncd_report2010/en/ (January 2013).

World Health Organization (2011). "Improving Coherence of Climate Change, Health, and Development Policy: Update and Policy Proposals for UNFCCC CoP17 in Durban". Geneva. http://www.who.int/globalchange/mediacentre/events/2011/WHO_Health_in_UNFCCC_COP17_.pdf (October 2013).

World Health Organization (2011). "TB/HIV Facts 2011–2012". Geneva. http://www.who.int/tb/publications/TBHIV_Facts_for_2011.pdf (June 2013).

World Health Organization (2011). "WHO Reform for a Healthy Future". July 20, Geneva. http://www.who.int/dg/reform/en_who_reform_overview.pdf (October 2013).

World Health Organization (2012). "World Malaria Report 2012". Geneva. http://www.who.int/malaria/publications/world_malaria_report_2012/report/en/index.html (September 2013).

World Health Organization (2013). "African Programme for Onchocerciasis Control (APOC)". Geneva. http://www.who.int/blindness/partnerships/APOC/en/ (September 2013).

World Health Organization (2013). "Cumulative Number of Confirmed Human Cases for Avian Influenza A(H5N1) Reported to WHO, 2003–2013". Geneva, August 29. http://www.who.int/influenza/human_animal_interface/EN_GIP_20130829CumulativeNumberH5N1cases.pdf (September 2013).

World Health Organization (2013). "Global Health Estimates Summary Tables: Deaths by Cause, Age, and Sex". Geneva, June. http://www.who.int/entity/healthinfo/global_burden_disease/GHE_DthGlobal_2000_2011.xls (September 2013).

World Health Organization (2013). "The Top 10 Causes of Death". Geneva, July. http://who.int/mediacentre/factsheets/fs310/en/ (September 2013).

World Health Organization (2013). "Trade, Foreign Policy, Diplomacy, and Health: Sovereignty". Geneva. http://www.who.int/trade/glossary/story082/en/index.html (October 2013).

World Health Organization (2013). "WHO Reform". Geneva. http://www.who.int/about/who_reform/en/ (October 2013).

World Health Organization (2013). "World Health Statistics 2013". Geneva. http://www.who.int/ghc/publications/world_health_statistics/EN_WHS2013_Full.pdf (January 2014).

World Health Organization (2013). "World Malaria Report 2013". Geneva. http://www.who.int/malaria/publications/world_malaria_report_2013/report/en/index.html (December 2013).

World Health Organization (2014). "Climate Change and Human Health: Publications". Geneva. http://www.who.int/globalchange/publications/en/ (January 2014).

World Health Organization and Health Care Without Harm (2009). "Healthy Hospitals, Healthy Planet, Healthy People: Addressing Climate Change in Healthcare Settings". Geneva. http://www.who.int/entity/globalchange/publications/climatefootprint_report.pdf (December 2013).

World Health Organization Regional Office for Africa (undated). "Clusters and Programs of WHO in the African Region". http://www.afro.who.int/en/clusters-a-programmes.html (December 2013).

World Health Organization Regional Office for Africa (undated). "Protection of the Human Environment: Overview". http://www.afro.who.int/en/clusters-a-programmes/hpr/protection-of-the-human-environment/overview.html (December 2013).

World Health Organization Regional Office for Europe (1999). "Strategy to Roll Back Malaria in the WHO European Region". Copenhagen. http://www.euro.who.int/__data/assets/pdf_file/0006/98790/E67133.pdf (January 2013).

World Health Organization Regional Office for Europe (2009). "EuroHEAT: Improving Public Health Responses to Extreme Weather/Heat-Waves". Copenhagen. http://www.euro.who.int/__data/assets/pdf_file/0009/95913/E92473.pdf (December 2013).

World Meteorological Organization (2007). "Report by the Task Team on Definitions of Extreme Weather and Climate Events". Geneva.

World Meteorological Organization (2013). "The Global Climate 2001–2010: A Decade of Climate Extremes". Geneva. http://library.wmo.int/pmb_ged/wmo_1103_en.pdf (January 2014).

World Trade Organization (1994). *The Results of the Uruguay Round of Multilateral Trade Negotiations: The Legal Texts*. Geneva: General Agreement on Tariffs and Trade.

World Trade Organization (2007). "World Trade Report 2007". Geneva. http://www.wto.org/english/res_e/booksp_e/anrep_e/world_trade_report07_e.pdf (October 2013).

World Trade Organization (2013). "Intellectual Property: Protection and Enforcement". Geneva. http://www.wto.org/english/thewto_e/whatis_e/tif_e/agrm7_e.htm (October 2013).

Zacher, Mark (1992). "The Decaying Pillars of the Westphalian Temple: Implications for International Order and Governance". In *Governance Without Government: Order and Change in Word Politics*, James N. Rosenau and Ernst-Otto Czemiel, eds. Cambridge: Cambridge University Press, pp. 58–101.

Zacher, Mark (2007). "The Transformation in Global Health Collaboration since the 1990s". In *Governing Global Health: Challenge, Response, Innovation*, Andrew F. Cooper, John J. Kirton, and Ted Schrecker, eds. Aldershot: Ashgate, pp. 15–27.

Zacher, Mark and Tania J. Keefe (2008). *The Politics of Global Health Governance: United by Contagion*. New York: Palgrave Macmillan.

Zacher, Mark W. (1999). "Global Epidemiological Surveillance: International Cooperation to Monitor Infectious Diseases". In *Global Public Goods: International Cooperation in the 21st Century*, Inge Kaul, Isabelle Grunberg, and Marc A. Stern, eds. New York: Oxford University Press for the United Nations Development Programme, pp. 266–83.

Žižek, Slavoj (1999). *The Ticklish Subject: The Absent Centre of Political Ontology*. London: Verso.

Zondi, Siphamandla (2012). *Public Health and African Initiative in South Africa: Aspects of the History of Public Health*. Saarbrucken: Lambert Academic Publishing.

Index

Page references to tables and figures are in **bold** type.

GLOBAL ENVIRONMENTAL GOVERNANCE SERIES

Full series list

Africa's Health Challenges
Sovereignty, Mobility of People
and Healthcare Governance
*Edited by Andrew F. Cooper, John J. Kirton,
Franklyn Lisk and Hany Besada*

Corporate Responses to
EU Emissions Trading
Resistance, Innovation or Responsibility?
*Edited by Jon Birger Skjærseth and
Per Ove Eikeland*

Renewable Energy Policy
Convergence in the EU
The Evolution of Feed-in Tariffs in
Germany, Spain and France
David Jacobs

The EU as International
Environmental Negotiator
Tom Delreux

Global Energy Governance in a
Multipolar World
*Dries Lesage, Thijs Van de Graaf
and Kirsten Westphal*

Innovation in Global Health Governance
Critical Cases
*Edited by Andrew F. Cooper
and John J. Kirton*

Environmental Skepticism
Ecology, Power and Public Life
Peter J. Jacques

Transatlantic Environment and
Energy Politics
Comparative and International Perspectives
*Edited by Miranda A. Schreurs, Henrik Selin,
and Stacy D. VanDeveer*

The Legitimacy of International Regimes
Helmut Breitmeier

Governing Agrobiodiversity
Plant Genetics and Developing Countries
Regine Andersen

The Social Construction of Climate Change
Power, Knowledge, Norms, Discourses
Edited by Mary E. Pettenger

Governing Global Health
Challenge, Response, Innovation
*Edited by Andrew Cooper, John Kirton
and Ted Schrecker*

Participation for Sustainability in Trade
*Edited by Sophie Thoyer and
Benoît Martimort-Asso*

Bilateral Ecopolitics
Continuity and Change in Canadian-
American Environmental Relations
*Edited by Philippe Le Prestre
and Peter Stoett*

Governing Global Desertification
Linking Environmental Degradation,
Poverty and Participation
*Edited by Pierre Marc Johnson,
Karel Mayrand and Marc Paquin*

Sustainability, Civil Society and
International Governance
Local, North American and
Global Contributions
Edited by John J. Kirton and Peter I. Hajnal

A World Environment Organization
Solution or Threat for Effective International
Environmental Governance?
Edited by Frank Biermann and Steffen Bauer

Hard Choices, Soft Law
Voluntary Standards in Global Trade,
Environment and Social Governance
*Edited by John J. Kirton and
Michael J. Trebilcock*

The Politics of Irrigation Reform
Contested Policy Formulation and Implementation in Asia, Africa and Latin America
Edited by Peter P. Mollinga and Alex Bolding

Governing Global Biodiversity
The Evolution and Implementation of the Convention on Biological Diversity
Edited by Philippe G. Le Prestre

Agricultural Policy Reform
Politics and Process in the EU and US in the 1990s
Wayne Moyer and Tim Josling

Linking Trade, Environment, and Social Cohesion
NAFTA Experiences, Global Challenges
Edited by John J. Kirton and Virginia W. Maclaren

International Equity and Global Environmental Politics
Power and Principles in US Foreign Policy
Paul G. Harris